Rare Kidney Diseases: Nephrology Essentials

Rare Kidney Diseases: Nephrology Essentials

Editor: Kevin Lewis

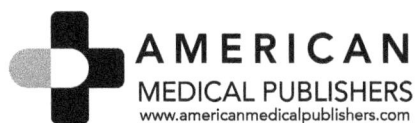

AMERICAN
MEDICAL PUBLISHERS
www.americanmedicalpublishers.com

AMERICAN
MEDICAL PUBLISHERS
www.americanmedicalpublishers.com

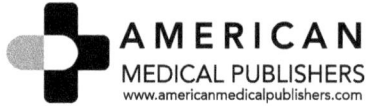

Cataloging-in-Publication Data

Rare kidney diseases : nephrology essentials / edited by Kevin Lewis.
    p. cm.
Includes bibliographical references and index.
ISBN 978-1-63927-793-3
1. Kidneys--Disease. 2. Nephrology. 3. Kidneys--Disease--Diagnosis.
4. Kidneys--Diseases--Treatment. I. Lewis, Kevin.
RC902 .R37 2023
616.61--dc23

American Medical Publishers,
41 Flatbush Avenue,
1st Floor, New York,
NY 11217, USA

ISBN 978-1-63927-793-3 (Hardback)

Contents

Preface

This book has been an outcome of determined endeavour from a group of educationists in the field. The primary objective was to involve a broad spectrum of professionals from diverse cultural background involved in the field for developing new researches. The book not only targets students but also scholars pursuing higher research for further enhancement of the theoretical and practical applications of the subject.

Kidney disease is refers to the damage or disease associated with the kidney. The major causes of kidney disease include the deposition of the immunoglobulin A antibodies in the glomerulus, toxicity of chemotherapy agents, xanthine oxidase deficiency, administration of analgesics and long-term exposure to lead or its salts. Rare kidney disease includes nephropathic cystinosis, acute kidney injury, nephrotic syndrome, etc. The common signs and symptoms of this disease include fatigue, feeling cold, shortness of breath, swelling in hands or feet, nausea, vomiting, and upset stomach. Patients with kidney disease have difficulty in urinating. The patients might also have foamy or bubbly, and dark colored urine. Diagnosis and management of kidney disease is performed by examining the medical history, physical examination, a urine test or an ultrasound. Dialysis and transplantation are major treatment methods for controlling the progression of end-stage renal disease. The book aims to shed light on some of the unexplored aspects of rare kidney diseases and the recent researches on this medical condition. It is appropriate for students seeking detailed information about these diseases as well as for experts.

It was an honour to edit such a profound book and also a challenging task to compile and examine all the relevant data for accuracy and originality. I wish to acknowledge the efforts of the contributors for submitting such brilliant and diverse chapters in the field and for endlessly working for the completion of the book. Last, but not the least; I thank my family for being a constant source of support in all my research endeavours.

Editor

Renal Tubular TRPA1 as a Risk Factor for Recovery of Renal Function from Acute Tubular Necrosis

Chung-Kuan Wu [1,2,3], **Chia-Lin Wu** [1,4,5], **Tzu-Cheng Su** [6], **Yu Ru Kou** [7], **Chew-Teng Kor** [8], **Tzong-Shyuan Lee** [9] **and Der-Cherng Tarng** [1,7,10,*]

1 Institute of Clinical Medicine, National Yang-Ming University, Taipei 11221, Taiwan; chungkuan.wu@gmail.com (C.-K.W.); 143843@cch.org.tw (C.-L.W.)
2 Division of Nephrology, Department of Internal Medicine, Shin-Kong Wu Ho-Su Memorial Hospital, Taipei 11101, Taiwan
3 School of Medicine, Fu-Jen Catholic University, New Taipei 24205, Taiwan
4 Division of Nephrology, Department of Internal Medicine, Changhua Christian Hospital, Changhua 50006, Taiwan
5 School of Medicine, Chung-Shan Medical University, Taichung 40201, Taiwan
6 Department of Pathology, Changhua Christian Hospital, Changhua 50006, Taiwan; 140062@cch.org.tw
7 Department of Physiology, School of Medicine, National Yang-Ming University, Taipei 11221, Taiwan; yrkou@ym.edu.tw
8 Internal Medicine Research Center, Changhua Christian Hospital, Changhua 50006, Taiwan; 179297@cch.org.tw
9 Department of Physiology, College of Medicine, National Taiwan University, Taipei 10617, Taiwan; ntutslee@ntu.edu.tw
10 Division of Nephrology, Department of Medicine, Taipei Veterans General Hospital, Taipei 11217, Taiwan
* Correspondence: dctarng@vghtpe.gov.tw

Abstract: Background: Transient receptor potential ankyrin 1 (TRPA1), a redox-sensing Ca^{2+}-influx channel, serves as a gatekeeper for inflammation. However, the role of TRPA1 in kidney injury remains elusive. Methods: The retrospective cohort study recruited 46 adult patients with acute kidney injury (AKI) and biopsy-proven acute tubular necrosis (ATN) and followed them up for more than three months. The subjects were divided into high- and low-renal-tubular-TRPA1-expression groups for the comparison of the total recovery of renal function and mortality within three months. The significance of TRPA1 in patient prognosis was evaluated using Kaplan–Meier curves and logistic regression analysis. Results: Of the 46 adult AKI patients with ATN, 12 totally recovered renal function. The expression level of tubular TRPA1 was detected by quantitative analysis of the immunohistochemistry of biopsy specimens from ATN patients. The AKI patients with high tubular TRPA1 expression showed a high incidence of nontotal renal function recovery than those with low tubular TRPA1 expression (OR = 7.14; 95%CI 1.35–37.75; p = 0.02). High TRPA1 expression was independently associated with nontotal recovery of renal function (adjusted OR = 6.86; 95%CI 1.26–37.27; p = 0.03). Conclusion: High tubular TRPA1 expression was associated with the nontotal recovery of renal function. Further mechanistic studies are warranted.

Keywords: acute kidney injury; acute tubular necrosis; TRPA1; recovery of renal function

1. Introduction

Acute kidney injury (AKI) is characterized by a sharp decline in the glomerular filtration rate and manifests as azotemia [1,2]. A large portion of patients with severe complications of AKI requires renal replacement therapy [3]. AKI also results in serious health burdens because of its association with high morbidity and mortality [4]. Patients with AKI are at risk of chronic kidney disease (CKD). Over the years, most severe CKD eventually proceeds to end-stage renal disease (ESRD) [5–7]. If available, immediate treatment of AKI would not only reduce morbidity and mortality, but also subsequent CKD.

Acute tubular necrosis (ATN), including renal tubular cell damage and death, is the most common cause of AKI in hospitalized patients. ATN can be precipitated by acute ischemic or toxic event or sepsis [8]. Oxidative stress plays a crucial role in the pathophysiology of ATN [9]. Oxidative stress characterized by increases in reactive oxygen species (ROS) and/or reactive nitrogen species after an insult to the kidneys can initiate a complex mechanism that directly or indirectly leads to tubular injury [10,11]. However, a valid antioxidant treatment for AKI remains lacking [12].

Transient receptor potential ankyrin 1 (TRPA1) is a nonselective transmembrane cation channel involving Ca^{2+} permeability, which can be activated by toxic or inflammatory mediators, such as ROS [13]. Previous studies reported that TRPA1 in neurons acts as a gatekeeper of inflammation [14]. Recent studies have shown that TRPA1 is expressed in various types of non-neuronal cells, including renal tubular cells [15]. Activation of TRPA1 in these non-neuronal cells may aggravate the inflammatory response [16,17]. However, two experimental animal studies suggested that TRPA1 protects against sepsis or angiotensin-II induced kidney injury [18,19]. Consequently, the role of renal TRPA1 in AKI is not exactly known.

The present study identified the association between renal tubular TRPA1 expression with oxidative stress, which is an activator of TRPA1, and the severity of renal injury in patients with ATN. It also investigated the association of tubular TRPA1 expression with total recovery of renal function and mortality.

2. Materials and Methods

2.1. Study Design and Participants

We retrospectively enrolled 52 adult inpatients with AKI and biopsy-proven ATN at Changhua Christian Hospital on 1 January 2000. The biopsy-proven ATN patients who meet the criteria of Acute Kidney Injury Network (AKIN) and were aged ≥18 years were included. The AKI inpatients admitted due to obstructive etiologies (as determined by renal ultrasound), chronic dialysis patients, kidney transplant recipients, and patients with active malignancy were excluded. Each patient was followed up for three months so that renal recovery from AKI could be assessed. Six patients who underwent follow-up for less than three months were excluded; hence, 46 patients were finally selected for further investigation. In addition, six patients with normal renal function and no other remarkable comorbidities underwent nephrectomy for localized circumscribed tumors and the uninvolved poles of their removed kidneys were regarded as normal renal tissues. The study was approved by the Institutional Review Board of Changhua Christian Hospital (approval number 150912). Written informed consent was obtained from all subjects.

Renal function was measured during follow-up visits until total recovery of estimated glomerular filtration rate (eGFR), death, or the end of follow-up. The endpoint was the total (return to baseline eGFR, within a 10% margin of error) recovery of eGFR within three months following AKI and mortality. Baseline renal function was determined from the last available serum creatinine value within one year before hospitalization or the lowest inpatient serum creatinine value after AKI if outpatient serum creatinine value was unavailable.

Demographic data, including gender, age, comorbidities, and medications, as well as urine protein excretion rate measured by the urine protein-to-creatinine ratio, were recorded at the time of AKI. Heart failure included the diagnoses of congestive or systolic heart failure, diastolic heart failure, or cardiomyopathy based on the manual review of medical charts before or at the time of AKI. The diagnosis of diabetes mellitus was based on the American Diabetes Association criteria, and hypertension was dependent on medical history and/or the use of antihypertensive medication.

2.2. Laboratory Data

Serum levels of hemoglobin, creatinine, albumin, total cholesterol, triglyceride, uric acid, sodium, and potassium and urine levels of creatinine and protein were measured in accordance with standardized procedures at the Department of Laboratory Medicine, Changhua Christian Hospital. eGFR, calculated using the Chronic Kidney Disease Epidemiology Collaboration (CKD-EPI) formula, was utilized to evaluate renal function.

2.3. Immunohistochemistry (IHC)

Formalin-fixed, paraffin-embedded renal tissue sections (4 μm) were placed on coated slides, dewaxed with xylene, and rehydrated in serial dilutions of alcohol, followed by washing with phosphate buffered saline solution. Activity of endogenous peroxidase was blocked by incubation in 3% H_2O_2. Antigen retrieval was performed by boiling in 10 mM citrate buffer for 20 min. The slides were washed three times with PBS after incubation with rabbit polyclonal anti-TRPA1 antibodies (Alomone Labs., Jerusalen, Israel) at 1:2000 dilution and mouse monoclonal 8-hydroxy-2′-deoxyguanosine antibodies (ab48508, Abcam, Cambridge, MA, USA) at 1:500 dilution for 30 min at room temperature, respectively. The reaction was visualized using the polymer-based MACH4 DAB Detection Kit (Biocare Medical, Concord, CA, USA) in accordance with the manufacturer's instructions, and the slides were incubated with horseradish peroxidase/Fab polymer conjugate for another 30 min. Finally, peroxidase activity was visualized by incubation with 3,3′-diaminobenzidine tetrahydrochloride (DAB) as the substrate for 5 min and hematoxylin as the counterstain.

Computer-assisted quantitative analysis was performed as previously described. In brief, we randomly selected at least five glomeruli and 10 nonoverlapping high-power fields for each renal cortical section and captured images by Olympus Microscope BX51 (Olympus, Tokyo, Japan) equipped with a digital color camera (DP21; Olympus, Tokyo, Japan). The captured images were then analyzed using Image Pro-Plus software (Version 6.0; Media Cybernetics, Silver Spring, MD, USA). Quantitative immunohistochemical staining value was calculated as the integrated optical density divided by the total area occupied by the DAB-stained and hematoxylin-stained cells of each slide [20].

2.4. Histopathology

Formalin-fixed, paraffin-embedded renal tissues including ATN and normal control were sectioned at 4 μm thickness and stained for histological examination. These sections were stained with a periodic acid-Schiff staining kit (Merck Millipore, Billerica, MA, USA) and Masson's trichrome Kit (American Master Tech Scientific, Lodi, CA, USA) to determine the severity of tubular injury and percentage of interstitial fibrosis, respectively. All sections were examined by a pathologist (T.-C.S.) unaware of the clinical and laboratory data. The characteristics of tubular injury included tubular cell swelling, loss of brush border, or nuclear condensation. The severity of tubular injury was scored from 0 to 4 according to the percentage of the injured area of the section (0—no change; 1—changes affecting 1–25%; 2—changes affecting 25–50%; 3—changes affecting 50–75%; 4—changes affecting 75–100% of the section).

2.5. Statistical Analysis

Results are expressed as a percentage, median (interquartile range, IQR), or mean ± standard deviation. Kolmogorov–Smirnov test was utilized for all variables to test normal distribution. Non-normally distributed variables were analyzed by nonparametric statistical tests. Mann–Whitney U test and Pearson's chi-squared test or Fisher's exact test were performed to compare two groups for continuous and categorical variables, respectively. We performed univariate logistic regression analysis to calculate the crude of odds ratio (OR) of nonrecovery of total renal function or death within three months after ATN for all variables. Subsequently, multivariate logistic regression analysis was performed to calculate the adjusted OR for age, sex, and each variable. We calculated the cumulative incidences of mortality and total recovery of renal function during the follow-up period by using the Kaplan–Meier method and compared the results between the high and low TRPA1 expression groups by using the log-rank test. All statistical analyses were performed using SAS 9.4 (SAS Institute Inc., Cary, NC, USA). Statistical significance was considered at $p < 0.05$ in two-tailed tests.

3. Results

3.1. Demographic and Clinical Characteristics of Patients

Fifty-two patients with biopsy-proven ATN were enrolled in the retrospective cohort study. Of the 52 patients, six were excluded because of follow-up less than three months. No patients started dialysis at the time of kidney biopsy. During the follow-up period, 12 patients (26.09%) completely recovered renal function. Among the 34 patients (73.91%) without complete recovery of renal function, 10 patients (21.74%) died, as seen in Figure 1. Table 1 shows the baseline demographic, laboratory data, and renal histopathology of the ATN patients. These patients are divided into patients with complete recovery of renal function (recovery group, $n = 12$) and those without complete recovery of renal function (nonrecovery or death group, $n = 34$). Patients of both groups were similar in age; gender distribution; presence of diabetic mellitus, hypertension, and heart failure; severity of AKI; levels of serum albumin, cholesterol, triglyceride, uric acid, sodium, and potassium; scores of tubular injury and interstitial inflammation; percentage of interstitial fibrosis; use of angiotensin-converting-enzyme inhibitors or angiotensin-II receptor blockers; and immunosuppressive treatment. Compared with the nonrecovery group, the complete recovery group had lower baseline serum creatinine level, higher baseline eGFR and hemoglobin levels, and lower percentage of tubular atrophy in the renal interstitium (all $p < 0.05$).

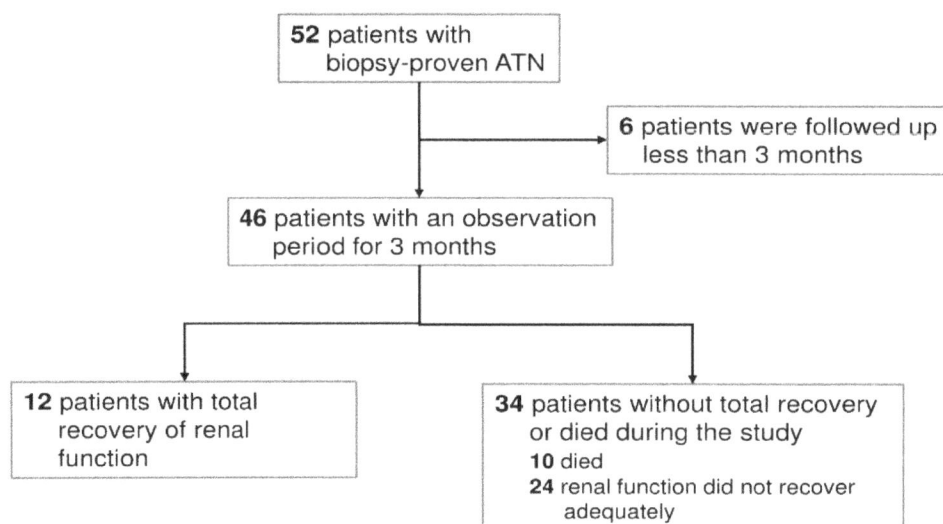

Figure 1. Flowchart presenting the selected biopsy-proven acute tubular necrosis (ATN) population.

Table 1. Baseline demographic and laboratory data and renal histopathology of acute tubular necrosis patients with and without total recovery of renal function within three months.

Characteristics	Total Recovery (n = 12)	Nonrecovery or Death [a] (n = 34)	p [b]
Demographics			
Age (years)	46.2 ± 21.7	56.8 ± 17.8	0.15 [b]
Male (n (%))	8 (66.7%)	21 (61.8%)	0.76 [c]
Diabetes mellitus (n (%))	1 (8.3%)	13 (38.2%)	0.05 [d]
Hypertension (n (%))	2 (16.7%)	10 (29.4%)	0.33 [d]
Heart failure (n (%))	0 (0%)	3 (8.8%)	0.39 [d]
Severity of AKI	3 (25%)	8 (23.5%)	0.60 [d]
AKIN stage I (n (%))	9 (75%)	26 (76.5%)	
AKIN stage II or III (n (%))	46.2 ± 21.7	56.8 ± 17.8	

Table 1. *Cont.*

Characteristics	Total Recovery (*n* = 12)	Nonrecovery or Death [a] (*n* = 34)	*p* [b]
Laboratory data			
Baseline serum creatinine (mg/dL)	1.0 (0.8–1.2)	1.5 (0.9–2.7)	0.03 [b]
Baseline eGFR (CKD-EPI) (mL/min/1.73m^2)	88.7 (64.7–113.5)	47.7 (20.7–87.5)	0.004 [b]
Urinary PCR (mg/g)	96.4 (30.0–976.0)	661.5 (100.0–5432.0)	0.05 [b]
Hemoglobin (g/dL)	11.7 (9.1–13.4)	9.6 (8.7–10.8)	0.03 [b]
Serum albumin (g/dL)	2.6 (1.8–3.2)	2.8 (2.2–3.3)	0.57 [b]
Serum cholesterol (mg/dL)	131 (119.0–260)	193 (157–252)	0.33 [b]
Serum triglyceride (mg/dL)	197.4 ± 132.6	165.6 ± 94.6	0.53 [b]
Serum uric acid (mg/dL)	8.6 (7.7–13.4)	8.4 (6.6–9.6)	0.44 [b]
Serum sodium (mmol/L)	137 (133.5–140.0)	133.5 (131–140)	0.51 [b]
Serum potassium (mmol/L)	4.4 (3.5–4.9)	3.9 (3.4–4.1)	0.15 [b]
Histopathology			
Tubular injury score	2 (1–3)	2 (1–4)	0.18 [b]
Tubular atrophy (%)	0 (0–1.5)	6 (3–10)	<0.001 [b]
Interstitial inflammation score	1 (0–1)	1 (1–1)	0.06 [b]
Interstitial fibrosis (%)	7.0 ± 4.9	10.4 ± 8.4	0.37 [b]
Medications			
ACEI or ARB (*n* (%))	2 (16.7%)	7 (20.6%)	0.57 [d]
Immunosuppressants (*n* (%))	2 (16.7%)	13 (38.2%)	0.16 [d]

Data are expressed as *n* (%) for categorical data and as mean ± standard deviation or median (interquartile range) for continuous data. AKI—acute kidney injury; AKIN—Acute Kidney Injury Network; CKD-EPI—Chronic Kidney Disease Epidemiology Collaboration; eGFR—estimated glomerular filtration rate; PCR—protein-to-creatinine ratio; ACEI—angiotensin-converting-enzyme inhibitors; ARB —angiotensin II receptor blockers. [a] Includes partial recoveries and nonrecoveries. [b] Mann–Whitney U test. [c] Pearson's chi-squared test. [d] Fisher's exact test.

3.2. Association of Tubular Expression of TRPA1 with Expression of 8-OHdG or Tubular Injury Score Among Patients with ATN and Normal Subjects

The expression of renal TRPA1 on renal biopsy specimen was significantly higher in the patients with ATN than in the normal controls, as seen in Figure 2A. These ATN patients with high expression of renal TRPA1 had higher expression of renal 8-OHdG than those with low expression of renal TRPA1, as seen in Figure 2A,B ($p = 0.033$). Moreover, the patients with ATN and high renal TRPA1 expression had severe tubular injury according to the tubular injury scoring scale compared with those with low renal TRPA1 expression, as seen in Figure 2A,C ($p = 0.006$).

3.3. Association of Tubular TRPA1 Expression with Complete Recovery of Renal Function

Our patients were divided into two groups according to renal tubular TRPA1 expression: those with high ($n = 22$) and low ($n = 24$) expression of renal tubular TRPA1. Kaplan–Meier analysis revealed a higher incidence of complete recovery of renal function during the three-month follow-up in the low TRPA1 expression group than in the high tubular TRPA1 expression group ($p = 0.02$), as seen in Figure 3. In univariable and age- and sex-adjusted logistical regression analysis, as seen in Table 2, high tubular TRPA1 expression remained significantly associated with noncomplete recovery of renal function during the three-month follow-up ($p = 0.02$, $p = 0.03$, respectively). Compared with the AKI patients with low tubular TRPA1 expression, the OR for noncomplete recovery of renal function during the three-month follow-up was 7.14 (95%CI 1.35–37.75) in the AKI patients with high tubular TRPA1 expression. After adjustment for age and gender, high expression of tubular TRPA1 remained a significant risk factor for noncomplete recovery of renal function during the three-month follow-up (adjusted OR 6.86; 95%CI 1.26–37.27). In addition to the high expression of TRPA1, univariable and age- and sex-adjusted logistical regression analysis found that high tubular atrophy, low baseline eGFR, and low level of hemoglobin were also significantly associated with noncomplete recovery of renal function during the three-month follow-up (all $p < 0.05$).

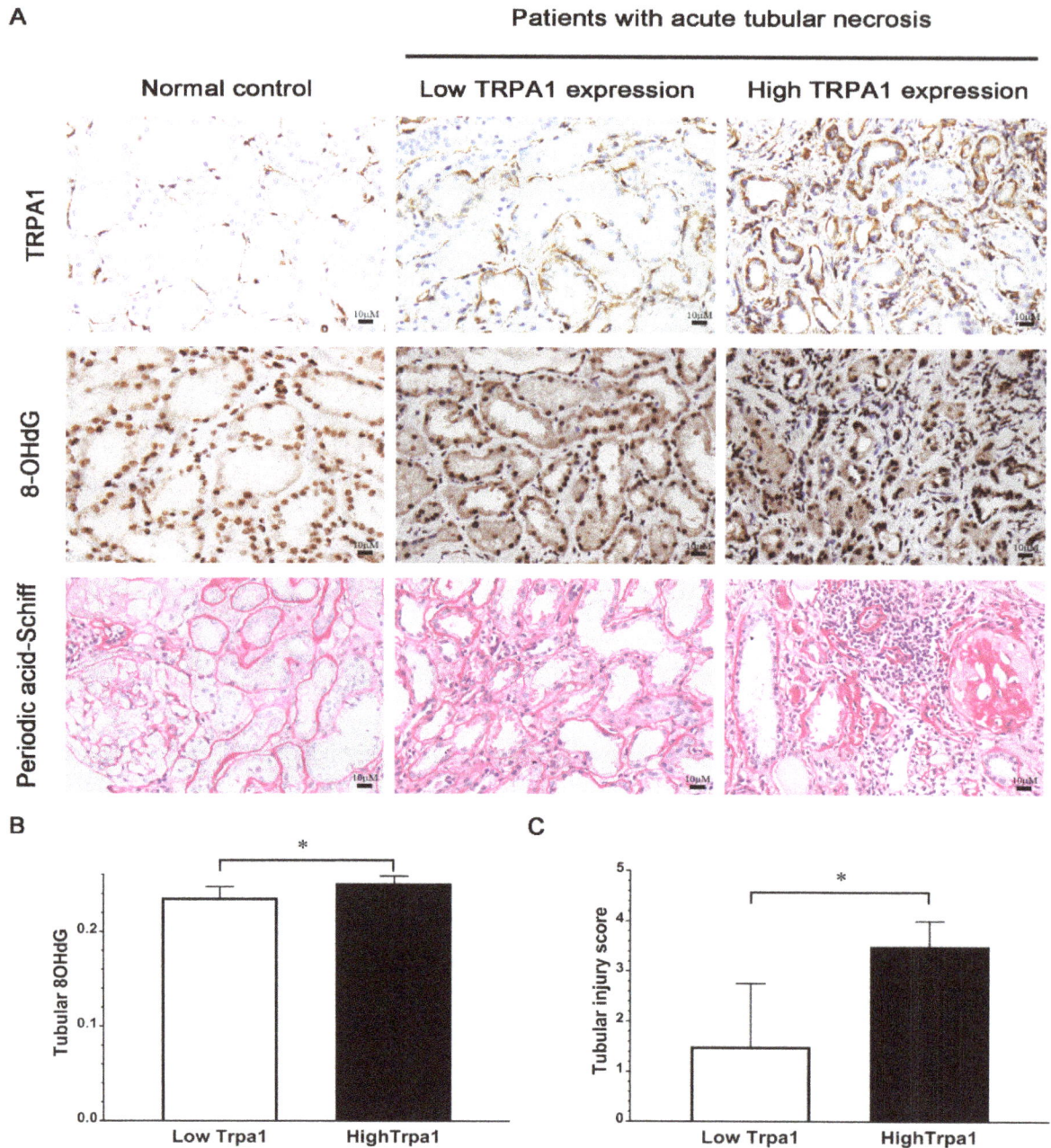

Figure 2. Different staining of kidney tissues from patients with ATN and association of TRPA1 expression with oxidative stress or tubular injury score. (**A**) Representative images of immunohistochemical staining of TRPA1, 8-OHdG, and periodic acid-Schiff staining of kidney tissues from patients with ATN and normal controls; 8-OHdG, an oxidative stress marker (**B**) QISV of tubular 8-OHdG (**C**) Tubular injury score. ATN patients were stratified into high and low expression groups by the cutoff value of 0.194 for tubular TRPA1 QISV based on the ROC curve analysis. Data are expressed as mean ± SD. * $p < 0.05$; TRPA1—Transient receptor potential ankyrin 1; 8-OHdG—8-hydroxy-2'-deoxyguanosine; QISV—quantitative immunohistochemical staining value; ROC—receiver operating characteristic; SD—standard deviation.

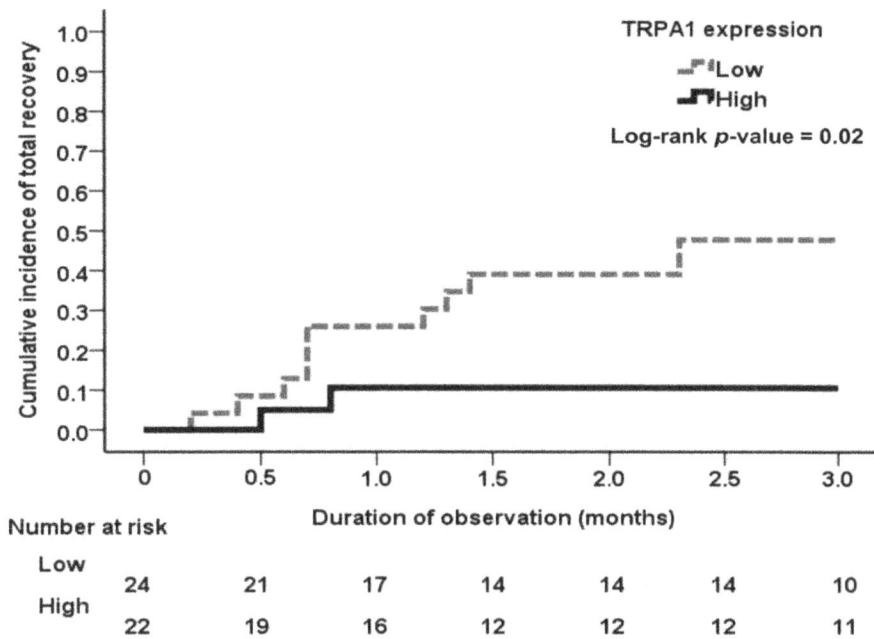

Figure 3. Cumulative incidence of total recovery of renal function among the ATN patients with different expression levels of tubular TRPA1. Incidence rate of the events of total recovery of renal function was significantly higher in the low tubular TRPA1 expression group than in the high tubular TRPA1 expression group during the follow-up period (log-rank test; $p = 0.02$).

Table 2. Logistical regression for nonrecovery of total renal function or death within three months after acute tubular necrosis.

Variables	Univariable		Model 1 (Adjusted for Age and Sex)	
	OR (95%CI)	*p* Value	OR (95%CI)	*p* Value
High tubular TRPA1 expression	7.14 (1.35–37.75)	0.02	6.86 (1.26–37.27)	0.03
Hypertension	2.08 (0.39–11.27)	0.39	1.84 (0.33–10.28)	0.49
Diabetes mellitus	6.81 (0.78–59.10)	0.08	5.34 (0.58–49.25)	0.14
Tubular atrophy (%)	1.96 (1.16–3.32)	0.01	2.01 (1.14–3.55)	0.02
Interstitial fibrosis (%)	1.08 (0.96–1.21)	0.19	1.06 (0.95–1.19)	0.29
Baseline eGFR (mL/min/1.73 m^2)	0.97 (0.94–0.99)	0.01	0.97 (0.95–0.99)	0.02
Urinary protein-to-creatinine ratio (10 mg/mg)	1.00 (1.00–1.01)	0.14	1.00 (1.00–1.01)	0.14
Hemoglobin (g/dL)	0.65 (0.45–0.93)	0.02	0.68 (0.47–0.99)	0.04
Concomitant use of ACEIs or ARBs	1.30 (0.23–7.32)	0.77	1.30 (0.22–7.80)	0.78
Concomitant use of immunosuppressants	3.10 (0.58–16.41)	0.18	4.41 (0.74–26.29)	0.10

OR—Odds ratio; CI—Confidence Interval; TRPA1—Transient receptor potential ankyrin 1; ACEI—Angiotensin-converting enzyme inhibitor; ARB—angiotensin-II receptor blocker; eGFR—estimated glomerular filtration rate.

3.4. Association of Tubular TRPA1 Expression with Mortality

Kaplan–Meier analysis revealed a higher incidence trend of mortality in ATN patients with high tubular TRPA1 expression during the three-month follow-up than in those with low tubular TRPA1 expression ($p = 0.07$), as seen in Figure 4.

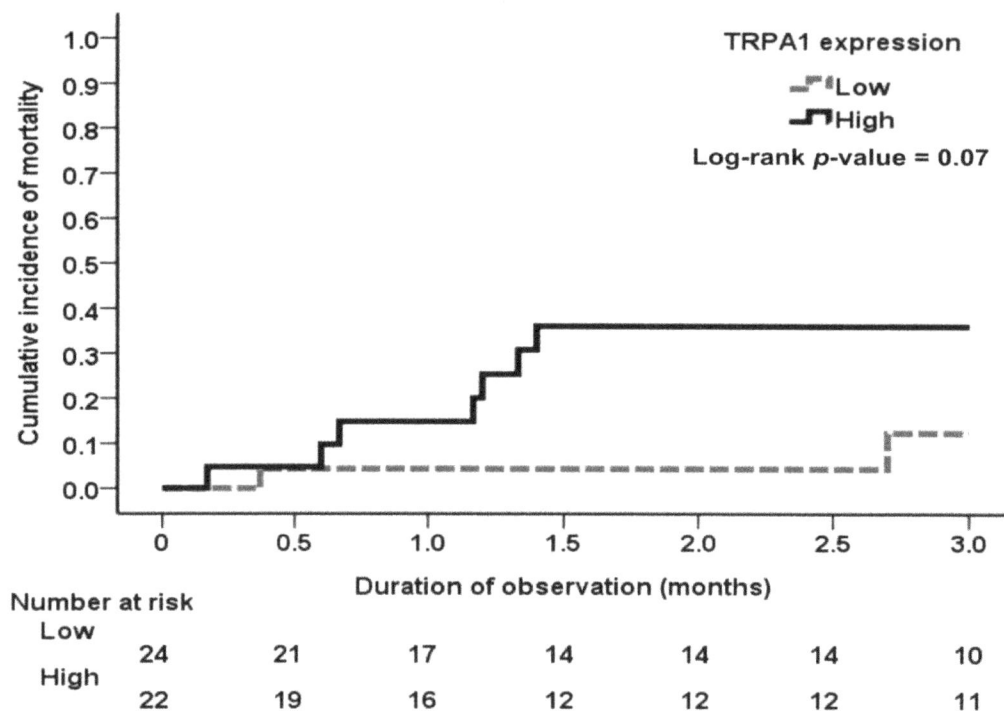

Figure 4. Cumulative incidence of mortality among the ATN patients with different expression levels of tubular TRPA1. Although ATN patients with high expression of tubular TRPA1 had a higher incidence of all-cause mortality than those with low expression of tubular TRPA1 during the follow-up period, the result was not statistically significant (log-rank test; $p = 0.07$). The severity of acute kidney injury may play a mediating role in all-cause mortality. Therefore, further research excluding the mediating factor is warranted.

4. Discussion

In this clinical observational study, TRPA1 was upregulated in the renal tubules of patients with ATN. In these patients with ATN, the tubular expression of TRPA1, a redox-sensing Ca^{2+}-influx channel [21], is positively associated with 8-hydroxydeoxyguanosine, a marker of oxidative DNA damage and oxidative stress [22]. We also have demonstrated the positive correlation of TRPA1 expression level with the severity of tubular injury.

The generation of oxidative stress after AKI is a major determinant of AKI; however, the effects of AKI on the renal redox system remains elusive [23]. TRPA1, an oxidative stress-sensitive Ca^{2+}-permeable channel, can be activated by endogenous inflammatory agents produced on oxidative stress, such as H_2O_2, 4-hydroxynonenal, 4-oxononenal, and cyclopentenone prostaglandin 15-deoxy-delta (12,14)-prostaglandin J (2) (15d-PGJ(2)) [24,25]. Therefore, the positive correlation between TRPA1 expression and oxidative stress is expected.

TRPA1 is an oxidative sensor and gatekeeper for inflammation. However, the role of TRPA1 in tissue inflammation and injury remains controversial. Some studies demonstrated that TRPA1 promotes inflammation and tissue injury in neurons or non-neuronal cells [13,17,26–29]. By contrast, a few studies suggested that TRPA1 exerts antioxidative, anti-inflammatory, organ-protective effects [30,31]. Literature with regard to TRPA1 and AKI is limited. A recent experimental animal study has suggested that TRPA1 plays a protective role in Ang II-induced renal injury possibly by inhibiting macrophage-mediated inflammation [19]. Another experimental animal study demonstrated TRPA1 may protect against sepsis-induced kidney injury by modulating mitochondrial biogenesis and mitophagy [18]. However, our previous study showed that renal tubular epithelial TRPA1 may act as an oxidative stress sensor to mediate ischemia-reperfusion-induced kidney injury through mitogen-activated protein kinases (MAPKs) and nuclear factor-kB (NF-kB) signaling. Thus, the role of TRPA1 in renal injury warrants further investigation.

In the present study, the AKI patients with high tubular TRPA1 expression had severe tubular injury. The result suggests that high TRPA1 expression in renal tubules may be a risk factor of tubular injury in AKI patients. However, the corresponding clinical role of renal tubular TRPA1 after AKI remains elusive. Therefore, we further investigated the association between clinical outcomes in AKI patients with ATN and TRPA1 expression in renal tubules.

The incidence of complete recovery of renal function was low in AKI patients with high expression of renal tubular TRPA1, and the patients with high expression of renal tubular TRPA1 had high odds of nonrecovery of renal function. This result suggests TRPA1 is associated with the progression of AKI to CKD. Progression of chronic kidney disease after acute kidney injury has a strong effect on long-term mortality [32]. As expected, the incidence of mortality in AKI patients with high TRPA1 expression was high because these patients had poor renal outcomes following AKI, although the result did not achieve statistical significance ($p = 0.07$) due to low case numbers.

The present study has several limitations. First, clinically, renal biopsy is not routinely performed in AKI patients, especially in AKI patients whose causes of AKI are known. Therefore, our results do not represent the association of TRPA1 with ATN in the total AKI population. Second, the relatively small sample size in the study lessens the statistical power of the results. Third, compared with prospective studies, retrospective cohort studies have lower statistical quality because of some unmeasured confounders. Fourth, although tubular 8-OHdG is an oxidative marker, it is not a direct activator of renal tubular TRPA1. Conversely, 4-hydroxy-2-nonenal (4-HNE) is an oxidative marker and a direct activator of renal tubular TRPA1 and thus requires further investigation to confirm the conclusion drawn from 8-OHdG staining. Fifth, this retrospective cohort study is correlational research, and thus cannot comprehensively elaborate on the causality of different expression levels of tubular TRPA1, tubular injury, and renal outcome. Therefore, the association of tubular TRPA1 expression with renal function or histopathology or clinical renal outcome of the different TRPA1 expression levels may be attributed to the severity of ATN. The role of tubular TRPA1 in AKI and its participatory mechanism in AKI remain to be elucidated. Further large prospective clinical studies or basic studies are warranted to investigate the biological role of TRPA1 in renal tubular injury after AKI.

In conclusion, high tubular TRPA1 expression was associated with a low probability of renal recovery in patients with ATN. High tubular TRPA1 expression was associated with the severity of tubular injury and poor renal outcomes following AKI. These findings suggest that tubular TRPA1 is a potential therapeutic target for AKI. The mechanism of TRPA1 in different AKI models warrants further investigation to confirm the roles of TRPA1 in AKI.

5. Conclusions

High renal tubular TRPA1 expression in AKI patients with biopsy-proven ATN was associated with the nontotal recovery of renal function.

Author Contributions: All authors reviewed the manuscript. C.-K.W. wrote the manuscript. C.-K.W., C.-L.W., Y.R.K., and D.-C.T. conceived and designed the experiments. C.-K.W., C.-L.W., and C.-T.K. performed the analyses. C.-K.W., C.-L.W., and T.-C.S. performed the experiments and collected the data. C.-K.W., C.-L.W., T.-C.S., T.-S.L., Y.R.K., and D.-C.T. contributed to the discussion and manuscript revision. Y.R.K. and D.-C.T. conceived the study and are the guarantors of this publication.

Acknowledgments: The authors are grateful for the assistance of KG Support-Academic Submission Services in the language editing of the manuscript. The authors thank Chung-Min Yeh from the Department of Pathology, Changhua Christian Hospital (Changhua, Taiwan) for their excellent assistance in staining human tissue samples.

References

1. Gameiro, J.; Agapito Fonseca, J.; Jorge, S.; Lopes, J.A. Acute kidney injury definition and diagnosis: A narrative review. *J. Clin. Med.* **2018**, *7*, E307. [CrossRef] [PubMed]
2. Thomas, M.E.; Blaine, C.; Dawnay, A.; Devonald, M.A.; Ftouh, S.; Laing, C.; Latchem, S.; Lewington, A.; Milford, D.V.; Ostermann, M. The definition of acute kidney injury and its use in practice. *Kidney Int.* **2015**, *87*, 62–73. [CrossRef] [PubMed]
3. Bagshaw, S.M.; Wald, R. Strategies for the optimal timing to start renal replacement therapy in critically ill patients with acute kidney injury. *Kidney Int.* **2017**, *91*, 1022–1032. [CrossRef] [PubMed]
4. Sawhney, S.; Fraser, S.D. Epidemiology of aki: Utilizing large databases to determine the burden of aki. *Adv. Chronic Kidney Dis.* **2017**, *24*, 194–204. [CrossRef] [PubMed]
5. Rangaswamy, D.; Sud, K. Acute kidney injury and disease: Long-term consequences and management. *Nephrology (Carlton)* **2018**, *23*, 969–980. [CrossRef]
6. Shiao, C.C.; Wu, P.C.; Wu, V.C.; Lin, J.H.; Pan, H.C.; Yang, Y.F.; Lai, T.S.; Huang, T.M.; Wu, C.H.; Yang, W.S.; et al. Nationwide epidemiology and prognosis of dialysis-requiring acute kidney injury (nep-aki-d) study: Design and methods. *Nephrology (Carlton)* **2016**, *21*, 758–764. [CrossRef]
7. Negi, S.; Koreeda, D.; Kobayashi, S.; Yano, T.; Tatsuta, K.; Mima, T.; Shigematsu, T.; Ohya, M. Acute kidney injury: Epidemiology, outcomes, complications, and therapeutic strategies. *Semin. Dial.* **2018**, *31*, 519–527. [CrossRef]
8. Hanif, M.O.; Ramphul, K. Acute renal tubular necrosis. In *Statpearls*; StatePearls Publishing: Treasure Island, FL, USA, 2019.
9. Pavlakou, P.; Liakopoulos, V.; Eleftheriadis, T.; Mitsis, M.; Dounousi, E. Oxidative stress and acute kidney injury in critical illness: Pathophysiologic mechanisms-biomarkers-interventions, and future perspectives. *Oxid. Med. Cell. Longev.* **2017**, *2017*, 6193694. [CrossRef]
10. Ratliff, B.B.; Abdulmahdi, W.; Pawar, R.; Wolin, M.S. Oxidant mechanisms in renal injury and disease. *Antioxid. Redox Signal.* **2016**, *25*, 119–146. [CrossRef]
11. Gorin, Y. The kidney: An organ in the front line of oxidative stress-associated pathologies. *Antioxid. Redox Signal.* **2016**, *25*, 639–641. [CrossRef]
12. de Caestecker, M.; Harris, R. Translating knowledge into therapy for acute kidney injury. *Semin. Nephrol.* **2018**, *38*, 88–97. [CrossRef] [PubMed]
13. Viana, F. Trpa1 channels: Molecular sentinels of cellular stress and tissue damage. *J. Physiol.* **2016**, *594*, 4151–4169. [CrossRef] [PubMed]
14. Bautista, D.M.; Pellegrino, M.; Tsunozaki, M. Trpa1: A gatekeeper for inflammation. *Ann. Rev. Physiol.* **2013**, *75*, 181–200. [CrossRef] [PubMed]
15. Dembla, S.; Hasan, N.; Becker, A.; Beck, A.; Philipp, S.E. Transient receptor potential a1 channels regulate epithelial cell barriers formed by mdck cells. *FEBS Lett.* **2016**, *590*, 1509–1520. [CrossRef] [PubMed]
16. Nassini, R.; Pedretti, P.; Moretto, N.; Fusi, C.; Carnini, C.; Facchinetti, F.; Viscomi, A.R.; Pisano, A.R.; Stokesberry, S.; Brunmark, C.; et al. Transient receptor potential ankyrin 1 channel localized to non-neuronal airway cells promotes non-neurogenic inflammation. *PLoS ONE* **2012**, *7*, e42454. [CrossRef] [PubMed]
17. Kanda, Y.; Yamasaki, Y.; Sasaki-Yamaguchi, Y.; Ida-Koga, N.; Kamisuki, S.; Sugawara, F.; Nagumo, Y.; Usui, T. Trpa1-dependent reversible opening of tight junction by natural compounds with an alpha,beta-unsaturated moiety and capsaicin. *Sci. Rep.* **2018**, *8*, 2251. [CrossRef] [PubMed]
18. Zhu, J.; Zhang, S.; Geng, Y.; Song, Y. Transient receptor potential ankyrin 1 protects against sepsis-induced kidney injury by modulating mitochondrial biogenesis and mitophagy. *Am. J. Transl. Res.* **2018**, *10*, 4163–4172.
19. Ma, S.; Zhang, Y.; He, K.; Wang, P.; Wang, D.H. Knockout of trpa1 exacerbates angiotensin ii-induced kidney injury. *Am. J. Physiol. Renal. Physiol.* **2019**, *317*, F623–F631. [CrossRef]
20. Tseng, W.C.; Yang, W.C.; Yang, A.H.; Hsieh, S.L.; Tarng, D.C. Expression of tnfrsf6b in kidneys is a novel predictor for progression of chronic kidney disease. *Mod. Pathol.* **2013**, *26*, 984–994. [CrossRef]
21. Nilius, B.; Appendino, G.; Owsianik, G. The transient receptor potential channel trpa1: From gene to pathophysiology. *Pflugers Arch.* **2012**, *464*, 425–458. [CrossRef]
22. Yokozawa, T.; Fujioka, K.; Oura, H. Increase in kidney 8-hydroxydeoxyguanosine level with the progression of renal failure. *Nephron* **1992**, *61*, 236–237. [CrossRef] [PubMed]
23. Kasuno, K.; Shirakawa, K.; Yoshida, H.; Mori, K.; Kimura, H.; Takahashi, N.; Nobukawa, Y.; Shigemi, K.;

Tanabe, S.; Yamada, N.; et al. Renal redox dysregulation in aki: Application for oxidative stress marker of aki. *Am. J. Physiol. Renal. Physiol.* **2014**, *307*, F1342–F1351. [CrossRef] [PubMed]

24. Sawada, Y.; Hosokawa, H.; Matsumura, K.; Kobayashi, S. Activation of transient receptor potential ankyrin 1 by hydrogen peroxide. *Eur. J. Neurosci.* **2008**, *27*, 1131–1142. [CrossRef] [PubMed]

25. Weng, Y.; Batista-Schepman, P.A.; Barabas, M.E.; Harris, E.Q.; Dinsmore, T.B.; Kossyreva, E.A.; Foshage, A.M.; Wang, M.H.; Schwab, M.J.; Wang, V.M.; et al. Prostaglandin metabolite induces inhibition of trpa1 and channel-dependent nociception. *Mol. Pain* **2012**, *8*, 75. [CrossRef] [PubMed]

26. Fernandes, E.S.; Fernandes, M.A.; Keeble, J.E. The functions of trpa1 and trpv1: Moving away from sensory nerves. *Br. J. Pharmacol.* **2012**, *166*, 510–521. [CrossRef]

27. Bautista, D.M.; Jordt, S.E.; Nikai, T.; Tsuruda, P.R.; Read, A.J.; Poblete, J.; Yamoah, E.N.; Basbaum, A.I.; Julius, D. Trpa1 mediates the inflammatory actions of environmental irritants and proalgesic agents. *Cell* **2006**, *124*, 1269–1282. [CrossRef]

28. Feng, J.; Yang, P.; Mack, M.R.; Dryn, D.; Luo, J.; Gong, X.; Liu, S.; Oetjen, L.K.; Zholos, A.V.; Mei, Z.; et al. Sensory trp channels contribute differentially to skin inflammation and persistent itch. *Nat. Commun.* **2017**, *8*, 980. [CrossRef]

29. Lin, A.H.; Liu, M.H.; Ko, H.K.; Perng, D.W.; Lee, T.S.; Kou, Y.R. Lung epithelial trpa1 transduces the extracellular ros into transcriptional regulation of lung inflammation induced by cigarette smoke: The role of influxed ca(2)(+). *Mediators Inflamm.* **2015**, *2015*, 148367. [CrossRef]

30. Kun, J.; Szitter, I.; Kemeny, A.; Perkecz, A.; Kereskai, L.; Pohoczky, K.; Vincze, A.; Godi, S.; Szabo, I.; Szolcsanyi, J.; et al. Upregulation of the transient receptor potential ankyrin 1 ion channel in the inflamed human and mouse colon and its protective roles. *PLoS ONE* **2014**, *9*, e108164. [CrossRef]

31. Lowin, T.; Apitz, M.; Anders, S.; Straub, R.H. Anti-inflammatory effects of n-acylethanolamines in rheumatoid arthritis synovial cells are mediated by trpv1 and trpa1 in a cox-2 dependent manner. *Arthritis Res. Ther.* **2015**, *17*, 321. [CrossRef]

32. An, J.N.; Hwang, J.H.; Kim, D.K.; Lee, H.; Ahn, S.Y.; Kim, S.; Park, J.T.; Kang, S.W.; Oh, Y.K.; Kim, Y.S.; et al. Chronic kidney disease after acute kidney injury requiring continuous renal replacement therapy and its impact on long-term outcomes: A multicenter retrospective cohort study in korea. *Crit. Care Med.* **2017**, *45*, 47–57. [CrossRef] [PubMed]

2

Use of Estimating Equations for Dosing Antimicrobials in Patients with Acute Kidney Injury Not Receiving Renal Replacement Therapy

Linda Awdishu [1,2,*], **Ana Isabel Connor** [1], **Josée Bouchard** [3], **Etienne Macedo** [2], **Glenn M. Chertow** [4] **and Ravindra L. Mehta** [2]

[1] Division of Clinical Pharmacy, UCSD Skaggs School of Pharmacy and Pharmaceutical Sciences, San Diego, CA 92093, USA; lehans158@msn.com

[2] Department of Medicine, Division of Nephrology, UCSD School of Medicine, San Diego, CA 92093, USA; emacedo@ucsd.edu (E.M.); rmehta@ucsd.edu (R.L.M.)

[3] Department of Medicine, University of Montreal, Montreal, QC H3T 1J4, Canada; joseebouchard123@yahoo.ca

[4] Department of Medicine, Division of Nephrology, Stanford University School of Medicine, Palo Alto, CA 94034, USA; gchertow@stanford.edu

*   Correspondence: lawdishu@ucsd.edu

Abstract: Acute kidney injury (AKI) can potentially lead to the accumulation of antimicrobial drugs with significant renal clearance. Drug dosing adjustments are commonly made using the Cockcroft-Gault estimate of creatinine clearance (CLcr). The Modified Jelliffe equation is significantly better at estimating kidney function than the Cockcroft-Gault equation in the setting of AKI. The objective of this study is to assess the degree of antimicrobial dosing discordance using different glomerular filtration rate (GFR) estimating equations. This is a retrospective evaluation of antimicrobial dosing using different estimating equations for kidney function in AKI and comparison to Cockcroft-Gault estimation as a reference. Considering the Cockcroft-Gault estimate as the criterion standard, antimicrobials were appropriately adjusted at most 80.7% of the time. On average, kidney function changed by 30 mL/min over the course of an AKI episode. The median clearance at the peak serum creatinine was 27.4 (9.3–66.3) mL/min for Cockcroft Gault, 19.8 (9.8–47.0) mL/min/1.73 m^2 for MDRD and 20.5 (4.9–49.6) mL/min for the Modified Jelliffe equations. The discordance rate for antimicrobial dosing ranged from a minimum of 8.6% to a maximum of 16.4%. In the event of discordance, the dose administered was supra-therapeutic 100% of the time using the Modified Jelliffe equation. Use of estimating equations other than the Cockcroft Gault equation may significantly alter dosing of antimicrobials in AKI.

Keywords: acute kidney injury; Cockcroft Gault; Jelliffe; MDRD; drug dosing; antimicrobials

1. Introduction

Acute kidney injury (AKI) has been reported to occur in approximately 6% of hospitalized patients [1]. Among patients admitted with AKI, infection is present in approximately 18% [2]. AKI is particularly common among critically ill patients and has been associated with increased morbidity and significant in-hospital mortality [2,3]. A decline in kidney function can potentially lead to the accumulation of antimicrobial and other therapeutic agents, with resultant adverse effects [4]. An accurate assessment of kidney function is important in order to optimize drug administration in this population [5–7].

The most accurate way to determine glomerular filtration rate (GFR) in chronic kidney disease (CKD) is by formal measurement using an intravenous injection of inulin or a radioisotope and subsequently collecting urine and serum samples at timed intervals [8,9]. However, the direct measurement of GFR is cumbersome, expensive and time consuming, and rarely performed in the acute hospital setting. These procedures are even more complicated in AKI. Pharmacists generally employ the Cockcroft-Gault (CG) equation to estimate kidney function, altering either or both the dose and frequency of drugs based on varying degrees of evidence in the setting of impaired kidney function and/or dialysis [10–16].

Several newer GFR estimating equations have been developed and used widely in epidemiological studies and clinical practice, including the Modification of Diet in Renal Disease (MDRD) study equation and the CKD-EPI equation. These equations were derived from varying populations who generally had stable kidney function. For example, the CG equation was derived from a hospitalized population including predominantly Caucasian men with stable serum creatinine concentrations (Scr) [17]. The MDRD study and CKD-EPI equations were largely derived from ambulatory populations with mild to moderate CKD and relatively stable Scr [12]. Additionally, acute changes in the Scr can invalidate conventional estimates of kidney function, where the estimates depend on the assumption that function is at steady state [18]. The Jelliffe equation was developed to estimate GFR in AKI, where kidney function is not in steady state [19]. Bouchard and colleagues demonstrated that the Jelliffe equation, modified by consideration of patient volume status, provided a more reliable and accurate assessment of kidney function when compared with timed urine collections in AKI [20]. While several studies have evaluated CG compared to MDRD estimates in patients with CKD, there is a paucity of data comparing whether alternative GFR estimating equations might alter dosing of drugs in AKI [11,21]. The objective of this study was to compare the theoretical influence of different estimating equations on drug dosing of antimicrobials in patients with AKI.

2. Experimental Section

The Program to Improve Care in Acute Renal Disease (PICARD) group included five academic medical centers in the United States. The study was approved by the ethics committees at each participating clinical site. A total of 618 subjects were enrolled over a 31-month period (February 1999 to August 2001), among who 398 required IHD or CRRT. We conducted a retrospective chart review of antimicrobial dosing for a subset of patients from one center in the PICARD data set. Complete descriptions of PICARD methods have been previously published [2,3].

AKI was defined differently depending on the baseline Scr. In patients with baseline Scr < 1.5 mg/dL, AKI was defined as an increase in Scr $\geq$ 0.5 mg/dL, whereas in those with baseline Scr $\geq$ 1.5 mg/dL and $\leq$ 5 mg/dL, as an increase in Scr $\geq$ 1 mg/dL. Patients with a baseline Scr > 5 mg/dL were not considered for study inclusion. Pertinent data elements from PICARD used for these analyses included age, sex, height, weight (to calculate body surface area), daily fluid balance, daily Scr and all dates on which patients received intermittent hemodialysis (IHD) or continuous renal replacement therapy (CRRT).

For inclusion in this study, patients were required to have complete laboratory information and must have received antimicrobials during some dates of enrollment in the PICARD study. We excluded the time period during which patients were on IHD or CRRT, including the days before and after dialysis. Drug dispensation records were retrieved electronically and included antibiotic name, dose, frequency, route, start and stop dates.

2.1. Estimation of GFR Using Cockroft-Gault, MDRD, Jelliffe and Modified Jelliffe Equations

Estimations of CLcr or GFR using CG [17], abbreviated MDRD (age, race, gender and Scr) [10], MDRD adjusted for BSA, Jelliffe [19] and Modified Jelliffe equations [20] were calculated for each patient during each date of admission that they received an antimicrobial agent (Table 1). For the CG equation, total body weight was used if this weight was less than 130% of ideal body weight. If total body weight was greater than 130% of ideal body weight, an adjusted body weight was calculated by adding 40% of the difference between the total and ideal body weights to the ideal body weight.

Table 1. Equations used to estimate renal function.

Name	Equation
Cockcroft Gault	CLcr = ((140 − age) × weight (kg))/(72 × Scr (mg/dL)) Multiply by 0.85 if female
MDRD	GFR = 186 × (SCr (mg/dL))$^{-1.154}$ × (age (years))$^{-0.203}$ × (0.742 if patient is female) × (1.21 if patient is black)
MDRD adjusted for BSA	GFR = MDRD × BSA / 1.73 m^2
Jelliffe	(((Volume of distribution × (Scr on day 1 − Scr on day 2)) + creatinine production) × 100/1440/average Scr
Modified Jelliffe	Substitute Adjusted SCr into Jelliffe equation Adjusted SCr = SCr (measured) × Correction Factor Correction Factor = ((admit weight (kg) × 0.6) + Sum (Daily fluid balance))/admit weight × 0.6

CLcr = creatinine clearance, MDRD = modification of diet in renal disease, GFR = glomerular filtration rate, BSA = body surface area.

Clearances were calculated at the peak and nadir Scr values to describe the severity and resolution of the AKI. The CG equation was used as the reference estimate for the analysis, as the CG equation is the most frequently used equation by pharmacists for drug dosing [18]. Timed urine collections were performed as part of routine medical care for a small subset of patients and the duration ranged from 4 to 24 h.

2.2. Evaluation of the Discordance in Drug Dosing Among Estimating Equations

Institutional guidelines from the University of California, San Diego on drug dosing in patients with impaired kidney function were utilized to assess dose appropriateness. These guidelines suggest using the CG equation for drug dosing and are based on modified FDA recommendations. An antimicrobial episode was defined as each day that the patient received the antimicrobial or any time the antimicrobial was altered (e.g., change in antimicrobial dose or frequency). The rate of discordance in drug dosing was calculated as the difference in the number of correctly dosed antimicrobial episodes between the CG and the other estimating equations (Table 1) divided by the total number of antimicrobial episodes (Equation (1)).

$$\frac{(\#\text{Correct Episodes CG} - \#\text{Correct Episodes comparison}) \times 100}{\text{Total \#Episodes}} \tag{1}$$

We used antimicrobial episodes for calculating discordance since a single patient may receive numerous antimicrobials for varied durations of therapy. Additionally, the potential for error could be different depending on the antimicrobial and dosing range. A chi square test of independence with Bonferroni correction for multiple comparisons was used to assess if there was a difference in number of antimicrobial episodes dosed correctly between estimating equations for each antimicrobial (R 2.8.1). Two-tailed p-values < 0.05 were considered statistically significant.

3. Results

A total of 719 antimicrobial episodes from 32 unique patients were included in the analysis. The median age was 49.5 (range 31 to 89) years, 12.5% had CKD and the most common etiology of AKI was acute tubular necrosis (ATN). Demographic characteristics are summarized in Table 2.

Daily Scr values were used to estimate clearance for the entire cohort (Table 3). In order to show the spectrum of AKI, we calculated the median clearance at peak and nadir Scr and this ranged from 19.8 to 27.4 and 46.9 to 58.8 mL/min, respectively (Figures 1 and 2). During the course of AKI, there was a clinically meaningful change in kidney function of approximately 30 mL/min, which would indicate the need for re-evaluation of drug dosing.

Table 2. Demographics.

Variable	n (%) or Median (Range)
Age (years)	49.5 (31–89)
Gender	
Male	14 (44%)
Female	18 (56%)
Weight (kg)	73.9 (45–99)
Height (cm)	169 (152–191)
BSA (m^2)	1.81 (1.38–2.26)
APACHE III Score *	90 (38–151)
History of CKD	4 (12.5)
Etiology of AKI	
ATN	14 (44%)
Nephrotoxicity	2 (6%)
Multifactorial	11 (34%)
Hepatorenal	3 (10%)
Prerenal	2 (6%)

* APACHE III scores available for 30 patients.

Table 3. Clearance estimates.

Parameter	Timed Urine Collection	CG (mL/min)	MDRD (mL/min/1.73 m^2)	MDRD – Adj BSA (mL/min)	Jelliffe (mL/min)	Modified Jelliffe (mL/min)
CL peak Scr Median (range)	-	27.4 (9.3–66.3)	19.8 (9.8–47.0)	21.2 (9.9–60.4)	21.2 (5.2–56.4)	20.5 (4.9–49.6)
CL Nadir Sc rMedian (range)	-	58.8 (18.4–88.9)	46.9 (24.8–85.8)	50.8 (22.0–92.1)	52.8 (17.3–79.0)	47.2 (14.3–79.0)
Median CL (range)	22.8 (13.4–26.2)	34.4 (9.3–88.9)	28.6 (9.8–85.8)	29.3 (9.9–92.1)	30.3 (4.5 78.9)	26.7 (4.6–78.9)

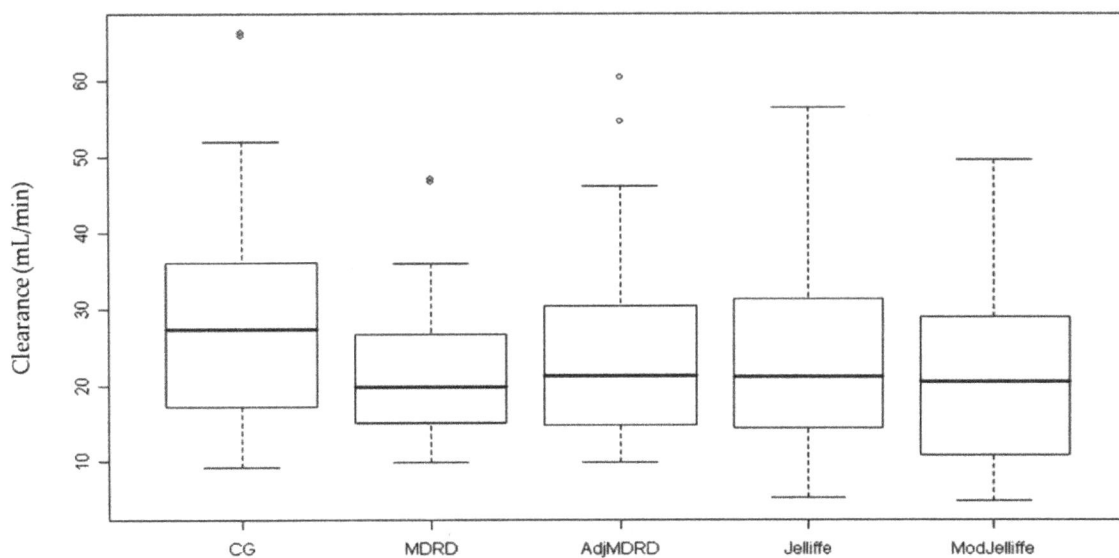

Figure 1. Clearance estimates at peak of kidney injury. This figure depicts the calculated median clearance using the peak serum creatinine value in each estimating equation. The circles represent outlier data points.

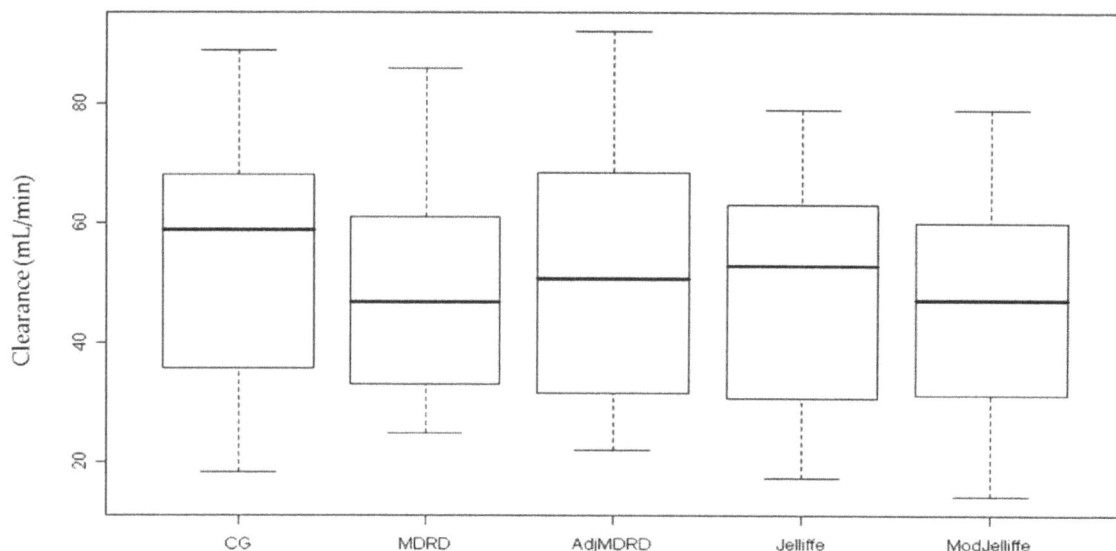

Figure 2. Clearance estimates at recovery of injury. This figure depicts the calculated median clearance at the time of injury recovery using the lowest serum creatinine value in each estimating equation.

3.1. Overall Impact on Drug Dosing Based on Individual Equations

Patients received at least one or more of the following antimicrobials whose disposition is influenced by kidney function: ampicillin, cefazolin, ceftazidime, ciprofloxacin, fluconazole, ganciclovir, metronidazole, piperacillin/tazobactam. Of the 719 dosing episodes, the appropriate dose of antimicrobials was administered at most 81% of the time (Table 4). Seventeen patients received a total of 139 episodes of inappropriate doses according to the CG equation, but after removing these inappropriate doses, 30 patients and 580 episodes remained. The discordance rate between the CG equation and the other estimation equations ranged from a minimum of 9% to a maximum of 16% (Table 4).

Table 4. Dose appropriateness for all drugs.

Estimating Equation	Number Dosed Correct (%) n = 719 episodes (32 patients)	Discordance Rate (%)	Number Dosed Correct (%) n = 580 episodes (30 patients)	Discordance Rate (%)
CG	580 (81)	-	580 (100)	-
MDRD	529 (74)	7	515 (89)	11
MDRD BSA	531 (74)	7	526 (91)	9
Jelliffe	531 (74)	7	530 (91)	9
Mod Jelliffe	488 (68)	12	485 (84)	16

3.2. Breakdown of Impact on Drug Dosing Based on Drug Administered

The most commonly prescribed drugs in our study population were ceftazidime, ciprofloxacin and fluconazole with 69%, 66% and 47% of patients receiving these medications. In the majority of cases, the discordance between estimating equations was statistically significant. The discordance rate for all episodes varied among the antimicrobial agents from 6 to 22% (Table 5).

Table 5. Dose appropriateness for specific antimicrobials.

Drug	# Patients Received (%)	# Correct CG (%)	# Correct Mod-Jelliffe (%)	Discordance Rate (%)	p Value
All drugs	-	580/719	488/719	13	<0.001
Ceftazidime	22 (69)	140/200 (70)	107/200 (54)	16	0.009
Ciprofloxacin	21 (66)	164/170 (96)	153/170 (90)	6	-
Fluconazole	15 (47)	104/129 (81)	91/129 (71)	10	-
Metronidazole	11 (34)	52/52 (100)	45/52 (87)	14	-
Cefazolin	7 (22)	31/36 (86)	23/36 (64)	22	-
Ganciclovir	7 (22)	59/92 (64)	41/92 (45)	20	-
Ampicillin	4 (13)	10/16 (63)	9/16 (56)	6	-
Piperacillin/ Tazobactam	4 (13)	16/16 (100)	15/16 (94)	6	-

The discordance in drug dosing between the CG and the Modified Jelliffe was highest for cefazolin (22%), ganciclovir (20%) and ceftazidime (16%). In patients who were not dosed correctly according to CG, we did not find any episodes of under-dosing. We analyzed the direction of error in dosing in the subset of episodes where the dose was correct based on the CG estimate of clearance (Table 6).

Table 6. Correct doses for Cockcroft Gault but overdosing for modified Jelliffe.

Antimicrobial	Number of Patients	Number of Dosing Episodes	Number of Overdosing Episodes	Median Daily Dose (Range)	Median Overdoseper Day (Range)
Acyclovir	2	4	0	2400 mg	0 mg
Ampicillin	3	10	1	3500 mg (3000–8000)	5000 mg
Cefazolin	7	31	7	3000 mg (2000–3000)	1000 mg
Ceftazidime	20	140	33	2000 mg (500–3000)	1000 mg (500–3000)
Ciprofloxacin	24	164	11	500 mg (400–1500)	400 mg (200–500)
Fluconazole	17	104	16	100 mg (50–400)	50 mg (50-100)
Ganciclovir	6	59	18	Oral: 3000 mg (1000–3000) IV: 100 mg (75–400)	Oral: 2000 mg (1000 2000) IV: 110 mg (45–200)
Metronidazole	11	52	7	1500 mg (1000–1500)	500 mg
Piperacillin/ Tazobactam	4	16	1	11,250 mg (6750–1,3500)	4500 mg

Depending on the frequency of antimicrobial administration, the percentage of over-dosing episodes was as high as 30%. Furthermore, in reviewing the doses administered, excess doses were clinically relevant for some antimicrobials (Table 6).

4. Discussion

In our study, we found that patients received an inappropriate dose of antimicrobials in approximately one in six dosing episodes. Almost half of the patients included in this study experienced a dosing error. The change in estimated clearance was clinically significant for the majority of patients, warranting a dosage adjustment of medications. The overall discordance rate between the CG equation and the other estimating equations was between 9% and 16%. Importantly, the difference in clearance between the estimating equations was approximately 8 mL/min or a 30% relative difference. This difference also crossed a cutoff value for our institutional guidelines for dosage adjustment (30 mL/min) resulting in antimicrobial dosing discordance. This presents a clinical challenge since physicians and pharmacists are faced with different kidney function estimates, which ultimately lead to variable doses of critical medications. We found that in cases of discordances between the CG and Modified Jelliffe equations, the dose of antimicrobial administered was supra-therapeutic when using the Modified Jelliffe estimate as the reference point.

Several factors can be attributed to the challenge of drug dosing in AKI. These include the delayed rise of Scr in response to injury, the accuracy of the various estimating equations in AKI, the lack of therapeutic drug monitoring for several antimicrobials, as well as the lack of published pharmacokinetic information on antimicrobial dosing in patients with AKI not receiving dialysis or hemofiltration.

Estimating kidney function in AKI remains controversial. Hoste and colleagues have demonstrated that in critically ill patients with normal Scr, urinary excretion of creatinine was markedly reduced [22]. They concluded that using Scr to predict kidney function was insensitive in the critically ill population and advocated for the use measured CLcr [22]. Clinicians often measure CLcr with urinary collections since patients may have an indwelling catheter and the collection can be completed by a nurse. However, urinary CLcrs have been shown to be inaccurate in the critically ill population. Robert and colleagues published results comparing the performance of 30 min urinary CLcr, 24 h urinary CLcr, and CG estimates to inulin clearance in 20 critically ill patients with stable Scr whose mean was 1.8 ± 1.5 mg/dL [16]. The 30 min collection performed similarly to the 24 h collection, but in a subset of patients, urinary CLcr over-predicted GFR by 30–300% [16]. Bragadottir and colleagues demonstrated that urinary CLcr had a low reproducibility compared to measured GFR [23]. Given the limitations of urinary collections in the critically ill population, estimating equations are attractive for routine bedside approximations of GFR. To date there are various studies comparing the ability of estimating equations to accurately predict measured CLcr or GFR in patients with stable renal function [8–17,24]. Analysis of these studies indicates that the most accurate equation varies according to the population studied [9,15]. Steady state equations such as CG will systematically over-estimate clearance and lead to over-dosing episodes in patients with AKI. Kirwan and colleagues compared the accuracy of the various steady state estimating equations to measured CLcr (4 h collection) in critically ill patients with AKI. They found that the accuracy of the various equations within 50% of measured CLcr to be 68, 78 and 81% for the CG, MDRD and CKD-EPI equations respectively [25]. The performance of these equations was not as good as in the setting of CKD. Poggio and colleagues examined the accuracy of the CG and MDRD equations in estimating GFR compared to measured GFR in hospitalized patients with kidney dysfunction [13]. They demonstrated that the MDRD and CG equations over-estimated GFR and the accuracy of the estimates within 50% of the measured GFR was 49% and 40%, respectively [13]. Bragadottir found that the MDRD, CKD-EPI and CG equations performed poorly when compared to measured GFR in critically ill patients with early AKI with biases of 7.39–11.58 mL/min [23]. This bias is consistent with other studies noting over-estimation of measured CLcr by approximately 6–17 mL/min [25,26]. These steady state equations are problematic for the estimation of kidney function in an intensive care setting or in AKI.

Non steady state equations such as Jelliffe will provide estimates of GFR that are closer to the true clearance [19]. Using data from PICARD, Bouchard and colleagues compared the accuracy of estimating GFR using CG, MDRD, Jelliffe and a modified Jelliffe equation to that of a 24-h measured urinary CLcr [20]. The authors found that among critically ill patients with AKI, traditional estimating equations (CG, MDRD) significantly overestimate kidney function compared to a modified Jelliffe equation adjusted for fluid balance [20].

One limitation of this study was the small sample size of 32 patients, as we could retrieve antimicrobial dosing data only on a small subset of patients from the PICARD database. In addition, the retrospective nature of the study is a limitation in capturing the dynamic nature of prescribing and pharmacist consulting on antimicrobial doses. This safety concern was unanticipated but provides strong rationale for electronic algorithms for drug dosage adjustments according to kidney function. Our retrospective study is limited in assessing the validity of the estimating equations for patients with AKI. We utilized the CG estimate as the criterion standard since this is the most commonly used equation for adjusting the doses of drugs [18]. We found discordance in kidney function estimates but we are limited in concluding which equation is most accurate and whether the use of the Modified Jelliffe equation would have resulted in appropriate antimicrobial concentrations.

Most clinicians feel that the therapeutic index is wide for many antimicrobials such as penicillins and cephalosporins. However, inappropriate dosing may contribute to the development of super-infections and increased costs.

Our study did not include antimicrobials in which therapeutic drug monitoring is available. If serum concentration monitoring is available, this guides dosage adjustments and little emphasis is placed on the renal estimating equation. The GFR estimating equations are used to calculate initial doses and subsequent dosing is based on serum concentrations.

Our study did not include patients on IHD or CRRT. In the setting of dialysis, a fixed clearance is prescribed. However, estimating CLcr from the prescribed effluent volumes may not be accurate since the clearance delivered is frequently less than that prescribed [27]. Dosing guidelines for many drugs in AKI are generally derived from experience in patients with CKD. This may not account for changes in drug metabolism, tubular function or drug transport in the setting of AKI [28–31]. Applying CLcr estimates from prescribed effluent volume, utilizing dosing guidelines derived from CKD and a lack of available therapeutic drug monitoring may create a potential for under-dosing antimicrobials in a critically ill population receiving IHD or CRRT [32].

The KDIGO position statement on drug dosing considerations indicates there is a lack of compelling evidence for the superiority of any one estimating equation for drug dosing [18]. The Acute Disease Quality Initiative (ADQI) recommends the use of short timed urine collections or the modified Jelliffe equation for estimating kidney function in persistent AKI [33]. Further research is needed on the quantification of kidney function in persistent AKI in the critically ill population.

5. Conclusions

Critically ill patients with AKI are at risk for significantly increased morbidity and mortality. It is essential that drugs be dosed as accurately as possible to minimize potential adverse effects and improve patient outcomes. The observations from our study indicate that there is discordance in drug dosing when using kidney function estimating equations. Prospective studies evaluating the Modified Jelliffe equation and other strategies for drug dosing in the setting of AKI should be undertaken.

Author Contributions: Conceptualization, L.A., A.I.C. and R.L.M.; Methodology, L.A., A.I.C., E.M. and J.B.; Software, L.A.; Validation, L.A., E.M. and J.B.; Formal Analysis, A.I.C. and L.A.; Investigation, L.A., A.I.C. J.B., E.M. and R.L.M.; Resources, R.L.M.; Data Curation, E.M. and J.B.; Writing-Original Draft Preparation, A.I.C., L.A., J.B., R.L.M. and G.M.C.; Writing-Review & Editing, A.I.C., L.A., J.B., R.L.M., E.M. and G.M.C.; Visualization, L.A.; Supervision, L.A.; Project Administration, L.A.; Funding Acquisition, L.A.

References

1. Uchino, S.; Kellum, J.A.; Bellomo, R.; Doig, G.S.; Morimatsu, H.; Morgera, S.; Schetz, M.; Tan, I.; Bouman, C.; Macedo, E.; et al. Acute renal failure in critically ill patients: A multinational, multicenter study. *JAMA* **2005**, *294*, 813–818. [CrossRef] [PubMed]
2. Chertow, G.M.; Burdick, E.; Honour, M.; Bonventre, J.V.; Bates, D.W. Acute kidney injury, mortality, length of stay, and costs in hospitalized patients. *J. Am. Soc. Nephrol.* **2005**, *16*, 3365–3370. [CrossRef] [PubMed]
3. Mehta, R.L.; Pascual, M.T.; Soroko, S.; Savage, B.R.; Himmelfarb, J.; Ikizler, T.A.; Paganini, E.P.; Chertow, G.M.; Program to Improve Care in Acute Renal Disease. Spectrum of acute renal failure in the intensive care unit: The PICARD experience. *Kidney Int.* **2004**, *66*, 1613–1621. [CrossRef] [PubMed]
4. Peyriere, H.; Branger, B.; Bengler, C.; Vecina, F.; Pinzani, V.; Hillaire-Buys, D.; Blayac, J.P. Neurologic toxicity caused by zelitrex (valaciclovir) in 3 patients with renal failure. Is overdose associated with improvement of product bioavailability improvement? *Rev. Med. Int.* **2001**, *22*, 297–303.
5. Matzke, G.R.; McGory, R.W.; Halstenson, C.E.; Keane, W.F. Pharmacokinetics of vancomycin in patients with various degrees of renal function. *Antimicrob. Agents Chemother.* **1984**, *25*, 433–437. [CrossRef] [PubMed]
6. Smith, C.R.; Moore, R.D.; Lietman, P.S. Studies of risk factors for aminoglycoside nephrotoxicity. *Am. J. Kidney Dis.* **1986**, *8*, 308–313. [CrossRef]

7.   Matzke, G.R.; Frye, R.F. Drug administration in patients with renal insufficiency. Minimising renal and extrarenal toxicity. *Drug Saf.* **1997**, *16*, 205–231. [CrossRef] [PubMed]

8.   Rosborough, T.K.; Shepherd, M.F.; Couch, P.L. Selecting an equation to estimate glomerular filtration rate for use in renal dosage adjustment of drugs in electronic patient record systems. *Pharmacotherapy* **2005**, *25*, 823–830. [CrossRef] [PubMed]

9.   Goerdt, P.J.; Heim-Duthoy, K.L.; Macres, M.; Swan, S.K. Predictive performance of renal function estimate equations in renal allografts. *Br. J. Clin. Pharmacol.* **1997**, *44*, 261–265. [CrossRef] [PubMed]

10. Levey, A.S.; Bosch, J.P.; Lewis, J.B.; Greene, T.; Rogers, N.; Roth, D. A more accurate method to estimate glomerular filtration rate from serum creatinine: A new prediction equation. Modification of Diet in Renal Disease Study Group. *Ann. Int. Med.* **1999**, *130*, 461–470. [CrossRef] [PubMed]

11. Wargo, K.A.; Eiland, E.H., 3rd; Hamm, W.; English, T.M.; Phillippe, H.M. Comparison of the modification of diet in renal disease and Cockcroft-Gault equations for antimicrobial dosage adjustments. *Ann. Pharmacother.* **2006**, *40*, 1248–1253. [CrossRef] [PubMed]

12. Lin, J.; Knight, E.L.; Hogan, M.L.; Singh, A.K. A comparison of prediction equations for estimating glomerular filtration rate in adults without kidney disease. *J. Am. Soc. Nephrol.* **2003**, *14*, 2573–2580. [CrossRef] [PubMed]

13. Poggio, E.D.; Nef, P.C.; Wang, X.; Greene, T.; Van Lente, F.; Dennis, V.W.; Hall, P.M. Performance of the Cockcroft-Gault and modification of diet in renal disease equations in estimating GFR in ill hospitalized patients. *Am. J. Kidney Dis.* **2005**, *46*, 242–252. [CrossRef] [PubMed]

14. le Riche, M.; Zemlin, A.E.; Erasmus, R.T.; Davids, M.R. An audit of 24-hour creatinine clearance measurements at Tygerberg Hospital and comparison with prediction equations. *S. Afr. Med. J.* **2007**, *97*, 968–970. [PubMed]

15. Kuan, Y.; Hossain, M.; Surman, J.; El Nahas, A.M.; Haylor, J. GFR prediction using the MDRD and Cockcroft and Gault equations in patients with end-stage renal disease. *Nephrol. Dial. Transplant.* **2005**, *20*, 2394–2401. [CrossRef] [PubMed]

16. Robert, S.; Zarowitz, B.J.; Peterson, E.L.; Dumler, F. Predictability of creatinine clearance estimates in critically ill patients. *Crit. Care Med.* **1993**, *21*, 1487–1495. [CrossRef] [PubMed]

17. Cockcroft, D.W.; Gault, M.H. Prediction of creatinine clearance from serum creatinine. *Nephron* **1976**, *16*, 31–41. [CrossRef] [PubMed]

18. Matzke, G.R.; Aronoff, G.R.; Atkinson, A.J., Jr.; Bennett, W.M.; Decker, B.S.; Eckardt, K.U.; Golper, T.; Grabe, D.W.; Kasiske, B.; Keller, F.; et al. Drug dosing consideration in patients with acute and chronic kidney disease—A clinical update from Kidney Disease: Improving Global Outcomes (KDIGO). *Kidney Int.* **2011**, *80*, 1122–1137. [CrossRef] [PubMed]

19. Jelliffe, R. Estimation of creatinine clearance in patients with unstable renal function, without a urine specimen. *Am. J. Nephrol.* **2002**, *22*, 320–324. [CrossRef] [PubMed]

20. Bouchard, J.; Macedo, E.; Soroko, S.; Chertow, G.M.; Himmelfarb, J.; Ikizler, T.A.; Paganini, E.P.; Mehta, R.L.; Program to Improve Care in Acute Renal Disease. Comparison of methods for estimating glomerular filtration rate in critically ill patients with acute kidney injury. *Nephrol. Dial. Transplant.* **2010**, *25*, 102–107. [CrossRef] [PubMed]

21. Gill, J.; Malyuk, R.; Djurdjev, O.; Levin, A. Use of GFR equations to adjust drug doses in an elderly multi-ethnic group—A cautionary tale. *Nephrol. Dial. Transplant.* **2007**, *22*, 2894–2899. [CrossRef] [PubMed]

22. Hoste, E.A.; Damen, J.; Vanholder, R.C.; Lameire, N.H.; Delanghe, J.R.; Van den Hauwe, K.; Colardyn, F.A. Assessment of renal function in recently admitted critically ill patients with normal serum creatinine. *Nephrol. Dial. Transplant.* **2005**, *20*, 747–753. [CrossRef] [PubMed]

23. Bragadottir, G.; Redfors, B.; Ricksten, S.E. Assessing glomerular filtration rate (GFR) in critically ill patients with acute kidney injury—True GFR versus urinary creatinine clearance and estimating equations. *Crit. Care* **2013**, *17*, R108. [CrossRef] [PubMed]

24. Marx, G.M.; Blake, G.M.; Galani, E.; Steer, C.B.; Harper, S.E.; Adamson, K.L.; Bailey, D.L.; Harper, P.G. Evaluation of the Cockcroft-Gault, Jelliffe and Wright formulae in estimating renal function in elderly cancer patients. *Ann. Oncol.* **2004**, *15*, 291–295. [CrossRef] [PubMed]

25. Kirwan, C.J.; Philips, B.J.; Macphee, I.A. Estimated glomerular filtration rate correlates poorly with four-hour creatinine clearance in critically ill patients with acute kidney injury. *Crit. Care Res. Pract.* **2013**, *2013*, 406075. [CrossRef] [PubMed]

26. Martin, J.H.; Fay, M.F.; Udy, A.; Roberts, J.; Kirkpatrick, C.; Ungerer, J.; Lipman, J. Pitfalls of using estimations of glomerular filtration rate in an intensive care population. *Int. Med. J.* **2011**, *41*, 537–543. [CrossRef] [PubMed]

27. Lyndon, W.D.; Wille, K.M.; Tolwani, A.J. Solute clearance in CRRT: Prescribed dose versus actual delivered dose. *Nephrol. Dial. Transplant.* **2012**, *27*, 952–956. [CrossRef] [PubMed]

28. Nolin, T.D.; Appiah, K.; Kendrick, S.A.; Le, P.; McMonagle, E.; Himmelfarb, J. Hemodialysis acutely improves hepatic CYP3A4 metabolic activity. *J. Am. Soc. Nephrol.* **2006**, *17*, 2363–2367. [CrossRef] [PubMed]

29. Dixon, J.; Lane, K.; Macphee, I.; Philips, B. Xenobiotic metabolism: The effect of acute kidney injury on non-renal drug clearance and hepatic drug metabolism. *Int. J. Mol. Sci.* **2014**, *15*, 2538–2553. [CrossRef] [PubMed]

30. Vilay, A.M.; Churchwell, M.D.; Mueller, B.A. Clinical review: Drug metabolism and nonrenal clearance in acute kidney injury. *Crit. Care* **2008**, *12*, 235. [CrossRef] [PubMed]

31. Eyler, R.F.; Mueller, B.A.; Medscap. Antibiotic dosing in critically ill patients with acute kidney injury. *Nat. Rev. Nephrol.* **2011**, *7*, 226–235. [CrossRef] [PubMed]

32. Goldstein, S.L.; Nolin, T.D. Lack of drug dosing guidelines for critically ill patients receiving continuous renal replacement therapy. *Clin. Pharmacol. Ther.* **2014**, *96*, 159–161. [CrossRef] [PubMed]

33. Chawla, L.S.; Bellomo, R.; Bihorac, A.; Goldstein, S.L.; Siew, E.D.; Bagshaw, S.M.; Bittleman, D.; Cruz, D.; Endre, Z.; Fitzgerald, R.L.; et al. Acute kidney disease and renal recovery: Consensus report of the Acute Disease Quality Initiative (ADQI) 16 Workgroup. *Nat. Rev. Nephrol.* **2017**, *13*, 241–257. [CrossRef] [PubMed]

3

Genetic Analyses in Dent Disease and Characterization of *CLCN5* Mutations in Kidney Biopsies

Lisa Gianesello [1,†], Monica Ceol [1,†], Loris Bertoldi [2,†], Liliana Terrin [1], Giovanna Priante [1], Luisa Murer [3], Licia Peruzzi [4], Mario Giordano [5], Fabio Paglialonga [6], Vincenzo Cantaluppi [7], Claudio Musetti [7], Giorgio Valle [2], Dorella Del Prete [1], Franca Anglani [1,2,*] and Dent Disease Italian Network [‡]

[1] Laboratory of Histomorphology and Molecular Biology of the Kidney, Clinical Nephrology, Department of Medicine—DIMED, University of Padua, 35128 Padua, Italy; lisa.gianesello@unipd.it (L.G.); monica.ceol@unipd.it (M.C.); liliana.terrin@gmail.com (L.T.); giovanna.priante@unipd.it (G.P.); dorella.delprete@unipd.it (D.D.P.)

[2] CRIBI Biotechnology Centre, University of Padua, 35131 Padua, Italy; loris.bertoldi@phd.unipd.it (L.B.); giorgio.valle@unipd.it (G.V.)

[3] Pediatric Nephrology, Dialysis and Transplant Unit, Department of Women's and Children's Health, Padua University Hospital, 35128 Padua, Italy; luisa.murer@aopd.veneto.it

[4] Pediatric Nephrology Unit, Regina Margherita Children's Hospital, 10126 CDSS Turin, Italy; licia.peruzzi@unito.it

[5] Pediatric Nephrology Unit, University Hospital, P.O. Giovanni XXIII, 70126 Bari, Italy; mario.giordano@policlinico.ba.it

[6] Pediatric Nephrology, Dialysis and Transplant Unit, Fondazione IRCCS, Ca' Granda Ospedale Maggiore Policlinico, 20122 Milan, Italy; fabio.paglialonga@policlinico.mi.it

[7] Nephrology and Kidney Transplantation Unit, Department of Translational Medicine, University of Piemonte Orientale (UPO), 28100 Novara, Italy; vincenzo.cantaluppi@med.uniupo.it (V.C.); claudio.musetti@med.uniupo.it (C.M.)

[*] Correspondence: franca.anglani@unipd.it

[†] These authors contributed equally to this work.

[‡] Membership of the Dent Disease Italian Network is provided in the Acknowledgments.

Abstract: Dent disease (DD), an X-linked renal tubulopathy, is mainly caused by loss-of-function mutations in *CLCN5* (DD1) and *OCRL* genes. *CLCN5* encodes the ClC-5 antiporter that in proximal tubules (PT) participates in the receptor-mediated endocytosis of low molecular weight proteins. Few studies have analyzed the PT expression of ClC-5 and of megalin and cubilin receptors in DD1 kidney biopsies. About 25% of DD cases lack mutations in either *CLCN5* or *OCRL* genes (DD3), and no other disease genes have been discovered so far. Sanger sequencing was used for *CLCN5* gene analysis in 158 unrelated males clinically suspected of having DD. The tubular expression of ClC-5, megalin, and cubilin was assessed by immunolabeling in 10 DD1 kidney biopsies. Whole exome sequencing (WES) was performed in eight DD3 patients. Twenty-three novel *CLCN5* mutations were identified. ClC-5, megalin, and cubilin were significantly lower in DD1 than in control biopsies. The tubular expression of ClC-5 when detected was irrespective of the type of mutation. In four DD3 patients, WES revealed 12 potentially pathogenic variants in three novel genes (*SLC17A1*, *SLC9A3*, and *PDZK1*), and in three genes known to be associated with monogenic forms of renal proximal tubulopathies (*SLC3A*, *LRP2*, and *CUBN*). The supposed third Dent disease-causing gene was not discovered.

Keywords: dent disease; *CLCN5* gene mutations; proximal tubular ClC-5 expression; megalin; cubilin; kidney biopsies; immunohistochemistry; whole exome sequencing

1. Introduction

The term Dent disease (DD) identifies a group of X-linked renal disorders characterized by features of incomplete Fanconi syndrome including low-molecular-weight proteinuria (LMWP), and more or less severe hypercalciuria, nephrocalcinosis and/or nephrolithiasis. This triad of symptoms has been variously named in the past as X-linked recessive nephrolithiasis with renal failure (OMIM 310468), X-linked recessive hypophosphatemic rickets (OMIM 300554), or the idiopathic LMWP of Japanese children (OMIM 308990), testifying to the disease's phenotypic variability [1,2]. DD usually presents in children or young adults, progressing to chronic kidney disease (CKD) between the third and fifth decades of life in 30–80% of cases [3,4].

The most common genetic cause of DD is a mutated *CLCN5* gene encoding the ClC-5 chloride channel Cl-/H+ antiporter (DD1; MIM#300009) [5–9]. In the kidney, ClC-5 is expressed primarily in the proximal tubular cells (PTCs) located mainly in the subapical endosomes. Together with megalin and cubilin synergistic receptors, it is involved in the endocytic reabsorption of albumin and LMW proteins [10,11]. ClC-5 expression levels are lower in the α intercalated cells of the cortical collecting duct and in the cortical and medullary thick ascending limb of Henle's loop [12].

DD1 features a marked allelic heterogeneity, with more than 200 *CLCN5* mutations described so far [9]. Functional investigations in Xenopus Levis oocytes and mammalian cells enabled these *CLCN5* mutations to be classified. The most common mutations lead to a defective protein folding and processing, resulting in endoplasmic reticulum (ER) retention of the mutant protein for further degradation by the proteasome [13–17]. Few studies have investigated ClC-5 expression in DD1 kidney biopsies.

OCRL gene mutations, which are usually associated with Lowe syndrome (OMIM #309000), have been identified in about 10–15% of DD patients (DD2; MIM#300555). Approximately 25% of DD patients (DD3) have neither *CLCN5* nor *OCRL* gene mutations [18–21].

This study aimed to investigate allelic and locus heterogeneity in DD and to analyze ClC-5, megalin, and cubilin expression in DD1 kidney biopsies. We further expanded the spectrum of *CLCN5* mutations in DD by describing 23 novel mutations. In DD1 kidney biopsies, we showed that the loss of ClC-5 tubular expression caused defective megalin and cubilin trafficking. In DD3, whole exome sequencing (WES) did not detect a new disease-causing gene. Instead, it revealed the concomitant presence of likely pathogenic variants in genes encoding proximal tubular (PT) endocytic apparatus components, suggesting that they may have had a role in determining the DD3 phenotype.

2. Results

2.1. CLCN5 Gene Mutation Analysis

The 85% of the 158 patients analyzed for the presence of *CLCN5* mutations were of Italian origin, 6% were non-Italian European (Balcanic and English), and the remaining 9% were extra-European (Figure 1).

DNA sequence analysis of the *CLCN5* gene revealed 50 different mutations in 56 unrelated patients. Six different mutations were found twice. Among the detected mutations, the most common types were missense mutations (21 cases), followed by frameshift mutations (14 cases), nonsense mutations (13 cases), and splicing mutations (eight cases) (Figure 2).

Twenty-three mutations were not previously described, which were judged potentially pathogenic by in silico tools and classified as pathogenic or likely pathogenic according to American College of Medical Genetics and American College of Pathologists (ACMG/AMP) guidelines [22] (Table 1). The novel frameshift, nonsense, and missense mutations were mapped onto ClC-5 protein domains (Table 1). Table S1 summarizes the clinical details of 20 patients with novel *CLCN5* mutations (clinical data were unavailable for three). LMWP and hypercalciuria were the most common signs at the time of their molecular diagnosis, and their clinical phenotypic variability reflected that of patients with known *CLCN5* mutations [9].

Population

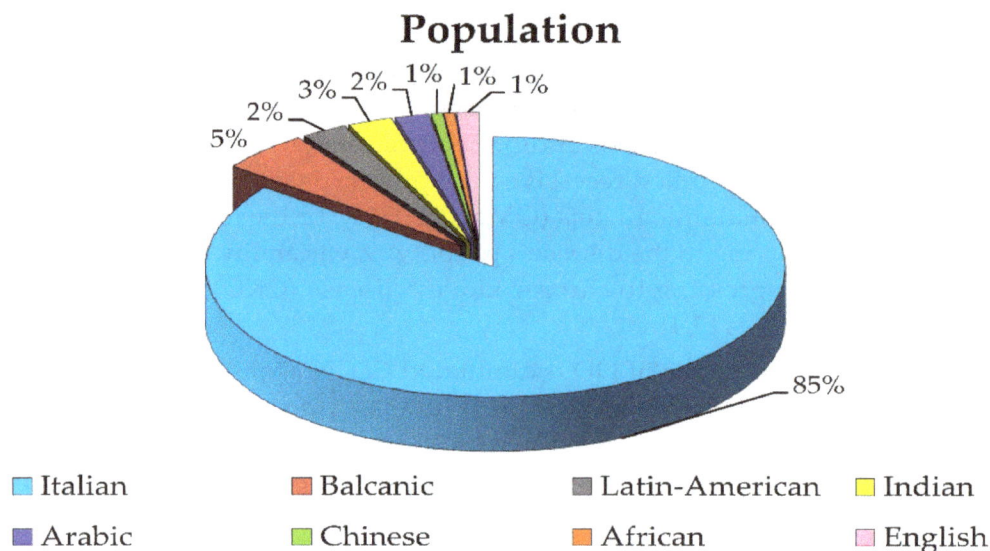

Figure 1. Ethnical distribution of the 158 analyzed patients.

CLCN5 mutations

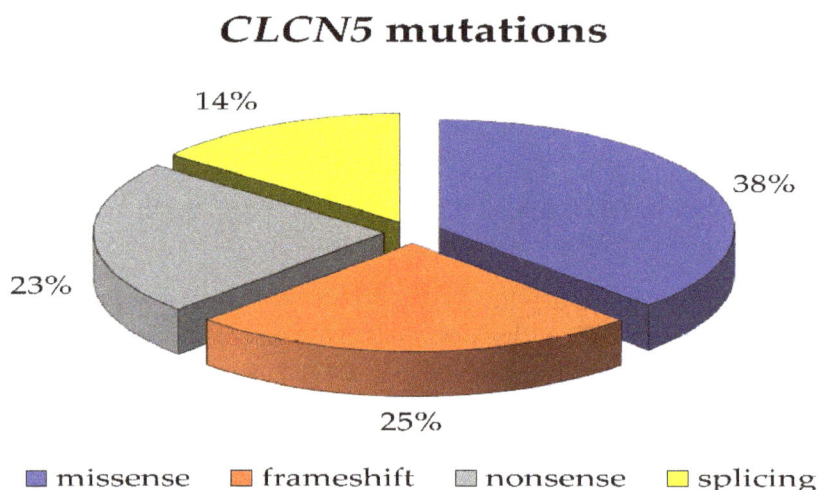

Figure 2. Percentages of mutations of *CLCN5* gene by type.

Table 1. Novel mutations in the *CLCN5* gene.

Type of Mutation	Nucleotide	Exon-Intron	Protein	Pathogenicity Assessment	Protein Domain
Frameshift	c.100_101insG	Exon 2	p.(Glu35fs)	Pathogenic (Ib)	A helix, stop in Loop A-B
Frameshift	c.125delA	Exon 3	p.(Glu42fs)	Pathogenic (Ib)	Loop A-B
Frameshift	c.266_267insT	Exon 4	p.(Ile89fs)	Pathogenic (Ib)	B helix, stop in Loop B-C
Frameshift	c.518delT	Exon 6	p.(Ile173fs)	Pathogenic (Ib)	D helix, stop in Loop D-E
Frameshift §	c.691delA	Exon 6	p.(Lys231fs)	Pathogenic (Ia)	Loop F-G, stop at the end of helix G
Frameshift	c.1164_1165insAG	Exon 8	p.(Lys388fs)	Pathogenic (Ib)	L helix, stop in helix M
Frameshift	c.1635_1638delCAAG	Exon 10	p.(Ser545fs)	Pathogenic (Ib)	Q helix, stop in cytoplasmic
Frameshift	c.1657delG	Exon 10	p.(Arg554fs)	Pathogenic (Ib)	Cytoplasmic, stop at the beginning of CBS1 cytoplasmic domain
Frameshift	c.1920delC	Exon 10	p.(Ile641fs)	Pathogenic (Ib)	CBS1 cytoplasmic domain, stop in cytoplasmic
Nonsense	c.1287G>A	Exon 8	p.(Trp429*)	Pathogenic (Ib)	M helix

Table 1. *Cont.*

Type of Mutation	Nucleotide	Exon-Intron	Protein	Pathogenicity Assessment	Protein Domain
Nonsense	c.2016C>G	Exon 11	p.(Tyr672*)	Pathogenic (Ib)	Cytoplasmic
Nonsense	c.2128C>T	Exon 11	p.(Gln710*)	Pathogenic (Ib)	Cytoplasmic-beta strand in CBS2 domain
Missense	c.262G>A	Exon 4	p.(Gly88Ser)	Likely pathogenic (IV)	B helix
Missense	c.305G>T	Exon 4	p.(Cys102Phe)	Likely pathogenic (V)	Loop B-C
Missense	c.518T>A	Exon 6	p.(Ile173Lys)	Likely pathogenic (V)	D helix
Missense §	c.608C>G	Exon 6	p.(Ser203Trp)	Pathogenic (II)	E helix
Missense	c.809G>A	Exon 8	p.(Ser270Asn)	Likely pathogenic (IV)	Loop H-I
Missense §	c.922G>A	Exon 8	p.(Val308Met)	Pathogenic (IIIb)	Loop I-J
Missense	c.1565T>A	Exon 10	p.(Val522Asp)	Likely pathogenic (V)	P helix
Missense	c.1619C>T	Exon 10	p.(Ala540Val)	Likely pathogenic (IV)	Q helix
Missense	c.2192A>C	Exon 12	p.(His731Pro)	Likely pathogenic (V)	Cytoplasmic-CBS2 domain
Splicing	c.105+5G>C	Intron 2-splice site	p.?	Likely pathogenic (II)	
Splicing	c.1348-1G>A	Intron 8-splice site	p.?	Pathogenic (Ic)	

§ *CLCN5* mutations also analyzed in patients' kidney biopsies.

2.2. ClC-5, Megalin, and Cubilin Immunolabeling in DD1 Kidney Biopsies

Renal tubular ClC-5 expression was analyzed by immunohistochemistry (IHC) in 10 patients carrying *CLCN5* stop codon (frameshift and nonsense mutations) or missense mutations (Table 2). In control biopsies, ClC-5 immunostaining was mainly apical and subapical (Figure 3). Our antibody has around 66% overall epitope sequence similarity to ClC-3 and ClC-4, which are both expressed in the membranes of intracellular organelles [23], so cross-reactivity can be expected. Immunolabeling for ClC-3, ClC-4, and ClC-5 in serial sections of a control sample showed that tubular apical staining was almost exclusively attributable to ClC-5 expression, while cytoplasmic staining was due largely to ClC-3 and ClC-5, and much less to ClC-4 (Figure S1).

In DD1 biopsies, ClC-5 apical immunolabeling was negligible in most tubules, whatever the type of mutation (Figure 3). As expected, ClC-5 expression was very significantly downregulated (Figure 4) in DD1 biopsies compared with control biopsies (median CTRL 8.69% [Interquartile range (IQR) 1.94–15.97%], DD1 0.01% [IQR 0.00–0.12%]; $p < 0.01$).

Table 2 shows the morphometric findings on ClC-5 immunostaining for each mutation. Notably, two patients (Pt3 and Pt4) carried the same very premature nonsense mutation p.(Arg34*), but with a completely different pattern of expression: ClC-5 immunolabeling was completely absent in one, while in the other, it stained 0.12% of the whole biopsy area, which was more than in any of the other biopsies analyzed (Figure 3).

Analyzing megalin and cubilin immunofluorescence (IF) in the same patients (Figure 5) revealed that both receptors were significantly downregulated by comparison with control biopsies (median megalin: CTRL 4.52% [IQR 3.64–8.39%], DD1 1.67% [IQR 0.09–3.91%], $p = 0.019$; median cubilin: CTRL 10.87% [IQR 1.54–19.85%], DD1 1.01% [IQR 0.83–2.67%], $p = 0.003$) (Figure 4).

Table 2. Morphometric evaluation of tubular ClC-5 immunolabeling in 10 DD1 patients' kidney biopsies.

Patient	CLCN5 Mutation	Age at Biopsy (Years)	Indication for Biopsy	Histopathological Findings	ClC-5 Immunolabeling Morphometric Evaluation (% Positive Area)
1	p.(Thr44fs)	2	Proteinuria	Minimal changes	0.01
2	p.(Lys231fs) (novel)	14	Proteinuria	Normal	0.00
3	p.(Arg34*)	11	Nephrotic syndrome	Chronic interstitial nephritis with global glomerulosclerosis	0.12
4	p.(Arg34*)	6	Proteinuria	Global glomerulosclerosis and IgM nephropathy	0.00
5	p.(Gln600*)	6	Proteinuria	Tubulointerstitial injury with focal glomerulosclerosis	0.05
6	p.(Ser203Trp) (novel)	3	Proteinuria	Normal	0.01
7	p.(Ser261Arg)	4	Heavy proteinuria	Proliferative mesangial glomerulonephritis	0.07
8	p.(Tyr272Cys)	NA	Proteinuria	Normal	0.01
9	p.(Val308Met) (novel)	9	Proteinuria and hematuria	Normal	0.08
10	p.(Trp547Arg)	1	Proteinuria	Normal	0.00

NA: not available.

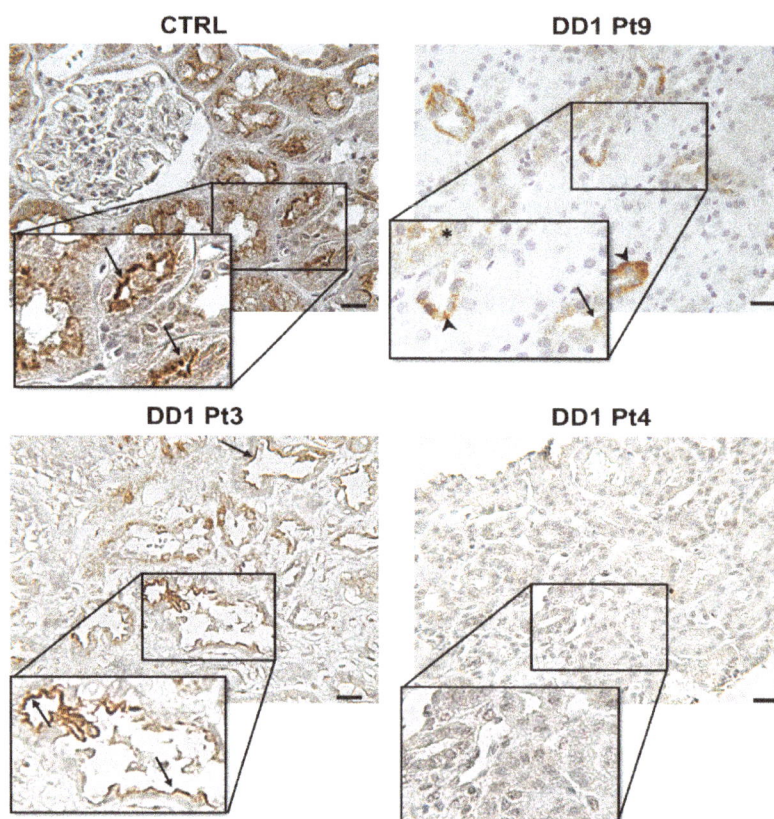

Figure 3. ClC-5 immunolabeling in control and DD1 kidneys. Representative images disclosing ClC-5 positivity in control and DD1 kidneys. In CTRL, ClC-5 staining was located mainly in tubular apical and subapical positions. In DD1 patients, some tubules presented basolateral or cytoplasmic ClC-5 positivity (Pt9), and very few showed apical staining (Pt9, Pt3). ClC-5 immunostaining was negligible in most DD1 tubules (Pt4), whatever the type of mutation. The asterisk indicates a cytoplasmic signal, arrows indicate apical and subapical signals, the arrowhead indicates a basolateral signal. Scale bar = 50 μm. CTRL= control, Pt = patient.

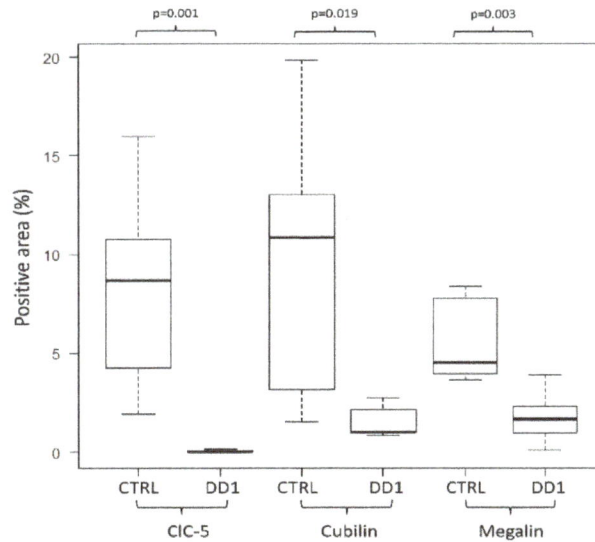

Figure 4. ClC-5, cubilin, and megalin quantitative analysis. Morphometric analysis showed a significant decrease in the percentage of positive area in kidneys of DD1 patients than in control kidneys for all molecules examined. Data were analyzed using the Mann–Whitney U-test. CTRL = control.

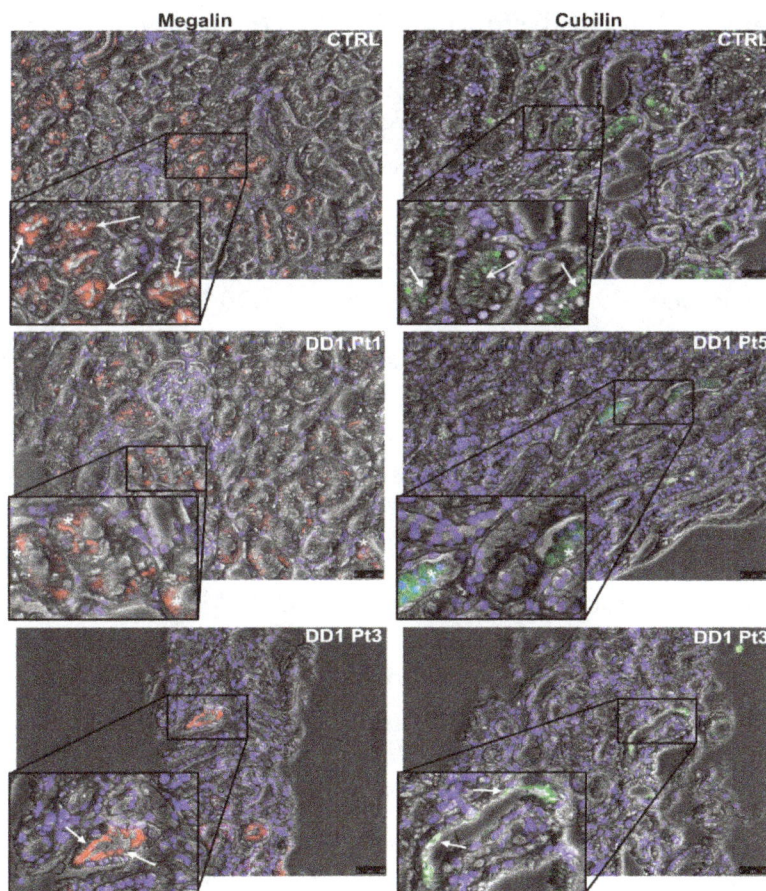

Figure 5. Megalin and cubilin immunolabeling in control and DD1 kidneys. Representative images disclosing megalin and cubilin positivity in control and DD1 kidneys. In CTRL, megalin (red) and cubilin (green) staining was located mainly in tubular apical and subapical positions. Immunolabeling for both receptors was rarely apical in DD1 patients (Pt3), while it was more frequently found in the cytoplasm (Pt1 and Pt5). The asterisk indicates a cytoplasmic signal, arrows indicate apical and subapical signals. Blue indicates counter-staining of nuclei with 4′,6-diamidino-2-phenylindole (DAPI). Scale bar = 50 μm. CTRL = control, Pt = patient.

2.3. Whole Exome Sequencing (WES) Study

Among *CLCN5* negative patients, 34 underwent mutational screening of the *OCRL* gene, and 19 patients were found to not carry mutations. In eight out of 19 *CLCN5* and *OCRL*-negative patients (four children and four adults), we performed WES.

We first searched for mutations in phenocopy genes. Known monogenic forms of nephrolithiasis and nephrocalcinosis as well as of proximal and distal tubulopathy, for a total of 62 genes including known genes of the PT endocytic pathway (Table S2), were firstly evaluated in these patients. Furthermore, the first 100 genes prioritized for their association with *CLCN5* or *OCRL* genes using the Scalable kernel-based gene prioritization (SCUBA) were investigated [24] (Table S3).

Unexpectedly, in two children, we detected *CLCN5* or *OCRL* known disease-causing mutations, p.(Lys231fs) and p.(Arg318Cys), respectively. If on one hand this finding was disturbing because it meant that by previous Sanger sequencing we had missed two causative mutations in the two known genes, on the other hand, it confirmed that our pool of DD3 cases was well representative of DD patients based on disease phenotype.

In four patients (three adults and one child), we detected 12 variants in three genes known to be associated either with monogenic forms of proximal renal tubulopathy (*SLC3A1*) or with monogenic syndromes involving proximal tubule dysfunction (*LRP2*, *CUBN*), as well as in novel genes not related to monogenic nephropathies (*SLC17A1*, *SLC9A3*, and *PDZK1*). These last genes could be candidates for DD-like phenotypes for their function in PT, and detected variants were predicted to be pathogenic or likely pathogenic by in silico tools (although with a different degree of concordance), except for one in the *SLC17A1* gene (Table 3). Table S4 summarizes the four patients' clinical phenotypes.

In two adults patients (AMS and BDA), we detected biallelic likely pathogenic variants in *SLC3A1* and *LRP2* genes whose mutations are responsible for the recessive diseases Cystinuria (MIM#220100) and Donnai–Barrow/Facio-oculo-acoustico-renal syndrome (DB/FOAR, MIM#222448), respectively.

In AMS, we also identified a very rare missense variant classified as a variant of uncertain significance (VUS) in the *SLC17A1* gene encoding sodium/phosphate cotransporter 1 (NPT1), which occurs at the apical pole of PTCs [25] and participates in renal urate export [26,27]. The same patient was found to be homozygous for the very rare nonsense variant p.(Arg8*) in the *PDKZ1* gene. This gene encodes the Na(+)/H(+) exchange regulatory cofactor NHE-RF3, which is a PDZ domain-containing scaffolding protein and one of the key molecules of the urate transportsome [28,29].

The already known pathogenic *LRP2* mutation p.(Asp2054Asn) [30] was detected in AMV. In this patient, we also found an in-frame indel variant of the *CUBN* gene encoding for cubilin. *CUBN* gene mutations are known to cause Imerslund–Gräsbeck syndrome (IGS, MIM#261100), which is an autosomal recessive disorder involving selective intestinal vitamin B12 malabsorption and LMWP. The p.(Val2347del) variant in *CUBN* is very rare (TOPmed 0.0000001); Mutation Taster (MT) and PROVEAN predicted its pathogenicity, and it was classified as VUS according to ACMG/AMP guidelines [22].

Among eight different *LRP2* uncommon coding variants with a minor allele frequency (MAF) < 0.05 detected in our DD3 patients, four were identified in one patient (AMT) of which two were predicted to be pathogenic by in silico tools (Table 3). Similar to AMV, this patient carried an uncommon *CUBN* missense variant that was considered pathogenic by MT, PROVEAN, and DANN, but classified as benign according to ACMG/AMP guidelines. He also harbored a very rare variant in the *SLC9A3* gene, which was predicted as pathogenic by in silico tools, and classified as VUS. The *SLC9A3* gene encodes sodium/hydrogen exchanger 3 (NHE3), which is the main apical Na+/H+ exchanger in adult kidneys [31], and part of the macromolecular endocytic complex at the brush border of PTCs [32,33].

Table 3. Candidate variants for DD3 phenotypes detected by whole-exome sequencing (WES).

Pt ID	Transcript Level Variation	Codon Substitution	Frequency ExAC (European)	Mutation Taster	PROVEAN	DANN	ClinVar	ACMG/AMP Variant Interpretation
				SLC17A1 (NM_005074.3)				
AMS	c.1309G>A	p.(Ala437Thr)	rs1189357572 0.000003 (GnomAD) (0.000008)	Polymorphism (1.000)	Neutral (−1.97)	0.967	NA	VUS
				PDZK1 (NM_002614.4)				
AMS	c.22C>T	p.(Arg8*) homozygous	rs191362962 0.0001157 (0.0001799)	Disease causing automatic	NA	0.998	NA	VUS
				LRP2 (NM_004525.2)				
BDA	c.6727C>T	p.(Arg2243*)	novel	Disease causing automatic (1.000)	NA	0.996	NA	Pathogenic (Ib)
BDA	c.242T>A	p.(Ile81Asn)	novel	Disease causing (1.000)	Damaging (−4.62)	0.993	NA	Likely pathogenic (V)
AMV	c.6160G>A	p.(Asp2054Asn)	rs138269726 0.0011 (0.0017)	Disease causing (1.000)	Neutral (−1.85)	0.999	Pathogenic allele	Likely pathogenic (II)
AMT	c.2006G>A	p.(Gly669Asp)	rs34291900 0.0285 (0.0434)	Disease causing (1.000)	Damaging (−5.44)	0.998	Likely benign allele	Likely benign
AMT	c.7894A>G	p.(Asn2632Asp)	rs17848169 0.02951 (0.0426)	Disease causing (1.000)	Neutral (−1.73)	0.452	Likely benign allele	Likely benign
				SLC3A1 (NM_000341.4)				
AMS	c.680G>A	p.(Arg227Gln)	rs142469446 0.0002 (0.0002)	Disease causing (1.000)	Neutral (−1.63)	1	NA	Likely pathogenic (IV)
AMS	c.797T>C	p.(Phe266Ser)	rs141587158 0.003 (0.004)	Disease causing (1.000)	Damaging (−4.7)	0.998	NA	Likely pathogenic (IIIb)
				CUBN (NM_001081.3)				
AMT	c.10265C>T	p.(Thr3422Ile)	rs1801230 0.01832 (0.02829)	Disease causing (1.000)	Damaging (−2.94)	0.985	Likely benign allele	Benign
AMV	c.7040_7042del	p.(Val2347del)	rs1279549461 (TOPmed) 0.0000001	Disease causing (0.998)	Deleterious (−9.81)	NA	NA	VUS
				SLC9A3 (NM_004174.3)				
AMT	c.848G>A	p.(Arg283His)	rs146899318 0.00033 (0.00036)	Disease causing (0.853)	Damaging (−3.85)	0.999	NA	VUS

Pt: patient, ACMG/AMP: American College of Medical Genetics and American College of Pathologists, NA: not available, VUS: Variant of uncertain significance.

3. Discussion

Dent disease 1 is a worldwide disease, and this is further confirmed by our cohort of patients which included persons from all over the word. More than 220 CLCN5 pathogenic mutations have been reported so far. Mutations were found scattered along all exons of the gene and in different protein domains [9,34–45]. Mansour-Hendili et al. [9] reported that the majority were missense and frameshift mutations (33.33% and 29.05% respectively) followed by nonsense mutations (17.52%), splicing mutations (12.39%), and large deletions (4.70%). In our cohort of patients, missense and frameshift mutations were also the most frequent, but with a lower proportion (38% and 25% respectively), while we observed more nonsense mutations compared to the previously reported data (23%).

In our study, DNA sequence analysis of the CLCN5 gene revealed 50 different mutations, 23 of which have never been described before. ACMG/AMP guidelines classify the nine missense novel mutations in CLCN5 as likely pathogenic. They were mapped onto ClC-5 protein domains (Table 1).

The p.(Ile173Lys) missense mutation is in the D helix, which is one of the four helixes (D, F, N, and R) brought together near the channel center to form the Cl-selectivity filter [46] and consequently believed to alter ClC-5 conductance.

The p.(His731Pro) missense mutation affects the ClC-5 carboxy-terminus cytoplasmic domain. All eukaryotic ClCs have a large cytoplasmic C-terminus containing a pair of cystathionine beta-synthase (CBS) domains. Several authors have shown that CBS domains are involved in regulating the activity of ClCs, including ClC-5 [47–49]. Mutations affecting the two CBS domains were reported correctly targeted to the plasma membrane and early endosomes, but with altered ClC-5 electrical activity [14]. The nonsense mutation p.(Arg718*) truncating the ClC-5 protein near the C-terminus reportedly results in ER retention, underscoring the importance of the C-terminus in passing protein quality control in ER [50]. These findings suggest that truncated ClC-5 proteins at the C-terminus could cause function loss through defective protein processing. However, three different truncated mutations at the C-terminus—p.(Tyr617*), p.(Arg648*), and p.(Arg704*)—targeted the cell surface (albeit only one with residual activity) [50], so we cannot say whether our stop codon mutations at the C-terminus of ClC-5 protein (Table 1) could exhibit residual activity targeting the plasma membrane.

The p.(Ser203Trp) missense mutation affects the E helix, whose role in ClC-5 function is still unclear. The nearby p.(Leu200Arg) mutation reportedly produced a loss of Cl- conductance [1], and the p.(Ser203Leu) was found to cause current failures due to ER retention [50]. Taken together, these findings indicate that the p.(Ser203Trp) mutation is probably pathogenic.

Six missense mutations map in the major helixes (B, H, I, O, P, and Q) involved in dimer interface formation [9,46], or in the intervening loops, suggesting an impaired physical contact between the two subunits that might disrupt proper pore configuration [50,51]. In addition, for the p.(Ala540Val), a pathogenic missense in the same position in a Dent family from New Zealand has already been reported [38], confirming the possible damaging role of the alteration of this residue. The p.(Ser270Asn) missense mutation maps in the loop between helixes H and I, near the "proton glutamate" (Glu 268), which is crucial to the Cl-/H+ transport function [9]. Since the p.(Ser270Arg) mutation was reportedly associated with chloride current abolition [52], we hypothesize a similar effect of this new mutation.

Very few studies investigated ClC-5 expression in kidney biopsies [10,53]. We analyzed ClC-5 protein expression in kidney biopsies from 10 patients carrying three novel and seven known CLCN5 mutations and in eight control biopsies. In controls, ClC-5 immunolabeling was mainly apical and subapical in tubular cells, and it was not co-localized with ClC-3 or ClC-4 staining. The few studies on ClC-5 expression in human kidney reported similar staining findings [10,53], which are justified by the well-accepted ClC-5 localization in early and recycling endosomes and the plasma membrane [54,55].

Our study is the first to demonstrate the loss of ClC-5 protein expression in DD1 kidneys. However, an apical staining was detected in very few tubules in 7/10 DD1 biopsies, including those with the novel p.(Val308Met) and p.(Ser203Trp) mutations. Therefore, we speculate that the expression of these ClC-5 mutants is regulated post-translationally, and mutated proteins can very rarely reach the plasma membrane. This is consistent with previous findings in ClC-5 mutant models. Both missense and nonsense ClC-5 mutants could be either targeted to early endosomes or plasma membrane, but with a limited activity, or confined to the ER [50]. In fact, some DD1 tubules were only labeled at the basolateral pole (probably a sign of ER retention) (Figure 3 Pt 9).

Apical staining was unexpectedly detected for the very premature truncated ClC-5 protein at codon 34. Premature stop codons (PSCs) account for one in two *CLCN5* mutations, and cause three distinct molecular alterations: (1) the production of a truncated, usually non-functional, protein; (2) degradation of the transcripts containing PSCs via the nonsense-mediated decay (NMD) pathway; and (3) exon skipping due to alternative cryptic acceptor or donor sites being used in the exon encompassing the stop codon [56]. The first molecular change can be excluded, because our ClC-5 antibody recognized an epitope at the C-terminus of the protein. The second and third might apply because (1) NMD may occasionally be bypassed when translational read-through allows the decoding of stop codons as sense codons, thus enabling protein translation; (2) PSCs can also prompt exon skipping by altering exonic splicing enhancer (ESE) or exonic splicing silencer (ESS) motifs. PSCs have even been found to be statistically inclined to induce exon skipping more than other exon mutations [57]. If this is true of the p.(Arg34*) mutation, we can expect exon skipping to be in frame, thus enabling complete protein synthesis and allowing the mutated protein to be detected by immunolabeling. However, such explanations for this ClC-5 mutant protein's presence in one biopsy should be considered with caution, as the ClC-5 protein was not found in most tubules, nor in another biopsy carrying the same mutation. This could mean that how PSCs are processed by cell transcriptional and translational apparatus might depend on the context (meaning the cell environment and/or the genomic context).

As in *Clcn5* knock-out (KO) animal models [58], ClC-5 loss in human kidney causes defective cubilin and megalin recycling, leading to LMWP. All the ClC-5 mutants studied here triggered both their defective expression at the brush border of PTCs and their downregulation. The presence of a megalin signal at the apical border of some tubules in the biopsy carrying the p.(Arg34*) mutation (Figure 5, Pt3) suggests a residual ClC-5 activity enabling a normal endocytic process and consequent megalin recycling.

Few studies have examined megalin and cubilin expression in DD1. Urinary megalin excretion was found to be significantly lower in DD1 patients than in normal individuals [59]. IHC on kidney biopsies from two patients carrying different *CLCN5* mutations revealed a defective megalin, cubilin, and Dab2 expression in PTCs [60,61]. Studies on megalin recycling in conditionally immortalized proximal tubular epithelial cell lines from three patients with *CLCN5* mutations showed defects in cell surface expression and internalization [62]. Our data definitively corroborate previous findings and suggest that a reduced intracellular megalin and cubilin synthesis may also contribute to their defective apical exposure.

Approximately one in four DD patients have no *CLCN5* or *OCRL* gene mutations. Whether mutations in a third, as yet unknown gene can cause DD3 remains to be seen, but—judging from our WES study on six DD3 patients—this seems unlikely. Instead, as we previously suggested [63], WES data point to DD3 patients having atypical phenotypes of known hereditary nephropathies or blended phenotypes. In fact, we identified in two patients (AMS and BDA) biallelic likely pathogenic variants in two genes (*SLC3A1*, *LRP2*) whose mutations are known to cause cystinuria and DB/FOAR. Our findings suggest that probably these patients were misdiagnosed as DD because of the presence renal Fanconi syndrome. Indeed, several disorders are caused by mutations of genes coding for components of the endolysosomal system in the PT. Besides *CLCN5* (DD1) and *OCRL* (Lowe syndrome and Dent disease type 2) genes, they include *LRP2* (DB/FOAR), *CUBN*, *AMN* (Imerslund–Gräsbeck syndrome), and *CTNS* (nephropathic cystinosis). Typically, these recessive disorders cause proximal tubular dysfunction and lead to inappropriate urinary loss of LMW proteins and solutes (e.g., phosphate, glucose, amino acids, urate), and they often lead to renal failure. The clinical entity of generalized proximal tubular dysfunction is referred to as renal Fanconi syndrome.

However, apart from BDA who was found to carry biallelic pathogenic variants in the *LRP2* gene and, for this reason, and after a careful clinical revaluation, was assessed to suffer from an atypical form of DB/FOAR syndrome [64], the other patient (AMS) did not suffer from cystinuria, despite carrying biallelic variants in the *SLC3A1* gene that were classified as likely pathogenic according to ACMG/AMP variant interpretation. Indeed, in this patient, the urinary level of cysteine was found to be normal even after repeated measurements. Two hypotheses may explain these findings: (1) the variants may be hypomorphic, thereby allowing a limited gene product activity, and (2) the two variants are in the same allele (complex allele), although their MAF was highly different, suggesting the absence of a linkage disequilibrium.

Instead, what appears relevant from this study is finding in three patients (comprising AMS) possible pathogenic variants in more than one gene connected in functional networks (*PDZK1*, *SLC17A1*, *CUBN*, *SLC3A9*, and *LRP2*), which we considered important for explaining patients' phenotypes, thus suggesting digenic or oligogenic disorders.

The major finding of WES study is the discovery in AMS of a homozygous truncating mutation in the *PDZK1* gene. This is a new gene that has never been related before to human diseases, although it is one of the loci of strongest effect on serum urate level and gut [65–67]. NHE-RF3 encoded by *PDZK1* is a major scaffolder protein in the brush border of kidney PTCs [68], interacting through its PDZ domain with key molecules of urate transport, including NPT1 [29]. Furthermore, NHE-RF3 is one of the several proteins interacting with the type-2a sodium phosphate cotransporter (NaPi-2a), which is the major inorganic phosphate cotransporter of the PTCs [69]. Targeted disruption of the *Pdzk1* gene by homologous recombination in mice induced modulation of the expression of selective ion channels in the kidney, including NaPi-2a. The steady-state levels of NaPi-2a were found to be reduced under a phosphorus (Pi)-rich diet, and this was paralleled by higher urinary total and fractional Pi excretion [69]. In these KO mice, serum urate was not measured, nor were urate transporters investigated. However, urine and serum analysis did not reveal any significant difference between KO and wild-type mice except for a significant increase in the cholesterol levels [69]. Interestingly, in *Pdzk1* KO mice under a high-Pi diet, the PDZ scaffolding protein NHE-RF1 was increased at the bush border of proximal tubules. NHE-RF1 was demonstrated to localize with megalin in the brush border, because it bounds to its internal C-terminal PDZ binding motif [70]. It was also showed that NHE-RF1 silencing in PTCs increased megalin expression [70].

In the same patient, we also detected a very rare missense variant in the *SLC17A1* gene, which is classified as VUS due to its extreme rarity in the human population (data from gnomAD: 1 allele out of 250846). The *SLC17A1* gene is one of the loci associated with serum urate level and gout [71] and encodes NPT1, which is a Cl-dependent urate transport interacting with NHE-RF3 encoded by the *PDZK1* gene [26]. The clinical phenotype of patient AMS involves multiple tubular defects (particularly hyperphosphaturia, hypercalciuria, and severe hypouricemia), which might be consistent with a partial renal Fanconi syndrome and had led to a clinical suspicion of renal hypouricemia (MIM#220150 and 612076) and atypical DD. By WES, we excluded the presence of pathogenic variants in both *SLC22A12* and *SLC2A9* genes encoding URAT1 and GLUT9, respectively. It is tempting to speculate that the *PDZK1* and the *SLC17A1* gene variants might have had a role in determining AMS clinical phenotype for their direct interaction with urate and phosphate transport. Family studies will help clarify these aspects.

Since megalin and cubilin PTC expression is altered in DD1, it is conceivable that *LRP2* and/or *CUBN* mutations can cause or contribute to a DD-like nephropathy. WES results seem to support this hypothesis. In addition to BDA, who has already been described as carrying biallelic mutations in the *LRP2* gene [64], AMV was also found to carry a known pathogenic *LRP2* allele and a very rare inframe deletion in the *CUBN* gene. *CUBN* variants have recently been associated with proteinuria with no signs of IGS. It was shown that a homozygous frameshift mutation in exon 53 of *CUBN* (p.Ser2785fs) only caused proteinuria [72]. Moreover, a missense variant in exon 57 (p.Ile2984Val) was associated with albuminuria [73]. Mutations in the *CUBN* gene cause IGS apparently only when they affect the cubilin–amnionless interaction domain (exons 1–20) or the IF-Cbl binding site (exons 21–29) [74]. In our patient, *CUBN* mutation is localized in exon 46. Follow-up showed that our patient's LMWP was intermittent while his proteinuria started at 1 year old and ranged between 0.4 and 1 g/24 h.

True digenic inheritance (DI) is the simplest form for oligogenic disease [75], but it is also encountered when pathogenic mutations responsible for two different diseases are co-inherited, leading to a blended phenotype [76]. The two heterozygous mutations in the *LRP2* and *CUBN* genes, encoding proteins working close together on the same endocytic pathway, might plausibly be responsible for patient AMV's disease phenotype. Further studies on his kidney biopsy and/or urinary proteoma might confirm this hypothesis. Family studies may help to solve these questions.

We detected two *LRP2* coding variants associated with two likely pathogenic missense variants in the *CUBN* and *SLC9A3* genes in the genome of a single patient (AMT). It is noteworthy that these genes respectively encode megalin, cubilin, and NHE3, which are located—together with ClC-5, amnionless, and Dab2—at the cell surface of PTCs, forming its endocytic apparatus [54,55].

SLC9A3 homozygous or compound heterozygous disease-causing mutations have recently been reported in nine patients from eight families with congenital secretory sodium diarrhea (MIM#616868) [77]. No association has been found as yet between *SLC9A3* variants and renal proximal tubulopathies, but a defective Nhe3 exposure was found in *Clcn5* KO mice [55,78]. Studies by Gekle et al. [33] support a crucial role for NHE3 in proximal tubular receptor-mediated endocytosis by demonstrating in Nhe3 KO mice that Nhe3 deficiency led to a reduced protein reabsorption: the urinary protein patterns resembled those of mice deficient in megalin or ClC-5. Recent evidence also highlights the importance of NHE3 for calcium reabsorption. Nhe3 KO mice revealed significant urinary calcium wasting and a low cortical bone mineral density and trabecular bone mass [79].

The genetic data of the AMT patient are puzzling and raise some questions. With the advent of high-throughput sequencing, we are bound to discover more patients suffering from oligogenic diseases and learn more about how complex interactions between allelic and locus heterogeneity affect disease phenotypes [80]. The presence of multiple coding variants in the same gene, either in cis or in trans, may also conceivably cause defective protein functioning, although this needs to be demonstrated in animal and in vitro models [81]. The genotype–phenotype correlation in the AMT patient is worth investigating, because it seems to reveal such an impact on disease phenotype. This patient was 26 years old when referred to a nephrologist for kidney stones. His height (158 cm) and weight (42 kg) were below the third percentile. His renal phenotype mainly featured proximal tubulopathy manifesting as Fanconi syndrome with LMWP, hypercalciuria, hyperphosphaturia, glycosuria, natriuresis, and hypercitraturia. Therefore, the patient's presenting phenotype was mainly related to an impaired renal calcium and phosphate metabolism. WES detected no relevant variants in genes known to be responsible for monogenic forms of nephrolithiasis and renal tubulopathies. We hypothesized that the AMT patient's phenotype was due to the variants in *LRP2*, *CUBN*, and *SLC9A3*, whose products work on the same cellular pathways as ClC-5, or pathways related thereto, but this hypothesis needs to be evaluated by in vitro studies. From the point of view of the referring clinicians, tubular abnormalities might be a real challenge: indeed, clinical characteristics of different diseases sometimes overlap, and a full-blown classical phenotype (in the case of AMS, a renal Fanconi syndrome) is rare. Therefore, when multiple tubular defects (i.e., alteration in tubular handling of 2–4 different solutes) coexist, the chance of a blended phenotype becomes more plausible, and a next-generation sequencing (NGS) approach might be a good strategy to identify multiple (and possibly interacting) genetic defects that may explain each individual phenotype.

4. Material and Methods

4.1. Patients

4.1.1. DNA Samples

From 2006 to 2018, DNA samples were collected from 158 unrelated pediatric and adult males with clinically suspected DD according to the criteria described in our previous study [82]. Patients should have encountered at least two of the above-mentioned criteria for being referred to our laboratory for a molecular diagnosis. Since proteinuria was recently reported as one of the DD symptoms in concomitance with signs of incomplete Fanconi tubulopathy [83], and because of the cost of urinary assessment of LMW proteins, we decided to include in the diagnostic workflow also patients presenting with proteinuria, although in the absence of documented LMWP. Informed consent to the genetic study was obtained from all probands or their parents.

DNA samples from eight patients (four children and four adults) with no detectable *CLCN5* or *OCRL* gene mutations underwent WES. The selection was based on the presence of a likely DD phenotype (i.e., the presence of LMWP and/or proteinuria, hypercalciuria, and at least one of the following: nephrocalcinosis, kidney stones, hypophosphataemia, renal failure, aminoaciduria, rickets, or a positive family history) with or without extra-renal symptoms. The study was approved by Padua University Hospital's Ethical Committee, protocol 0028285 (11 May 2016)

4.1.2. Biopsies

Ten kidney biopsies were collected from patients carrying nine different *CLCN5* mutations (Table 2). All biopsies were performed for diagnostic purposes and available for immunolabeling studies subject to informed consent.

Eight control cortical tissues were obtained from nephrectomies for renal cancer (sites remote from the tumor-bearing renal tissue), disclosing a normal morphology and no immunofluorescence. The study was approved by Padua University Hospital's Ethical Committee, protocol 0007452 (1 February 2018).

4.2. Sanger Sequencing

CLCN5 gene mutation analysis was performed by Sanger sequencing. Genomic DNA was extracted from peripheral blood using the QIAamp DNA Blood Minikit (Qiagen, Milan, Italy) according to the manufacturer's instructions. The primers and PCR conditions for amplifying the *CLCN5* gene-coding region and intron–exon boundaries are described elsewhere [82]. The PCR products were analyzed using the Bioanalyzer 2100 (Agilent Technologies, Milan, Italy) and purified with the MinElute PCR Purification Kit (Qiagen, Milan, Italy). Sanger sequencing was done with the BigDye Terminator v1.1 Cycle Sequencing Kit (ThermoFisher Scientific, Milan, Italy) and the ABI-PRISM 3100 Genetic Analyzer (ThermoFisher Scientific, Milan, Italy). The nomenclature of mutations is based on the *CLCN5* cDNA sequence NM_0000844. Missense and splicing mutations were interpreted using the Mutation Taster (MT) [84], and classified according to the American College of Medical Genetics and American College of Pathologists (ACMG/AMP) variant classification guidelines [22]. Mutations were confirmed by sequencing a second independent PCR product.

4.3. Whole-Exome Sequencing (WES)

WES was performed at Padua University's Centro di Ricerca Interdipartimentale per le Biotecnologie Innovative (CRIBI) sequencing center using the Ion Proton System (ThermoFisher Scientific, Milan, Italy), obtaining an average reads coverage of 80X for each sample. Data were analyzed as suggested by the manufacturer, with read alignment using TMAP and variant calling with TSVC, which are both included in the Ion Proton Suite (v 5.0). QueryOR (http://queryor.cribi.unipd.it, accessed on 27 November 2019) [85] was used to analyze and prioritize short-nucleotide variants (SNV). This web-based query platform enables quick, easy, in-depth variant prioritization by aggregating several functional annotations of both genes and variants. The prioritization strategy entails a ranking that sorts results by the number and weight of the criteria met (see below).

Two main approaches were initially used to identify the most promising variants: (1) a gene-centered search, considering known details of genes and associated pathways, and information about the disease and related disorders; and (2) a variant-centered search, focusing on the intrinsic characteristics of variants, such as type (indel, snp, mnp), codon effect (frameshift, missense, and nonsense variants), and genomic position.

In a subsequent prioritization step, variants were ranked by sequencing coverage, minor allele frequency (MAF) values ≤ 0.05, and predicted possible–probable deleteriousness. For this purpose, QueryOR provides coding variant predictions based on several tools, including the well-known SIFT, PolyPhen2, and MT, and the more recent PROVEAN, CADD, and DANN scores [84,86–90]. Sanger sequencing was used to validate variants identified by the in silico prioritization strategy during WES. Table S5 shows the gene names, NCBI reference sequences, primers, and PCR amplification conditions.

Identified variants were checked against relevant database such as Clinvar (https://www.ncbi. nlm.nih.gov/clinvar/, accessed on 27 November 2019) and The Human Gene Mutation Database (HGMD) (http://www.hgmd.cf.ac.uk/ac/index.php, accessed on 27 November 2019), and were classified according to ACMG/AMP guidelines [22].

4.4. Immunohistochemistry (IHC)

IHC was conducted on formalin-fixed, paraffin-embedded sections using an indirect immunoperoxidase method. Specimens were treated as previously described [91], and incubated overnight with rabbit anti-human ClC-5 (Sigma-Aldrich, Milan, Italy, cat. HPA000401) diluted 1:200, goat anti-human ClC-3 (Santa Cruz Biotechnologies, Heidelberg, Germany, cat. sc-17572) diluted 1:150, and rabbit anti-human ClC-4 (Sigma-Aldrich, Milan, Italy, cat. HPA063637) diluted 1:50 in PBS at 4 °C in a humidified chamber. A donkey anti-goat IgG-HRP secondary antibody (Santa Cruz Biotechnologies, Heidelberg, Germany, cat. sc-2020) diluted 1:100 was used for ClC-3. Immunolabeling specificity was confirmed by incubating without any primary antibody. Images were acquired with the Diaplan light microscope (Leitz, Como, Italy) and 20X/0.45 objective using a Micropublisher 5.0 RTV camera (Teledyne QImaging, Surrey, BC, Canada).

4.5. Immunofluorescence (IF)

IF analyses were performed on serial sections of kidney biopsies. Samples were treated as previously described [92] and incubated overnight with primary antibody (sheep anti-human cubilin [R&D Systems, Minneapolis, MN, USA, cat. AF3700], rabbit anti-human megalin [LS-Bio, Seattle, WA, USA, cat. LS-B105]) diluted 1:100 in PBS 5% BSA at 4 °C. Sections were incubated with the appropriate fluorescent secondary antibody [92]. Nuclei were counterstained with 4′,6-diamidino-2-phenylindole (DAPI). Negative controls were run by omitting the primary antibody. Images were acquired with a DMI6000CS-TCS SP8 fluorescence microscope (Leica Microsystems, Milan, Italy) with a 20X/0.4 objective using a DFC365FX camera (Leica Microsystems, Milan, Italy) and analyzed with the LAS-AF software (Leica Microsystems, Milan, Italy).

4.6. Morphometric Analysis

ClC-5, megalin, and cubilin signals on kidney biopsies were quantified by morphometric analysis using Image-Pro Plus 7.0 (Media Cybernetics, Abingdon, United Kingdom). Signals were acquired at 200X with the same time exposure, gain, and intensity for all patients, and quantified excluding the glomerular compartment. For ClC-5, only apical or subapical tubular staining was considered as positive. Quantities were expressed as the mean area covered by pixels (%).

4.7. Statistical Analysis

Non-parametric tests (Mann–Whitney U-test) were used due to the small sample size. Results with $p < 0.05$ were considered significant and given as median ± IQR. All analyses were performed with R software version 3.5.1 (R Foundation for Statistical Computing, Vienna, Austria) [93].

5. Conclusions

By describing 23 novel *CLCN5* mutations, this study extends the allelic heterogeneity of DD1. Our results on DD1 kidney biopsies provide evidence that ClC-5 is lost in PTCs, and this, in turn, leads to a defective trafficking of megalin and cubilin in these cells.

Using WES to investigate DD3 patients, we did not identify the supposed third Dent disease-causing gene. Instead, our study suggests that likely pathogenic variants in genes encoding components of the endocytic apparatus of tubular cells (megalin, cubilin, NHE3, and NHE-RF3) may have determined DD3 phenotypes. However, except for one patient in whom we identified a known monogenic disease, in the other patients, the presence of variants in more than one gene related in functional networks suggest that we are probably facing oligogenic disorders. Furthermore, our study suggests that DD3 patients are a pool of patients with DD-like phenotypes, which may present atypical phenotypes of known hereditary nephropathies or blended phenotypes.

Supplementary Materials:
Figure S1: ClC-5, ClC-4 and ClC-3 immunolabeling in serial sections of a control kidney. Tubular staining was almost exclusively apical (arrows) for ClC-5, while cytoplasmic staining (arrowheads) was seen for ClC-3, and ClC-5 and much less for ClC-4. Scale bar = 50 μm. Table S1: Clinical phenotypes of 20 patients carrying novel CLCN5 mutations. Table S2: List of phenocopy genes. Table S3: List of the genes prioritized according to scalable kernel-based gene prioritization (SCUBA) [24]. Table S4: DD-like phenotype of patients carrying likely pathogenic variants as detected by whole exome sequencing. Table S5: PCR primer sequences and amplification conditions.

Author Contributions: Study conception, design of experiments, and critical review of the results: F.A., G.V., M.C., L.B.; WES experiments: L.B.; WES data analyses: F.A., L.B., and L.T.; Sanger experiments: L.G., L.T., and M.C.; IHC experiments: M.C. and G.P.; IF experiments: L.G. and G.P.; Statistical analysis: L.G.; Morphometric analysis: M.C. and D.D.P.; Drafting of the paper: F.A., L.B., L.G., and M.C.; Supervision of clinical cases and clinical data collection: D.D.P., V.C. and C.M.; Histopathological data reporting on kidney biopsies: L.M., M.G., L.P., F.P., and F.A. F.A. conceived the paper's structure, supervised its writing, and thoroughly reviewed all content. All authors have read and agreed to the published version of the manuscript.

Acknowledgments: This work was performed with the contribution of the Italian Network of Dent Disease researchers: Gian Marco Ghiggeri and Giancarlo Barbano (Division of Nephrology, Dialysis and Kidney Transplantation, G. Gaslini Pediatric Institute, Genova), Francesco Emma and Gianluca Vergine (Division of Nephrology and Dialysis, Bambin Gesù Pediatric Hospital, Rome), Giuseppe Vezzoli (Division of Nephrology, Dialysis and Hypertension, IRCCS San Raffaele Hospital, Milan), Marilena Cara (Nephrology Division, Camposampiero General Hospital, Camposampiero) Gabriele Ripanti (Pediatrics and Neonatology Division, San Salvatore Hospital, Pesaro), Anita Ammenti (Pediatric Institute, University of Parma), Licia Peruzzi (Division of Nephrology, Dialysis and Transplantation, Regina Margherita Hospital, Turin), Giacomo Colussi (Nephrology Unit, Varese Hospital, Varese), Mario Giordano (Nephrology and Pediatric Dialysis, Pediatric Hospital, Bari) Maria Rosa Caruso (Nephrology Unit, Bergamo Hospital, Bergamo), Ilse Maria Ratsch (Pediatric Institute, University of Ancona), Giuseppina Marra and Fabio Paglialonga (Nephrology Unit, IRCCS Foundation, Ca' Granda Ospedale Maggiore Policlinico, University of Milan), Angela La Manna (Department of Pediatrics, 2nd University of Napoli), Caterina Canavese (Nephrology and Kidney Transplantation Unit, Department of Translational Medicine, University of Piemonte Orientale (UPO), Novara), Diego Bellino (Division of Nephrology, Dialysis and Kidney Transplantation, San Martino University Hospital, Genova), Luisa Murer (Pediatric Nephrology, Dialysis and Transplant Unit, Department of Women's and Children's Health, Padua University Hospital), Milena Brugnara (Pediatric Division, Department of Life and Reproduction Sciences, University of Verona), Andrea Pasini and Claudio La Scola (Nephrology and Dialysis Unit, Department of Pediatrics, Azienda Ospedaliero Universitaria Sant'Orsola-Malpighi, Bologna).

References

1. Lloyd, S.E.; Pearce, S.H.; Fisher, S.E.; Steinmeyer, K.; Schwappach, B.; Scheinman, S.J.; Harding, B.; Bolino, A.; Devoto, M.; Goodyer, P.; et al. A common molecular basis for three inherited kidney stone diseases. *Nature* **1996**, *379*, 445–449. [CrossRef] [PubMed]

2. Thakker, R.V. Pathogenesis of Dent's disease and related syndromes of X-linked nephrolithiasis. *Kidney Int.* **2000**, *57*, 787–793. [CrossRef] [PubMed]

3. Wrong, O.M.; Norden, A.G.; Feest, T.G. Dent's disease; a familial proximal renal tubular syndrome with low-molecular-weight proteinuria, hypercalciuria, nephrocalcinosis, metabolic bone disease, progressive renal failure and a marked male predominance. *Q. J. Med.* **1994**, *87*, 473–493.

4. Reinhart, S.C.; Norden, A.G.; Lapsley, M.; Thakker, R.V.; Pang, J.; Moses, A.M.; Frymoyer, P.A.; Favus, M.J.; Hoepner, J.A.; Scheinman, S.J. Characterization of carrier females and affected males with X-linked recessive nephrolithiasis. *J. Am. Soc. Nephrol.* **1995**, *5*, 1451–1461. [CrossRef] [PubMed]

5. Lloyd, S.E.; Gunther, W.; Pearce, S.H.; Thomson, A.; Bianchi, M.L.; Bosio, M.; Craig, I.W.; Fisher, S.E.; Scheinman, S.J.; Wrong, O.; et al. Characterization of renal chloride channel, CLCN5, mutations in hypercalciuric nephrolithiasis (kidney stones) disorders. *Hum. Mol. Genet.* **1997**, *6*, 1233–1239. [CrossRef] [PubMed]

6. Jentsch, T.J.; Günther, W.; Pusch, M.; Schwappach, B. Properties of voltage-gated chloride channels of the ClC gene family. *J. Physiol.* **1995**, *482*, 19S–25S. [CrossRef]

7. Thakker, R.V. Chloride channels cough up. *Nat. Genet.* **1997**, *17*, 125. [CrossRef]

8. Picollo, A.; Pusch, M. Chloride/proton antiporter activity of mammalian CLC proteins ClC-4 and ClC-5. *Nature* **2005**, *436*, 420–423. [CrossRef]

9. Mansour-Hendili, L.; Blanchard, A.; Le Pottier, N.; Roncelin, I.; Lourdel, S.; Treard, C.; González, W.; Vergara-Jaque, A.; Morin, G.; Colin, E.; et al. Mutation update of the CLCN5 gene responsible for Dent disease 1. *Hum. Mutat.* **2015**, *36*, 743–752. [CrossRef]

10. Jouret, F.; Igarashi, T.; Gofflot, F.; Wilson, P.D.; Karet, F.E.; Thakker, R.V.; Devuyst, O. Comparative ontogeny; processing; and segmental distribution of the renal chloride channel; ClC-5. *Kidney Int.* **2004**, *65*, 198–208. [CrossRef]

11. Christensen, E.I.; Devuyst, O.; Dom, G.; Nielsen, R.; Van Der Smissen, P.; Verroust, P.; Leruth, M.; Guggino, W.B.; Courtoy, P.J. Loss of chloride channel ClC-5 impairs endocytosis by defective trafficking of megalin and cubilin in kidney proximal tubules. *Proc. Natl. Acad. Sci. USA* **2003**, *100*, 8472–8477. [CrossRef] [PubMed]

12. Gunther, W.; Luchow, A.; Cluzeaud, F.; Vandewalle, A.; Jentsch, T.J. ClC-5, the chloride channel mutated in Dent's disease; colocalizes with the proton pump in endocytically active kidney cells. *Proc. Natl. Acad. Sci. USA* **1998**, *95*, 8075–8080. [CrossRef] [PubMed]

13. D'Antonio, C.; Molinski, S.; Ahmadi, S.; Huan, L.J.; Wellhauser, L.; Bear, C.E. Conformational defects underlie proteasomal degradation of Dent's disease-causing mutants of ClC-5. *Biochem. J.* **2013**, *452*, 391–400. [CrossRef] [PubMed]

14. Lourdel, S.; Grand, T.; Burgos, J.; González, W.; Sepúlveda, F.V.; Teulon, J. ClC-5 mutations associated with Dent's disease: A major role of the dimer interface. *Pflug. Arch.* **2012**, *463*, 247–256. [CrossRef] [PubMed]

15. Grand, T.; L'Hoste, S.; Mordasini, D.; Defontaine, N.; Keck, M.; Pennaforte, T.; Genete, M.; Laghmani, K.; Teulon, J.; Lourdel, S. Heterogeneity in the processing of CLCN5 mutants related to Dent disease. *Hum. Mutat.* **2011**, *32*, 476–483. [CrossRef] [PubMed]

16. Smith, A.J.; Reed, A.A.; Loh, N.Y.; Thakker, R.V.; Lippiat, J.D. Characterization of Dent's disease mutations of CLC-5 reveals a correlation between functional and cell biological consequences and protein structure. *Am. J. Physiol. Ren. Physiol.* **2009**, *296*, F390–F397. [CrossRef]

17. Ludwig, M.; Doroszewicz, J.; Seyberth, H.W.; Bökenkamp, A.; Balluch, B.; Nuutinen, M.; Utsch, B.; Waldegger, S. Functional evaluation of Dent's disease-causing mutations: Implications for ClC-5 channel trafficking and internalization. *Hum. Genet.* **2005**, *117*, 228–237. [CrossRef]

18. Hoopes, R.R., Jr.; Raja, K.M.; Koich, A.; Hueber, P.; Reid, R.; Knohl, S.J.; Scheinman, S.J. Evidence for genetic heterogeneity in Dent's disease. *Kidney Int.* **2004**, *65*, 1615–1620. [CrossRef]

19. Hoopes, R.R., Jr.; Shrimpton, A.E.; Knohl, S.J.; Hueber, P.; Reed, A.A.; Christie, P.T.; Igarashi, T.; Lee, P.; Lehman, A.; White, C.; et al. Dent disease with mutations in OCRL1. *Am. J. Hum. Genet.* **2005**, *76*, 260–267. [CrossRef]

20. Hichri, H.; Rendu, J.; Monnier, N.; Coutton, C.; Dorseuil, O.; Poussou, R.V.; Baujat, G.; Blanchard, A.; Nobili, F.; Ranchin, B.; et al. From Lowe syndrome to Dent disease: Correlations between mutations of the OCRL1 gene and clinical and biochemical phenotypes. *Hum. Mutat.* **2011**, *32*, 379–388. [CrossRef]

21. Shrimpton, A.E.; Hoopes, R.R., Jr.; Knohl, S.J.; Hueber, P.; Reed, A.A.; Christie, P.T.; Igarashi, T.; Lee, P.; Lehman, A.; White, C.; et al. OCRL1 mutations in Dent 2 patients suggest a mechanism for phenotypic variability. *Nephron Physiol.* **2009**, *112*, 27–36. [CrossRef] [PubMed]

22. Richards, S.; Aziz, N.; Bale, S.; Bick, D.; Das, S.; Gastier-Foster, J.; Grody, W.W.; Hegde, M.; Lyon, E.; Spector, E.; et al. ACMG Laboratory Quality Assurance Committee. Standards and guidelines for the interpretation of sequence variants: A joint consensus recommendation of the American College of Medical Genetics and Genomics and the Association for Molecular Pathology. *Genet. Med.* **2015**, *17*, 405–424. [CrossRef] [PubMed]

23. Jentsch, T.J. Chloride channels are different. *Nature* **2002**, *415*, 276–277. [CrossRef] [PubMed]

24. Zampieri, G.; Tran, D.V.; Donini, M.; Navarin, N.; Aiolli, F.; Sperduti, A.; Valle, G. Scuba: Scalable kernel-based gene prioritization. *BMC Bioinform.* **2018**, *19*, 23. [CrossRef]

25. Merriman, T.R.; Dalbeth, N. The genetic basis of hyperuricaemia and gout. *Jt. Bone Spine* **2011**, *78*, 35–40. [CrossRef]

26. Iharada, M.; Miyaji, T.; Fujimoto, T.; Hiasa, M.; Anzai, N.; Omote, H.; Moriyama, Y. Type 1 sodium-dependent phosphate transporter (SLC17A1 Protein) is a Cl(-)-dependent urate exporter. *J. Biol. Chem.* **2010**, *285*, 26107–26113. [CrossRef] [PubMed]

27. Chiba, T.; Matsuo, H.; Kawamura, Y.; Nagamori, S.; Nishiyama, T.; Wei, L.; Nakayama, A.; Nakamura, T.; Sakiyama, M.; Takada, T.; et al. NPT1/SLC17A1 is a renal urate exporter in humans and its common gain-of-function variant decreases the risk of renal under-excretion gout. *Arthritis Rheumatol.* **2015**, *67*, 281–287. [CrossRef]

28. Higashino, T.; Matsuo, H.; Sakiyama, M.; Nakayama, A.; Nakamura, T.; Takada, T.; Ogata, H.; Kawamura, Y.; Kawaguchi, M.; Naito, M.; et al. Common variant of PDZ domain containing 1 (PDZK1) gene is associated with gout susceptibility: A replication study and meta-analysis in Japanese population. *Drug Metab. Pharm.* **2016**, *31*, 464–466. [CrossRef]

29. Anzai, N.; Kanai, Y.; Endou, H. New insights into renal transport of urate. *Curr. Opin. Rheumatol.* **2007**, *19*, 151–157. [CrossRef]

30. De Ligt, J.; Willemsen, M.H.; van Bon, B.W.; Kleefstra, T.; Yntema, H.G.; Kroes, T.; Vulto-van Silfhout, A.T.; Koolen, D.A.; de Vries, P.; Gilissen, C.; et al. Diagnostic exome sequencing in persons with severe intellectual disability. *N. Engl. J. Med.* **2012**, *367*, 1921–1929. [CrossRef]

31. Alexander, R.T.; Dimke, H.; Cordat, E. Proximal tubular NHEs: Sodium, protons and calcium? *Am. J. Physiol. Ren. Physiol.* **2013**, *305*, F229–F236. [CrossRef] [PubMed]

32. Biemesderfer, D.; Nagy, T.; DeGray, B.; Aronson, P. Specific association of megalin and the Na+/H+ exchanger isoform NHE3 in the proximal tubule. *J. Biol. Chem.* **1999**, *274*, 17518–17524. [CrossRef]

33. Gekle, M.; Völker, K.; Mildenberger, S.; Freudinger, R.; Shull, G.E.; Wiemann, M. NHE3 Na+/H+ exchanger supports proximal tubular protein reabsorption in vivo. *Am. J. Physiol. Ren. Physiol.* **2004**, *287*, F469–F473. [CrossRef] [PubMed]

34. Szczepanska, M.; Zaniew, M.; Recker, F.; Mizerska-Wasiak, M.; Zaluska-Lesniewska, I.; Kilis-Pstrusinska, K.; Adamczyk, P.; Zawadzki, J.; Pawlaczyk, K.; Ludwig, M.; et al. Dent disease in children: Diagnostic and therapeutic considerations. *Clin. Nephrol.* **2015**, *84*, 222–230. [CrossRef] [PubMed]

35. Tang, X.; Brown, M.R.; Cogal, A.G.; Gauvin, D.; Harris, P.C.; Lieske, J.C.; Romero, M.F.; Chang, M.H. Functional and transport analyses of CLCN5 genetic changes identified in Dent disease patients. *Physiol. Rep.* **2016**, *4*, e12776. [CrossRef] [PubMed]

36. Li, F.; Yue, Z.; Xu, T.; Chen, M.; Zhong, L.; Liu, T.; Jing, X.; Deng, J.; Hu, B.; Liu, Y.; et al. Dent Disease in Chinese Children and Findings from Heterozygous Mothers: Phenotypic Heterogeneity, Fetal Growth, and 10 Novel Mutations. *J. Pediatr.* **2016**, *174*, 204–210.e1. [CrossRef]

37. Kubo, K.; Aizawa, T.; Watanabe, S.; Tsugawa, K.; Tsuruga, K.; Ito, E.; Joh, K.; Tanaka, H. Does Dent disease remain an underrecognized cause for young boys with focal glomerulosclerosis? *Pediatr. Int.* **2016**, *58*, 747–749. [CrossRef]

38. Wong, W.; Poke, G.; Stack, M.; Kara, T.; Prestidge, C.; Flintoff, K. Phenotypic variability of Dent disease in a large New Zealand kindred. *Pediatr. Nephrol.* **2017**, *32*, 365–369. [CrossRef]

39. Guven, A.; Al-Rijjal, R.A.; BinEssa, H.A.; Dogan, D.; Kor, Y.; Zou, M.; Kaya, N.; Alenezi, A.F.; Hancili, S.; Tarım, Ö.; et al. Mutational analysis of PHEX, FGF23 and CLCN5 in patients with hypophosphataemic rickets. *Clin. Endocrinol.* **2017**, *87*, 103–112. [CrossRef]

40. Günthner, R.; Wagner, M.; Thurm, T.; Ponsel, S.; Höfele, J.; Lange-Sperandio, B. Identification of co-occurrence in a patient with Dent's disease and ADA2-deficiency by exome sequencing. *Gene* **2018**, *649*, 23–26. [CrossRef]

41. Sancakli, O.; Kulu, B.; Sakallioglu, O. A novel mutation of Dent's disease in an 11-year-old male with nephrolithiasis and nephrocalcinosis. *Arch. Argent. Pediatr.* **2018**, *116*, e442–e444.

42. Bignon, Y.; Alekov, A.; Frachon, N.; Lahuna, O.; Jean-Baptiste Doh-Egueli, C.; Deschênes, G.; Vargas-Poussou, R.; Lourdel, S. A novel CLCN5 pathogenic mutation supports Dent disease with normal endosomal acidification. *Hum. Mutat.* **2018**, *39*, 1139–1149. [CrossRef] [PubMed]

43. Wen, M.; Shen, T.; Wang, Y.; Li, Y.; Shi, X.; Dang, X. Next-Generation Sequencing in Early Diagnosis of Dent Disease 1: Two Case Reports. *Front. Med.* **2018** *5*, 347. [CrossRef] [PubMed]

44. Matsumoto, A.; Matsui, I.; Mori, T.; Sakaguchi, Y.; Mizui, M.; Ueda, Y.; Takahashi, A.; Doi, Y.; Shimada, K.; Yamaguchi, S.; et al. Severe Osteomalacia with Dent Disease Caused by a Novel Intronic Mutation of the CLCN5 gene. *Intern. Med.* **2018**, *57*, 3603–3610. [CrossRef] [PubMed]

45. Ye, Q.; Shen, Q.; Rao, J.; Zhang, A.; Zheng, B.; Liu, X.; Shen, Y.; Chen, Z.; Wu, Y.; Hou, L.; et al. Multicenter study of the clinical features and mutation gene spectrum of Chinese children with Dent disease. *Clin. Genet.* **2019**. [CrossRef]

46. Wu, F.; Roche, P.; Christie, P.T.; Loh, N.Y.; Reed, A.A.; Esnouf, R.M.; Thakker, R.V. Modeling study of human renal chloride channel (hCLC-5) mutations suggests a structural-functional relationship. *Kidney Int.* **2003**, *63*, 1426–1432. [CrossRef]

47. Meyer, S.; Savaresi, S.; Forster, I.C.; Dutzler, R. Nucleotide recognition by the cytoplasmic domain of the human chloride transporter ClC-5. *Nat. Struct. Mol. Biol.* **2007**, *14*, 60–67. [CrossRef]

48. Wellhauser, L.; Luna-Chavez, C.; D'Antonio, C.; Tainer, J.; Bear, C.E. ATP induces conformational changes in the carboxylterminal region of ClC-5. *J. Biol. Chem.* **2011**, *286*, 6733–6741. [CrossRef]

49. Zifarelli, G.; Pusch, M. Intracellular regulation of human ClC-5 by adenine nucleotides. *EMBO Rep.* **2009**, *10*, 1111–1116. [CrossRef]

50. Grand, T.; Mordasini, D.; L'Hoste, S.; Pennaforte, T.; Genete, M.; Biyeyeme, M.J.; Vargas-Poussou, R.; Blanchard, A.; Teulon, J.; Lourdel, S. Novel CLCN5 mutations in patients with Dent's disease result in altered ion currents or impaired exchanger processing. *Kidney Int.* **2009**, *76*, 999–1005. [CrossRef]

51. Pusch, M.; Ludewig, U.; Jentsch, T.J. Temperature dependence of fast and slow gating relaxations of CLC-0 chloride channels. *J. Gen. Physiol.* **1997**, *109*, 105–116. [CrossRef] [PubMed]

52. Igarashi, T.; Günther, W.; Sekine, T.; Inatomi, J.; Shiraga, H.; Takahashi, S.; Suzuki, J.; Tsuru, N.; Yanagihara, T.; Shimazu, M.; et al. Functional characterization of renal chloride channel, CLCN5, mutations associated with Dent's Japan disease. *Kidney Int.* **1998**, *54*, 1850–1856. [CrossRef] [PubMed]

53. Devuyst, O.; Christie, P.T.; Courtoy, P.J.; Beauwens, R.; Thakker, R.V. Intra-renal and subcellular distribution of the human chloride channel, CLC-5, reveals a pathophysiological basis for Dent's disease. *Hum. Mol. Genet.* **1999**, *8*, 247–257. [CrossRef] [PubMed]

54. Wang, Y.; Cai, H.; Cebotaru, L.; Hryciw, D.H.; Weinman, E.J.; Donowitz, M.; Guggino, S.E.; Guggino, W.B. ClC-5: Role in endocytosis in the proximal tubule. *Am. J. Physiol. Ren. Physiol.* **2005**, *289*, F850–F862. [CrossRef]

55. Hryciw, D.H.; Wang, Y.; Devuyst, O.; Pollock, C.A.; Poronnik, P.; Guggino, W.B. Cofilin interacts with ClC-5 and regulates albumin uptake in proximal tubule cell lines. *J. Biol. Chem.* **2003**, *278*, 40169–40176. [CrossRef]

56. Kellermayer, R. Translational readthrough induction of pathogenic nonsense mutations. *Eur. J. Med. Genet.* **2006**, *49*, 445–450. [CrossRef]

57. Oren, Y.S.; Pranke, I.M.; Kerem, B.; Sermet-Gaudelus, I. The suppression of premature termination codons and the repair of splicing mutations in CFTR. *Curr. Opin. Pharmacol.* **2017**, *34*, 125–131. [CrossRef]

58. Piwon, N.; Günther, W.; Schwake, M.; Bösl, M.R.; Jentsch, T.J. ClC-5 Cl$^-$-channel disruption impairs endocytosis in a mouse model for Dent's disease. *Nature* **2000**, *408*, 369–373. [CrossRef]

59. Norden, A.G.; Lapsley, M.; Igarashi, T.; Kelleher, C.L.; Lee, P.J.; Matsuyama, T.; Scheinman, S.J.; Shiraga, H.; Sundin, D.P.; Thakker, R.V.; et al. Urinary megalin deficiency implicates abnormal tubular endocytic function in Fanconi syndrome. *J. Am. Soc. Nephrol.* **2002**, *13*, 125–133.

60. Tanuma, A.; Sato, H.; Takeda, T.; Hosojima, M.; Obayashi, H.; Hama, H.; Iino, N.; Hosaka, K.; Kaseda, R.; Imai, N.; et al. Functional characterization of a novel missense CLCN5 mutation causing alterations in proximal tubular endocytic machinery in Dent's disease. *Nephron Physiol.* **2007**, *107*, p87–p97. [CrossRef]

61. Santo, Y.; Hirai, H.; Shima, M.; Yamagata, M.; Michigami, T.; Nakajima, S.; Ozono, K. Examination of megalin in renal tubular epithelium from patients with Dent disease. *Pediatr. Nephrol.* **2004**, *19*, 612–615. [CrossRef] [PubMed]

62. Gorvin, C.M.; Wilmer, M.J.; Piret, S.E.; Harding, B.; van den Heuvel, L.P.; Wrong, O.; Jat, P.S.; Lippiat, J.D.; Levtchenko, E.N.; Thakker, R.V. Receptor-mediated endocytosis and endosomal acidification is impaired in proximal tubule epithelial cells of Dent disease patients. *Proc. Natl. Acad. Sci. USA* **2013**, *110*, 7014–7019. [CrossRef] [PubMed]

63. Anglani, F.; D'Angelo, A.; Bertizzolo, L.M.; Tosetto, E.; Ceol, M.; Cremasco, D.; Bonfante, L.; Addis, M.A.; Del Prete, D. Dent Disease Italian Network. Nephrolithiasis; kidney failure and bone disorders in Dent disease patients with and without CLCN5 mutations. *SpringerPlus* **2015**, *4*, 492. [CrossRef]

64. Anglani, F.; Terrin, L.; Brugnara, M.; Battista, M.; Cantaluppi, V.; Ceol, M.; Bertoldi, L.; Valle, G.; Joy, M.P.; Pober, B.R.; et al. Hypercalciuria and nephrolithiasis: Expanding the renal phenotype of Donnai-Barrow syndrome. *Clin. Genet.* **2018**, *94*, 187–188. [CrossRef] [PubMed]

65. Köttgen, A.; Albrecht, E.; Teumer, A.; Vitart, V.; Krumsiek, J.; Hundertmark, C.; Pistis, G.; Ruggiero, D.; O'Seaghdha, C.M.; Haller, T.; et al. Genome-wide association analyses identify 18 new loci associated with serum urate concentrations. *Nat. Genet.* **2013**, *45*, 145–154. [CrossRef] [PubMed]

66. Phipps-Green, A.J.; Merriman, M.E.; Topless, R.; Altaf, S.; Montgomery, G.W.; Franklin, C.; Jones, G.T.; van Rij, A.M.; White, D.; Stamp, L.K.; et al. Twenty-eight loci that influence serum urate levels: Analysis of association with gout. *Ann. Rheum. Dis.* **2016**, *75*, 124–130. [CrossRef] [PubMed]

67. Ketharnathan, S.; Leask, M.; Boocock, J.; Phipps-Green, A.J.; Antony, J.; O'Sullivan, J.M.; Merriman, T.R.; Horsfield, J.A. A non-coding genetic variant maximally associated with serum urate levels is functionally linked to HNF4A-dependent PDZK1 expression. *Hum. Mol. Genet.* **2018**, *27*, 3964–3973. [CrossRef]

68. Gisler, S.M.; Pribanic, S.; Bacic, D.; Forrer, P.; Gantenbein, A.; Sabourin, L.A.; Tsuji, A.; Zhao, Z.S.; Manser, E.; Biber, J.; et al. PDZK1: I. a major scaffolder in brush borders of proximal tubular cells. *Kidney Int.* **2003**, *64*, 1733–1745. [CrossRef]

69. Capuano, P.; Bacic, D.; Stange, G.; Hernando, N.; Kaissling, B.; Pal, R.; Kocher, O.; Biber, J.; Wagner, C.A.; Murer, H. Expression and regulation of the renal Na/phosphate cotransporter NaPi-IIa in a mouse model deficient for the PDZ protein PDZK1. *Pflug. Arch.* **2005**, *449*, 392–402. [CrossRef]

70. Slattery, C.; Jenkin, K.A.; Lee, A.; Simcocks, A.C.; McAinch, A.J.; Poronnik, P.; Hryciw, D.H. Na+-H+ exchanger regulatory factor 1 (NHERF1) PDZ scaffold binds an internal binding site in the scavenger receptor megalin. *Cell. Physiol. Biochem.* **2011**, *27*, 171–178. [CrossRef]

71. Sakiyama, M.; Matsuo, H.; Nagamori, S.; Ling, W.; Kawamura, Y.; Nakayama, A.; Higashino, T.; Chiba, T.; Ichida, K.; Kanai, Y.; et al. Expression of a human NPT1/SLC17A1 missense variant which increases urate export. *Nucleosides Nucleotides Nucleic Acids* **2016**, *35*, 536–542. [CrossRef] [PubMed]

72. Böger, C.A.; Chen, M.H.; Tin, A.; Olden, M.; Köttgen, A.; de Boer, I.H.; Fuchsberger, C.; O'Seaghdha, C.M.; Pattaro, C.; Teumer, A.; et al. CUBN is a gene locus for albuminuria. *J. Am. Soc. Nephrol.* **2011**, *22*, 555–570. [CrossRef] [PubMed]

73. Ovunc, B.; Otto, E.A.; Vega-Warner, V.; Saisawat, P.; Ashraf, S.; Ramaswami, G.; Fathy, H.M.; Schoeb, D.; Chernin, G.; Lyons, R.H.; et al. Exome sequencing reveals cubilin mutation as a single-gene cause of proteinuria. *J. Am. Soc. Nephrol.* **2011**, *22*, 1815–1820. [CrossRef] [PubMed]

74. Tanner, S.M.; Sturm, A.C.; Baack, E.C.; Liyanarachchi, S.; de la Chapelle, A. Inherited cobalamin malabsorption. Mutations in three genes reveal functional and ethnic patterns. *Orphanet J. Rare Dis.* **2012**, *7*, 56. [CrossRef] [PubMed]

75. Schäffer, A.A. Digenic inheritance in medical genetics. *J. Med. Genet.* **2013**, *50*, 641–652. [CrossRef] [PubMed]

76. Deltas, C. Digenic inheritance and genetic modifiers. *Clin. Genet.* **2018**, *93*, 429–438. [CrossRef]

77. Janecke, A.R.; Heinz-Erian, P.; Yin, J.; Petersen, B.S.; Franke, A.; Lechner, S.; Fuchs, I.; Melancon, S.; Uhlig, H.H.; Travis, S.; et al. Reduced sodium/proton exchanger NHE3 activity causes congenital sodium diarrhea. *Hum. Mol. Genet.* **2015**, *24*, 6614–6623. [CrossRef]

78. Lin, Z.; Jin, S.; Duan, X.; Wang, T.; Martini, S.; Hulamm, P.; Cha, B.; Hubbard, A.; Donowitz, M.; Guggino, S.E. Chloride channel (Clc)-5 is necessary for exocytic trafficking of Na+/H+ exchanger 3 (NHE3). *J. Biol. Chem.* **2011**, *286*, 22833–22845. [CrossRef]

79. Pan, W.; Borovac, J.; Spicer, Z.; Hoenderop, J.G.; Bindels, R.J.; Shull, G.E.; Doschak, M.R.; Cordat, E.; Alexander, R.T. The epithelial sodium/proton exchanger; NHE3; is necessary for renal and intestinal calcium (re)absorption. *Am. J. Physiol. Ren. Physiol.* **2012**, *302*, F943–F956. [CrossRef]

80. Katsanis, N. The continuum of causality in human genetic disorders. *Genome Biol.* **2016**, *17*, 233. [CrossRef]

81. Cooper, D.N.; Krawczak, M.; Polychronakos, C.; Tyler-Smith, C.; Kehrer-Sawatzki, H. Where genotype is not predictive of phenotype: Towards an understanding of the molecular basis of reduced penetrance in human inherited disease. *Hum. Genet.* **2013**, *132*, 1077–1130. [CrossRef] [PubMed]

82. Tosetto, E.; Ghiggeri, G.M.; Emma, F.; Barbano, G.; Carrea, A.; Vezzoli, G.; Torregrossa, R.; Cara, M.; Ripanti, G.; Ammenti, A.; et al. Phenotypic and genetic heterogeneity in Dent's disease: The results of an Italian collaborative study. *Nephrol. Dial. Transplant.* **2006** *21*, 2452–2463. [CrossRef] [PubMed]

83. Van Berkel, Y.; Ludwig, M.; van Wijk, J.A.E.; Bökenkamp, A. Proteinuria in Dent disease: A review of the literature. *Pediatr. Nephrol.* **2017**, *32*, 1851–1859. [CrossRef]

84. Schwarz, J.M.; Cooper, D.N.; Schuelke, M.; Seelow, D. MutationTaster2: Mutation prediction for the deep-sequencing age. *Nat. Methods* **2014**, *11*, 361–362. [CrossRef] [PubMed]

85. Bertoldi, L.; Forcato, C.; Vitulo, N.; Birolo, G.; De Pascale, F.; Feltrin, E.; Schiavon, R.; Anglani, F.; Negrisolo, S.; Zanetti, A.; et al. QueryOR: A comprehensive web platform for genetic variant analysis and prioritization. *BMC Bioinform.* **2017**, *18*, 225. [CrossRef] [PubMed]

86. Kumar, P.; Henikoff, S.; Ng, P.C. Predicting the effects of coding non-synonymous variants on protein function using the SIFT algorithm. *Nat. Protoc.* **2009**, *4*, 1073–1081. [CrossRef] [PubMed]

87. Adzhubei, I.; Jordan, D.M.; Sunyaev, S.R. Predicting functional effect of human missense mutations using PolyPhen-2. *Curr. Protoc. Hum. Genet.* **2013**, *7*, 7.20.1–7.20.41. [CrossRef]

88. Yongwook, C.; Agnes, P.C. PROVEAN web server: A tool to predict the functional effect of amino acid substitutions and indels. *Bioinformatics* **2015**, *31*, 2745–2747.

89. Kircher, M.; Witten, D.M.; Jain, P.; O'Roak, B.J.; Cooper, G.M.; Shendure, J. A general framework for estimating the relative pathogenicity of human genetic variants. *Nat. Genet.* **2014**, *46*, 310–315. [CrossRef]

90. Quang, D.; Chen, Y.; Xie, X. DANN: A deep learning approach for annotating the pathogenicity of genetic variants. *Bioinformatics* **2015**, *31*, 761–763. [CrossRef]

91. Ceol, M.; Tiralongo, E.; Baelde, H.J.; Vianello, D.; Betto, G.; Marangelli, A.; Bonfante, L.; Valente, M.; Della Barbera, M.; D'Angelo, A.; et al. Involvement of the tubular ClC-type exchanger ClC-5 in glomeruli of human proteinuric nephropathies. *PLoS ONE* **2012**, *7*, e45605. [CrossRef] [PubMed]

92. Gianesello, L.; Priante, G.; Ceol, M.; Radu, C.M.; Saleem, M.A.; Simioni, P.; Terrin, L.; Anglani, F.; Del Prete, D. Albumin uptake in human podocytes: A possible role for the cubilin-amnionless (CUBAM) complex. *Sci. Rep.* **2017**, *7*, 13705. [CrossRef] [PubMed]

93. R Development Core Team. *R: A Language and Environment for Statistical Computing*; R Foundation for Statistical Computing: Vienna, Austria, 2008; ISBN 3-900051-07-0.

4

Safety Lapses Prior to Initiation of Hemodialysis for Acute Kidney Injury in Hospitalized Patients: A Patient Safety Initiative

Adrianna Douvris [1], Khalid Zeid [1], Swapnil Hiremath [2], Pierre Antoine Brown [2], Manish M. Sood [2], Rima Abou Arkoub [1], Gurpreet Malhi [1] and Edward G. Clark [2,*]

[1] Department of Medicine, University of Ottawa, Ottawa, ON K1H 7W9, Canada; adouvris@toh.ca (A.D.); kzeid027@uottawa.ca (K.Z.); rima-n82@hotmail.com (R.A.A.); gmalh035@uottawa.ca (G.M.)

[2] Division of Nephrology, Department of Medicine and Kidney Research Centre, Ottawa Hospital Research Institute, University of Ottawa, Ottawa, ON K1H 7W9, Canada; shiremath@toh.ca (S.H.); pibrown@toh.ca (P.A.B.); msood@toh.ca (M.M.S.)

* Correspondence: edclark@toh.ca

Abstract: Background: Safety lapses in hospitalized patients with acute kidney injury (AKI) may lead to hemodialysis (HD) being required before renal recovery might have otherwise occurred. We sought to identify safety lapses that, if prevented, could reduce the need for unnecessary HD after AKI; **Methods:** We conducted a retrospective observational study that included consecutive patients treated with HD for AKI at a large, tertiary academic center between 1 September 2015 and 31 August 2016. Exposures of interest were pre-specified iatrogenic processes that could contribute to the need for HD after AKI, such as nephrotoxic medication or potassium supplement administration. Other outcomes included time from AKI diagnosis to initial management steps, including Nephrology referral; **Results:** After screening 344 charts, 80 patients were included for full chart review, and 264 were excluded because they required HD within 72 h of admission, were deemed to have progression to end-stage kidney disease (ESKD), or required other renal replacement therapy (RRT) modalities in critical care settings such as continuous renal replacement therapy (CRRT) or sustained low efficiency dialysis (SLED). Multiple safety lapses were identified. Sixteen patients (20%) received an angiotensin converting enzyme inhibitor or angiotensin receptor blocker after AKI onset. Of 35 patients with an eventual diagnosis of pre-renal AKI due to hypovolemia, only 29 (83%) received a fluid bolus within 24 h. For 28 patients with hyperkalemia as an indication for starting HD, six (21%) had received a medication associated with hyperkalemia and 13 (46%) did not have a low potassium diet ordered. Nephrology consultation occurred after a median (IQR) time after AKI onset of 3.0 (1.0–5.7) days; **Conclusions:** Although the majority of patients had multiple indications for the initiation of HD for AKI, we identified many safety lapses related to the diagnosis and management of patients with AKI. We cannot conclude that HD initiation was avoidable, but, improving safety lapses may delay the need for HD initiation, thereby allowing more time for renal recovery. Thus, development of automated processes not only to identify AKI at an early stage but also to guide appropriate AKI management may improve renal recovery rates.

Keywords: acute kidney injury; patient safety; hemodialysis

1. Introduction

Acute kidney injury (AKI) is a frequent and serious complication of hospitalization, affecting up to 20% of hospitalized patients, and conferring a four-fold increased risk of in-hospital mortality [1]. In-hospital mortality increases with increasing severity of AKI, with the highest mortality observed in patients that require renal replacement therapy (RRT) [2,3]. Systematic reviews have shown that AKI is associated with long term consequences including increased mortality, chronic kidney disease (CKD), and progression to end-stage kidney disease (ESKD) [4,5]. Although the use of RRT for AKI is life-sustaining when urgently indicated, it is costly [6,7] and may be harmful for renal recovery [8].

Currently, there are no effective pharmacological interventions for AKI, [9] and management is aimed at limiting further kidney injury and reducing the likelihood that acute indications for RRT will develop prior to renal recovery [8]. The progression of AKI may be limited by timely diagnostic workup if worsening renal injury (and the consequent need for RRT) is prevented by limiting the use of nephrotoxic medications [10], and iodinated contrast dye [11], although there is debate in the literature surrounding the association between intravenous iodinated contrast and AKI in hospitalized patients [12]. Limiting excess dietary or intravenous potassium may increase the likelihood of recovery prior to hyperkalemia becoming an indication for RRT, however there is a paucity of data in this area. Nonetheless, there is some evidence that safety lapses in the care of hospitalized patients with AKI are frequent [13].

Early identification of AKI in hospitalized patients using electronic alerts has the potential to reduce the likelihood of AKI progression and need for RRT [14–16], however, this has not been supported by the literature up to now. A large single-center randomized controlled trial assessing automated electronic clinician notifications did not reduce death or need for RRT [17]. In addition, a recent systematic review of six studies of electronic alerts for AKI found no improvement in survival or need for RRT, with variable impact on processes of care [18]. The lack of efficacy of these early alerts may relate to AKI being a syndrome of many causes that require different interventions. Another issue is that alerts may not trigger significant changes in care processes, such as medication review with cessation of nephrotoxic medications, or IV fluid administration [19]. Consequently, to improve outcomes and reduce the need for unnecessary RRT, it may be first necessary to identify the processes that are most likely to lead to iatrogenic harm.

As such, we undertook a study to characterize safety lapses that might have contributed to the need for potentially avoidable hemodialysis (HD) for AKI patients at our center. Given that patients who initiate forms of RRT for AKI other than HD (e.g., continuous renal replacement therapy (CRRT) or slow low-efficiency dialysis (SLED)/prolonged intermittent RRT (PIRRT)) typically do so in the intensive care unit (ICU) setting due to hemodynamic instability, we sought to focus on more stable patients initiating HD for AKI with respect to their preceding exposure to nephrotoxic oral medications and incorrect dietary orders (while still including patients if their HD for AKI was ultimately initiated in the ICU setting).

2. Experimental Section

2.1. Study Design and Setting

We conducted a retrospective chart review of patients who started treatment with HD for AKI while hospitalized at The Ottawa Hospital (TOH) between 1 September 2015 and 31 August 2016. TOH is a tertiary care academic medical center with 1061 inpatient beds that services a population of approximately 1.2 million people across Eastern Ontario, Canada [20]. TOH has over 50,000 patient admissions annually at three campuses (Ottawa General Hospital; Ottawa Civic Hospital and University of Ottawa Heart Institute) [20]. At the time of this study, TOH did not have computer physician order entry (CPOE) for medications or investigations other than imaging studies.

Prior to the start of the study, approval for waived patient consent was obtained from TOH research ethics board.

2.2. Patient Population, Inclusion and Exclusion Criteria

Patients were identified retrospectively for screening using consecutive nephrology billing codes that had been submitted for new, inpatient hemodialysis starts.

Inclusion criteria were: hospitalized patients; aged 18 years or older; with AKI (as defined below); who required initiation of RRT in the form of intermittent HD. We excluded patients who: required HD within 72 h of admission (as such cases were considered to be more likely reflective of severe AKI at the outset of hospitalization in which RRT was less likely to be avoidable); patients with ESKD; RRT started for a reason other than AKI (e.g., intoxication, hypothermia); or if RRT was started using a modality other than HD (i.e., CRRT or SLED). For patients re-admitted to hospital requiring HD on re-admission, we gathered data from both admissions to capture the initial AKI that did not resolve.

2.3. Data Sources and Data Collection

Data was collected through a retrospective chart review of electronic medical records. Electronic medical records included relevant investigations (labs and imaging), as well as consultation notes, scanned progress notes, physician orders and medication administration records.

Two investigators (AD, KZ) independently screened charts then reviewed the electronic charts of included patients and collected data on their baseline demographics, co-morbidities and iatrogenic processes. All charts were reviewed by both investigators and disagreements between the two primary chart reviewers on aspects of data collection were resolved by a third investigator (E.C.) for consistency of data collection.

Data was extracted from the inpatient chart, and recorded on data collection forms before being entered into an Excel database. The onset of AKI was determined as the first instance that patients fulfilled the serum creatinine (SCr)-based Kidney Disease Improving Global Outcomes (KDIGO) criteria for AKI, which corresponds to a rise in SCr of ≥1.5 times baseline over 7 days or an increase in SCr by at least 26.5 μmol/L [21] within 48 h. Baseline SCr was calculated using the lowest available outpatient SCr within 12 months [22]. When none was available, the first SCr following hospitalization was used [22].

2.4. Outcomes and Analysis

Our outcomes of interest were the frequency with which specific iatrogenic processes may have contributed to the need for RRT in our population (described below). Other outcomes included time from AKI diagnosis to initial management steps, including Nephrology referral (which occurred at some point for all included patients as it is a necessary pre-requisite to receiving HD at our institution).

To identify delays in AKI identification and initial management, the timing of Nephrology consultation and HD initiation relative to the onset of AKI was reported as the median number of days with interquartile ranges. The possible causes of AKI were determined from admission notes, Nephrology consultations, and progress notes. Renal investigations post-AKI, including urine studies and imaging, were recorded. IV fluid administration within 24 h of AKI onset when AKI was recorded to be 'pre-renal' from hypovolemia, was recorded. We did not differentiate between a bolus or infusion of IV crystalloid as ordering practices varied between prescribing physicians depending on clinical context. The number and type of iodinated contrast imaging studies after AKI were recorded. The indications for first HD were obtained from Nephrology consult and progress notes.

Iatrogenic events and processes relating to AKI and hyperkalemia were recorded. This included the administration of certain medications after the onset of AKI including non-steroidal anti-inflammatory drugs (NSAIDs), angiotensin converting enzyme inhibitors (ACEi), angiotensin receptor antagonists (ARBs) and potassium-sparing diuretics or aldosterone inhibitors. The administration of oral K^+ supplements, and IV solutions containing at least 10 mmol/L of potassium after the onset of AKI and when serum potassium was ≥5.0 mmol/L was also recorded. Ordered diets were recorded, including failure to order 'renal' or low potassium diet after onset of AKI who were ultimately dialyzed with hyperkalemia (defined as potassium ≥ 5.5 mmol/L). The frequency of iatrogenic events was calculated.

The collected data was also analyzed qualitatively and selected cases that were felt by the investigators to be representative of particular patient safety lapses in this population are reported in a narrative synthesis.

3. Results

3.1. Patient Demographics and AKI Information

We reviewed 344 charts and excluded 264 patients for a total of 80 consecutive patients, over a one-year period, treated with at least one HD session for AKI while hospitalized. The process is outlined in Figure 1.

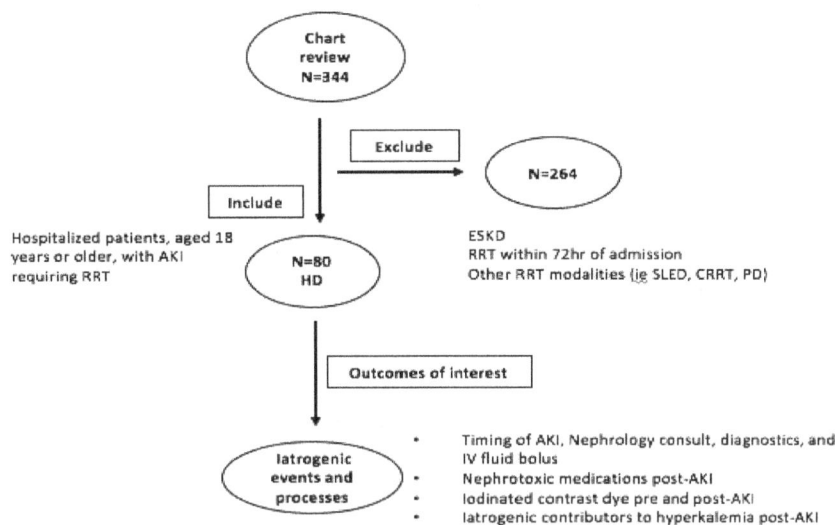

Figure 1. Summary of study design for this retrospective chart review. A total of 344 electronic inpatient records were reviewed, and 80 consecutive hospitalized patients meeting inclusion criteria were included. Data was collected for qualitative assessment of iatrogenic events and processes that may have contributed to the need for RRT (in the form of HD) for AKI. AKI, acute kidney injury; RRT, renal replacement therapy; HD, intermittent hemodialysis; ESKD, end-stage kidney disease; SLED, slow low efficiency dialysis; PD, peritoneal dialysis.

Table 1 summarizes baseline patient characteristics. The mean age of patients was 65 years old and over half were documented to have CKD. The average baseline serum creatinine (SCr) was 1.9 mg/dL (138 μmol/L). All patients were initiated on HD for AKI at the Ottawa Hospital (TOH), but 19 patients (23.7%) were initially admitted to other hospitals and transferred to TOH for specialty or intensive care. In-hospital mortality was 26% (21 patients) and the median length of stay in hospital was 28.0 days [IQR 16.3–53.5]. Overall, 64 patients (80%) were initially admitted to a medical service and 16 (20%) to a surgical service. Thirty patients (38%) required critical care (in an intensive care unit (ICU), cardiac care unit, or cardiac surgery ICU) by the time of HD initiation. The most common admission diagnosis was sepsis (in 25 patients (31%)) but cardiac causes were listed for 27 patients (34%) (classified as acute coronary syndrome in 13 patients (16%) and CHF in 14 patients (18%) overall).

Supplementary Figure S1 details the etiology of AKI for included patients, as determined by documentation in each patient's chart from admitting services and Nephrology consultants. More than one etiology was implicated in 51 patients (64%).

Timing of AKI recognition, work-up, and management is reported in Table 2. As summarized in Table 2, half of our patients met criteria for AKI at the time of admission. Of those who developed AKI in hospital, the median time to AKI was 4.5 days. The time from AKI to Nephrology consultation and HD initiation was 3 days and 6 days, respectively. With respect to diagnostic work up for AKI, urinalysis with microscopy and urine electrolytes were assessed for 61 patients (76%) and 45 patients (56%), respectively. The median time between AKI and obtaining urine electrolytes was 3 days. Fifty-three (66%) patients underwent renal ultrasonography or another form of abdominal imaging that could rule out hydronephrosis. Lastly, of the 35 patients with pre-renal AKI secondary to hypovolemia, 29 (83%) received an IV fluid administration of crystalloid or colloid within 24 h of AKI onset.

Table 1. Baseline patient characteristics (*n* = 80).

Mean age in years (SD)	65.5 (+/− 15.4)
Male sex, *n* (%)	50 (62)
Mean baseline serum creatinine in mg/dL (SD)	1.6 (+/− 0.9)
Co-morbidities, *n* (%)	
Hypertension	54 (68)
Diabetes mellitus	47 (59)
Chronic kidney disease	43 (54)
Congestive heart failure	33 (41)
Peripheral vascular disease	13 (16)
Home medications, *n* (%)	
Thiazide diuretic or furosemide	(54)
ACEi or ARB	(50)
Metformin	(23)
Spironolactone	(15)
Admission diagnoses *	
Sepsis	26 (33)
Congestive heart failure	17 (21)
Acute coronary syndrome	14 (18)
Acute kidney injury	15 (19)
Malignancy	8 (10)
Hospitalization and outcomes	
Admitted upon hospital transfer, *n* (%)	(23.7)
Median hospital length of stay, days (IQR)	28.0 (16.3–53.5)
In-hospital mortality, *n* (%)	(26.2)

* Patients could have more than one diagnosis recorded as the reason for admission. SD, standard deviation; IQR, interquartile range; ACEi, angiotensin converting enzyme inhibitor; ARB, angiotensin receptor blocker

Table 2. Diagnosis and management of Acute Kidney Injury, *n* = 80 *.

AKI present at admission, *n* (%)	40 (50.0)
Median time from admission to AKI, days (IQR)	4.5 (2.0–11.2)
Median time from AKI to Nephrology consult, days (IQR)	3.0 (1.0–5.7)
Median time from AKI to first hemodialysis, days (IQR)	6.0 (4.0–11.0)
Tests and initial management, *n* (%)	
IV fluid administration within 24 h for pre-renal AKI, *n* = 35	29 (83)
Urinalysis and routine microscopy	61 (76)
Renal ultrasound	53 (66)
Urine electrolytes	45 (56)

* Unless otherwise specified. AKI, acute kidney injury; IQR, interquartile range

3.2. Nephrotoxins, Medications, Hyperkalemia and Indications for Dialysis

Table 3 summarizes the frequency of selected medications and exposure to contrast dye after the onset of AKI and prior to HD. Either an ACEi or ARB was given post-AKI in 16 patients (20%) and 11 patients (14%) were given spironolactone. Three patients (4%) received both ACEi or ARB plus spironolactone after AKI. One patient (1%) received NSAIDs post-AKI. In the post-AKI period, 15 patients (19%) and 9 patients (11%) received either intravenous or intra-arterial contrast, respectively.

Figure 2 illustrates the frequency of the presence of indications for initiation of HD at the time it was started. Volume overload was the most common indication, present in 69 patients (86%). Uremia was cited as an indication in 40 patients (50%). Hyperkalemia (with a serum potassium $\geq$ 5.5 mmol/L in all such cases) was documented as an indication for HD in 28 patients (35%). Most patients had multiple indications for HD initiation, and hyperkalemia was only an isolated indication for 2 patients (3%). For the 28 patients dialyzed with hyperkalemia as an indication for initiation of HD, all had serum potassium $\geq$ 5.5 mmol/L and 6 (21%) had serum potassium $\geq$ 6.0 mmol/L at HD initiation.

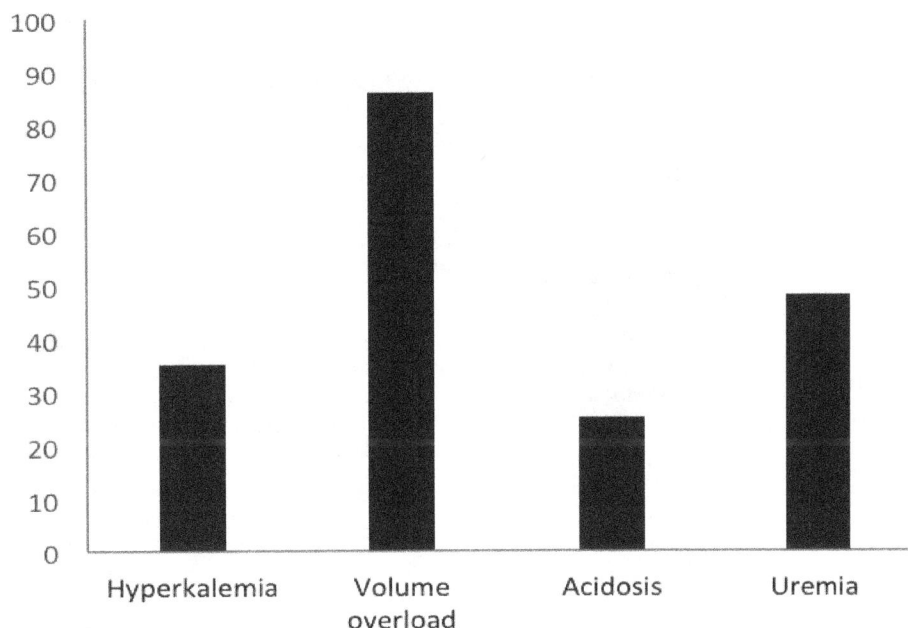

Figure 2. Indications for initiation of hemodialysis ($n = 80$). Legend: Percentage of patients with a particular indication for initiation of hemodialysis. Fifty-one patients (64%) had two or more indications present.

Table 3. Selected iatrogenic medications and contrast exposure after Acute Kidney Injury.

Medications, n (%)	
ACEi or ARB	16 (20)
Spironolactone	11 (14)
NSAIDs	1 (1)
Aminoglycoside antibiotic	1 (1)
Contrast exposure, n (%)	24 (30)
Intravenous	15 (19)
Intra-arterial	9 (11)

ACEi, angiotensin converting enzyme inhibitor; ARB, angiotensin receptor blocker; NSAIDs, nonsteroidal anti-inflammatory drug.

Table 4 highlights iatrogenic contributors to hyperkalemia. Of the 28 patients dialyzed with hyperkalemia, 13 (46%) were not given a low potassium diet and 3 (11%) were receiving either an ACEi, ARB or spironolactone; one (4%) received potassium supplements in addition to spironolactone. Further, of the 6 patients with serum potassium $\geq$ 6.0 mmol/L at HD initiation, 3 were not provided with low potassium diets, and 2 received potassium supplements or potassium sparing diuretics.

Table 4. Iatrogenic contributors to hyperkalemia after Acute Kidney Injury.

Occurrence of hyperkalemia ($n = 80$), n (%)	
During admission, after AKI	33 (41)
As an indication for dialysis	28 (35)
Safety lapses in patients with hyperkalemia as a subsequent indication for hemodialysis ($n = 28$), n (%)	
Low potassium diet not ordered	13 (46)
Oral potassium supplements given while serum potassium $\geq$ 5.0 mmol/L	2 (7)
ACEi, ARB and/or spironolactone given while serum potassium $\geq$ 5.0 mmol/L	6 (21)

AKI, acute kidney injury; ACEi, angiotensin converting enzyme inhibitor; ARB, angiotensin receptor blocker.

3.3. Summary of Representative Cases

Table 5 summarizes four cases that highlight safety lapses that may have contributed to the need to initiate HD after the onset of AKI.

Table 5. Selected cases that highlight safety lapses in patients requiring hemodialysis after Acute Kidney Injury.

Admission Diagnoses	Indication(s) for HD	Summary of Events after AKI and Prior to Initiation of HD
Lymphoma, AKI	Hyperkalemia, Volume overload	• Diuresis then IV contrast for CT scan; worsening AKI • Spironolactone and potassium supplements continued despite serum potassium 5.5 mmol/L.
Sepsis, NSTEMI and AKI	Volume overload	• Long-acting CCB, BB and nitropatch continued despite relative hypotension; CT with IV contrast • Given 9 L of IV crystalloid for refractory hypotension while oligoanuric with subsequent development of pulmonary edema.
NSTEMI, then AKI *	Volume overload Hyperkalemia	• CKD with baseline Cr 200 • Discharged 24 h after coronary angiogram with Cr 210, K 5.6. Was continued on ARB and started on NSAID at discharge. • Re-admitted 48 h later with oliguric AKI, serum potassium up to 6.3 mmol/L, volume overload.
Anemia, AKI	Respiratory failure	• Late Nephrology referral (9 days post-admission with AKI non-responsive to IV fluids • Urinalysis at admission showed microscopic hematuria, proteinuria with hypoalbuminemia. • GN work up initiated by Nephrology, including renal biopsy. • Transfer to ICU for respiratory failure; initiated HD, and started plasmapheresis, cyclophosphamide, steroids for microscopic polyangiitis.

AKI, acute kidney injury; CT, computed tomography; IV, intravenous; CCB, Calcium channel blocker; BB, beta-blocker; ARB, angiotensin receptor blocker; NSAID, non-steroidal anti-inflammatory drug; GN, glomerulonephritis; HD, intermittent hemodialysis. * This case was excluded from our study cohort because this patient was initiated on hemodialysis within 48 h of admission. It has been included in this table to highlight a patient safety issue around this patient's discharge post-angiogram that was still detected on chart review.

4. Discussion

Our study of 80 consecutive inpatients who required hemodialysis for AKI after at least 72 h of hospitalization revealed that safety lapses occur frequently and may have contributed to the need for initiation of HD in some instances. This is consistent with previous studies that have demonstrated safety lapses occur frequently in patients who die in hospital with a primary admission diagnosis of AKI [13] and in end-stage kidney disease patients admitted to surgical services [23].

Our results suggest deficiencies in diagnostic testing to determine the etiology of acute kidney injury. In particular, it was notable that only 61 patients (76%) had urinalysis testing after AKI while the KDIGO Clinical Practice Guidelines for AKI [21] suggest that urinalysis testing is necessary to ensure a complete diagnostic work-up for AKI. Another safety lapse we discovered was the frequent failure to order low potassium diets in patients with AKI who ultimately started dialysis with elevated serum potassium levels. Low potassium diets were ordered in less than half of such patients. Although there is no published data in the literature on low potassium diets and RRT initiation in patients with AKI, we feel this is a low risk intervention that has the potential to delay HD in the AKI population. As well, supplemental potassium or medications known to increase the serum potassium level were continued in many such patients. This suggests that our institution might improve care through an automated trigger to review these particular medications after the onset of AKI and/or elevated serum potassium. For potassium supplements, automatic substitution to a *prn* order restricted according to serum potassium values could also be useful.

Another issue that our study identified is that Nephrology consultation was often delayed, with a median time from AKI to consultation of three days. Studies of hospitalized patients with AKI, including a recent systematic review and meta-analysis [24], have shown that delayed Nephrology consultation for AKI is associated with increased in-hospital mortality in both non-critically ill [25] and critically ill patients [24,26,27], increased risk of requiring RRT [25], and increased dialysis dependence rates upon hospital discharge [26]. One particular study found that for hospital-acquired AKI (using the same KDIGO definition [21] as our study), nephrology assessment within 18 h was associated with significantly fewer patients progressing to a 2.5-fold increase in SCr level from admission [28]. We also found that, for patients who had urine electrolyte testing performed, it was done a median of three days after the AKI onset. Although the clinical utility of urine electrolyte testing for AKI is itself debatable, it does suggest a substantial time lapse between the onset of AKI and investigations related to AKI and that AKI may be under-recognized. Further evidence that AKI is under-recognized is that only 29 of the 35 patients (83%) with a pre-renal element to their AKI received IV fluids as a bolus or infusion within 24 h of AKI. Overall, our findings suggest that an automated trigger for nephrology assessment (and initial diagnostic testing, including serial SCr measurements, urinalysis, microscopy, ultrasound, and initial management strategies including medication review and volume status) might be one avenue to reducing the likelihood of AKI patients progressing to require RRT initiation at our institution. We recognize that this could add substantial burden to the existing inpatient Nephrology service and may require a dedicated team to address assessments.

The main strength of our study is that it involved a comprehensive case-by-case review to capture clearly defined, pre-specified, safety lapses. However, there are many important limitations. The study was not comprehensive and did not evaluate a myriad of other possible medication or treatment-related safety lapses that could have a bearing on AKI progression to HD initiation. As well, our study was not able to determine the clinical significance of any safety lapses with respect to whether they impacted the subsequent requirement for HD as we did not assess a comparator group of AKI patients who did not progress to require HD. Furthermore, many 'iatrogenic' processes are likely unavoidable. For example, although it was not possible to quantify, on the basis of our case-by-case analysis, the vast majority of contrast imaging was clearly indicated in the overall context of patients' clinical management despite its potential nephrotoxicity. As briefly discussed earlier, there is also controversy in the literature regarding the association between IV iodinated contrast dye and AKI [12]. A final limitation relates to generalizability: some of the lapses in safety might be less likely to occur in institutions utilizing CPOE. Furthermore, our experience might not be generalizable to the community hospital setting where specialist consultations or subspecialty admitting services are less likely to be available.

Despite its limitations, this study clearly highlights several care processes to target for improvement. The development of an automated trigger to ensure discontinuation of medications that are either nephrotoxic and/or promote hyperkalemia could be beneficial. As well, an automated review of diet orders (to ensure a low potassium diet, when indicated) and automated triggers for nephrology referral soon after AKI onset could increase the frequency with which renal recovery occurs prior to hemodialysis being required.

Author Contributions: A.D. and K.Z. performed data acquisition. E.G.C. and A.D. undertook statistical analysis and manuscript creation. All authors revised the manuscript. E.G.C. conceived and supervised the project. S.H., P.A.B., M.M.S. and G.M. provided critical intellectual input. All authors have read and approved the manuscript.

References

1.   Wang, H.E.; Muntner, P.; Chertow, G.M.; Warnock, D.G. Acute Kidney Injury and Mortality in Hospitalized Patients. *Am. J. Nephrol.* **2012**, *35*, 349–355. [CrossRef] [PubMed]

2.   Uchino, S.; Bellomo, R.; Goldsmith, D.; Bates, S.; Ronco, C. An assessment of the RIFLE criteria for acute renal failure in hospitalized patients. *Crit. Care Med.* **2006**, *34*, 1913–1917. [CrossRef] [PubMed]

3.   Metnitz, P.G.H.; Krenn, C.G.; Steltzer, H.; Lang, T.; Ploder, J.; Lenz, K.; Gall, J.-R.L.; Druml, W. Effect of acute renal failure requiring renal replacement therapy on outcome in critically ill patients. *Crit. Care Med.* **2002**, *30*, 2051–2058. [CrossRef] [PubMed]

4.   Coca, S.G.; Yusuf, B.; Shlipak, M.G.; Garg, A.X.; Parikh, C.R. Long-Term Risk of Mortality and Other Adverse Outcomes After Acute Kidney Injury: A Systematic Review and Meta-analysis. *Am. J. Kidney Dis.* **2009**, *53*, 961–973. [CrossRef] [PubMed]

5.   Coca, S.G.; Singanamala, S.; Parikh, C.R. Chronic kidney disease after acute kidney injury: A systematic review and meta-analysis. *Kidney Int.* **2012**, *81*, 442–448. [CrossRef] [PubMed]

6.   Chertow, G.M.; Burdick, E.; Honour, M.; Bonventre, J.V.; Bates, D.W. Acute kidney injury, mortality, length of stay, and costs in hospitalized patients. *J. Am. Soc. Nephrol.* **2005**, *16*, 3365–3370. [CrossRef] [PubMed]

7.   Kerr, M.; Bedford, M.; Matthews, B.; O'Donoghue, D. The economic impact of acute kidney injury in England. *Nephrol. Dial. Transplant.* **2014**, *29*, 1362–1368. [CrossRef] [PubMed]

8.   Clark, E.G.; Bagshaw, S.M. Unnecessary Renal Replacement Therapy for Acute Kidney Injury is Harmful for Renal Recovery. *Semin. Dial.* **2015**, *28*, 6–11. [CrossRef] [PubMed]

9.   Jo, S.K.; Rosner, M.H.; Okusa, M.D. Pharmacologic Treatment of Acute Kidney Injury: Why Drugs Haven't Worked and What Is on the Horizon. *Clin. J. Am. Soc. Nephrol.* **2007**, *2*, 356–365. [CrossRef] [PubMed]

10. Perazella, M.A. Renal vulnerability to drug toxicity. *Clin. J. Am. Soc. Nephrol.* **2009**, *4*, 1275–1283. [CrossRef] [PubMed]

11. Ozkok, S.; Ozkok, A. Contrast-induced acute kidney injury: A review of practical points. *World J. Nephrol.* **2017**, *6*, 86–99. [CrossRef] [PubMed]

12. Aycock, R.D.; Westafer, L.M.; Boxen, J.L.; Majlesi, N.; Schoenfeld, E.M.; Bannuru, R.R. Acute kidney injury after computed tomography: A meta-analysis. *Ann. Emerg. Med.* **2018**, *71*, 44–53. [CrossRef] [PubMed]

13. Stewart, J.; Findlay, G.; Smith, N.; Kelly, K.; Mason, M. *Adding Insult to Injury: A Review of the Care of Patients Who Died in Hospital with a Primary Diagnosis of Acute Kidney Injury (Acute Renal Failure)*; National Confidential Enquiry into Patient Outcome and Death: London, UK, 2009.

14. Handler, S.M.; Kane-Gill, S.L.; Kellum, J.A. Optimal and early detection of acute kidney injury requires effective clinical decision support systems. *Nephrol. Dial. Transplant.* **2014**, *29*, 1802–1803. [CrossRef] [PubMed]

15. Kirkendall, E.S.; Spires, W.L.; Mottes, T.A.; Schaffzin, J.K.; Barclay, C.; Goldstein, S.L. Development and perfmance of acute kidney injury triggers to identuify pediatric patients at risk for nephrotoxic medication-associated harm. *Appl. Clin. Inform.* **2014**, *5*, 313–333. [PubMed]

16. Porter, C.J.; Jurrlink, I.; Bisset, L.H.; Bavakunji, R.; Mehta, R.L.; Devonald, M.A. A real-time electronic alert to improve detection of acute kidney injury in a large teaching hospital. *Nephrol. Dial. Transplant.* **2014**, *29*, 1888–1893. [CrossRef] [PubMed]

17. Wilson, F.P.; Shashaty, M.; Testani, J. Automated, electronic alerts for acute kidney injury: A single-blind, parallel-group, randomised controlled trial. *Lancet* **2015**, *385*, 1966–1974. [CrossRef]

18. Lachance, P.; Villeneuve, P.-M.; Rewa, O.G.; Wilson, F.P.; Selby, N.M.; Featherstone, R.M.; Bagshaw, S.M. Association between e-alert implementation for detection of acute kidney injury and outcomes: A systematic review. *Nephrol. Dial. Transplant.* **2017**, *32*, 265–272. [CrossRef] [PubMed]

19. Laing, C. On the alert for outcome improvement in acute kidney injury. *Lancet* **2015**, *385*, 1924–1926. [CrossRef]

20. About Our Hospital. Available online: http://www.ottawahospital.on.ca/en/about-us (accessed on 20 November 2017).

21. Kidney Disease Improving Global Outcomes (KDIGO); Acute Kidney Injury Work Group. KDIGO Clinical Practice Guidelines for Acute Kidney Injury. *Nephron Clin. Pract.* **2012**, *120*, c179–c184.

22. Ricci, Z.; Cruz, D.N.; Ronco, C. Classification and staging of acute kidney injury: Beyond the RIFLE and AKIN criteria. *Nat. Rev. Nephrol.* **2011**, *7*, 201–208. [CrossRef] [PubMed]

23. Harel, Z.; Wald, R.; Liu, J.J.; Bell, C.M. Lapses in safety in end-stage renal disease patients admitted to surgical services. *Hemodial. Int.* **2012**, *16*, 286–293. [CrossRef] [PubMed]

24. Soares, D.M.; Pessanha, J.F.; Sharma, A.; Brocca, A.; Ronco, C. Delayed Nephrology Consultation and High Mortality on Acute Kidney Injury: A. Meta-Analysis. *Blood Purif.* **2017**, *43*, 57–67. [CrossRef] [PubMed]

25. Meier, P.; Bonfils, R.M.; Vogt, B.; Burnand, B.; Burnier, M. Referral Patterns and Outcomes in Noncritically Ill Patients with Hospital-Acquired Acute Kidney Injury. *Clin. J. Am. Soc. Nephrol.* **2011**, *6*, 2215–2225. [CrossRef] [PubMed]

26. E Silva, V.T.C.; Liaño, F.; Muriel, A.; Díez, R.; de Castro, I.; Yu, L. Nephrology Referral and Outcomes in Critically Ill Acute KIdney Injury Patients. *PLoS ONE* **2013**, *8*, e70482.

27. Ponce, D.; Zorzenon, C.D.P.F.; Santos, N.Y.D.; Balbi, A.L. Early nephrology consultation can have an impact on outcome of acute kidney injury patients. *Nephrol. Dial. Transplant.* **2011**, *26*, 3202–3206. [CrossRef] [PubMed]

28. Balasubramanian, G.; Al-Aly, Z.; Moiz, A.; Rauchman, M.; Zhang, Z.; Gopalakrishnan, R.; Balasubramanian, S.; El-Achkar, T.M. Early nephrologist involvement in hospital-acquired acute kidney injury: A pilot study. *Am. J. Kidney Dis.* **2011**, *57*, 228–234. [CrossRef] [PubMed]

5

Acute Kidney Injury Definition and Diagnosis

Joana Gameiro *, Jose Agapito Fonseca, Sofia Jorge and Jose Antonio Lopes

Division of Nephrology and Renal Transplantation, Department of Medicine Centro Hospitalar Lisboa Norte, EPE, Av. Prof. Egas Moniz, 1649-035 Lisboa, Portugal; jose.nuno.agapito@gmail.com (J.A.F.); sofiacjorge@sapo.pt (S.J.); jalopes93@hotmail.com (J.A.L.)

* Correspondence: joana.estrelagameiro@gmail.com

Abstract: Acute kidney injury (AKI) is a complex syndrome characterized by a decrease in renal function and associated with numerous etiologies and pathophysiological mechanisms. It is a common diagnosis in hospitalized patients, with increasing incidence in recent decades, and associated with poorer short- and long-term outcomes and increased health care costs. Considering its impact on patient prognosis, research has focused on methods to assess patients at risk of developing AKI and diagnose subclinical AKI, as well as prevention and treatment strategies, for which an understanding of the epidemiology of AKI is crucial. In this review, we discuss the evolving definition and classification of AKI, and novel diagnostic methods.

Keywords: acute kidney injury; definition; incidence; classification

1. Introduction

Acute kidney injury (AKI) is a complex syndrome characterized by a decrease in renal function, associated with numerous etiologies and pathophysiological mechanisms [1,2]. It is a common diagnosis in hospitalized patients, associated with poorer short- and long-term outcomes and increased health care costs [3].

The incidence of AKI has increased in recent years [2,3]. However, there is significant variability in the reported incidence of AKI, which is associated with the different characteristics of the populations studied, cause of AKI, and diagnostic criteria used [1–4]. Additionally, the lack of studies assessing AKI in community settings and comparing critically ill and non-critical patients hampers the characterization of the epidemiology of AKI [2–4].

The importance of recognizing AKI applies to pediatric and adult patients, as well as ambulatory, hospitalized, and critically ill patients in multiple clinical settings, due to its prognostic impact [4–6]. The incidence of AKI is lowest in ambulatory patients and higher in critically ill and patients which need dialysis [4–8]. In literature reviews, AKI is most commonly reported in surgical and critical settings, where patients are systematically monitored by assessing hourly urinary output and daily creatinine. Despite the lack of extensive data, this syndrome has undeniable importance also in internal medicine wards, where cardiorenal syndrome plays a substantial role [1–3,9]. Indeed, AKI occurs in up to 40% of acute decompensated heart failure hospitalizations, which differs according to the criteria used to define AKI [10]. This is known as cardiorenal syndrome type 1 and is an important prognostic factor [10]. Importantly, with the increase in patients with heart failure, the prevalence of this syndrome is also estimated to rise in the near future [9,10]. Mortality rates have declined in critically ill patients, although an increase has been reported in patients with dialysis-requiring AKI [5–11].

AKI is more common in older patients and those with predisposing factors, who present with a higher rate of comorbidities and higher probability of developing severe disease [12]. Sepsis is the leading cause of AKI in critically ill patients, accounting for 50% of cases [13,14]. Furthermore, the differences in patient characteristics, setting, pathophysiology, and outcomes distinguish septic AKI as a separate clinical entity from non-septic AKI [14]. Indeed, septic AKI patients are more likely to require mechanically assisted ventilation and vasoactive drugs, and have longer hospital stays, a higher likelihood of dialysis-requiring AKI, and higher in-hospital mortality rates. Moreover, they have an increased probability of renal function recovery [15,16].

Surgery is another important cause of AKI that accounts for up to 40% of in-hospital AKI cases [17,18]. The highest rates of AKI are found after cardiac (18.7%), general (13.2%), and thoracic (12.0%) surgeries, representing the impact of surgical settings on the incidence variability [19,20].

Recently, the Acute Disease Quality Initiative Workgroup proposed the term acute kidney disease (AKD) to reflect the continuing pathological processes and adverse events developing after AKI [20]. AKD is defined by presenting Kidney Disease Improving Global Outcomes (KDIGO) stage 1 criteria for longer than 7 days after an AKI initiating event [20]. This definition includes the post-AKI period in which critical interventions potentially alter the progression of kidney disease, therefore recognizing a population at risk of chronic kidney disease (CKD) development, cardiovascular events, and mortality [20].

Considering the impact of AKI on patient prognosis, research has focused on methods to assess patients at risk for developing AKI and diagnose subclinical AKI, as well as prevention and treatment strategies, for which it is crucial to have an understanding of the epidemiology of AKI. In this review, we discuss the evolving definition and classification of AKI, and its novel diagnostic methods.

2. Definitions and Classification

Over the last century, the definition of AKI has evolved significantly [21]. In fact, the diagnosis of AKI has changed from a clinical and biochemical level to a molecular level, with the most recent advances in tubular damage biomarkers increasing the accuracy of the diagnosis [21]. The use of standard classifications to define and stratify AKI has helped to increase the recognition of this disease in clinical practice and epidemiological research, which has led to defining the incidence of AKI in different settings and assessing its association with adverse outcomes [20,21]. This highlighted the importance of prevention, early diagnosis, and prompt treatment of AKI.

2.1. Risk, Injury, Failure, Loss of Kidney Function, End-Stage Kidney Disease (RIFLE) Classification

The RIFLE classification was first published in 2004, resulting from the Acute Dialysis Quality Initiative (ADQI) group conference, which aimed to determine a consensual AKI definition [22]. This classification defines AKI based on variations in serum creatinine (SCr) or estimated glomerular filtration rate (eGFR) and/or urine output (UO), and contemplates three severity levels (risk, injury, and failure) and two outcomes (loss of kidney function and end-stage kidney disease) in AKI [22]. The criteria to use are those that lead to the most negative classification, meaning the maximum RIFLE. The deterioration of renal function from baseline must occur within 7 days and persist for more than 24 h. When baseline SCr is unknown and there is no history of chronic kidney disease, the Modification of Diet in Renal Disease (MDRD) equation should be used to calculate the baseline SCr [23].

The RIFLE classification has been used for determining the incidence of AKI, stratifying AKI severity in multiple settings, and establishing the association between AKI severity and mortality [3,8,24,25]. Despite some limitations, this classification was vital in standardizing the criteria of AKI and confirming AKI severity as an outcome predictor [26].

2.2. Acute Kidney Injury Network (AKIN) Classification

In 2007, the AKIN classification was proposed and published by the AKIN working group [27]. There was cumulative evidence demonstrating that small increases in SCr were associated with poor outcomes and that there was variation between hospitals regarding the start of renal replacement therapy, leading to the importance of revising the RIFLE classification [28–30].

The AKIN classification depends only on SCr and not on eGFR changes, and does not require baseline SCr, but needs at least two values of SCr obtained within a period of 48 h, thus defining AKI as an increase in SCr of at least 0.3 mg/dL or a percentage increase in SCr equal to or higher than 50%, or by a decrease in UO lower than 0.5 mL/kg/h for more than 6 h. The diagnosis of AKI is only to be considered after achieving an adequate hydration status and excluding urinary obstruction. This classification also excluded the two outcome classes [27].

Both the AKIN and RIFLE classifications led to the identification and stratification of AKI in hospitalized patients, which was independently associated with outcome [31–34]. The AKIN classification, despite improving diagnostic sensitivity and specificity, shows no evidence of better prognostic acuity [34–39].

2.3. Kidney Disease Improving Global Outcomes (KDIGO) Classification

Recently, the KDIGO work group has developed a classification by merging the RIFLE and AKIN classifications to provide simplified and integrated criteria that could be applied in clinical practice and research (Table 1) [40].

Table 1. Risk, Injury, Failure, Loss of kidney function, End-stage kidney disease (RIFLE) [22], Acute Kidney Injury Network (AKIN) [27], and Kidney Disease Improving Global Outcomes (KDIGO) [40] classifications.

Class/Stage	SCr/GFR			UO		
	RIFLE	AKIN	KDIGO	RIFLE	AKIN	KDIGO
Risk/1 *	↑ SCr X 1.5 or ↓ GFR > 25%	↑ SCr ≥ 26.5 µmol/L (≥0.3 mg/dL) or ↑ SCr ≥ 150 to 200% (1.5 to 2X)	↑ SCr ≥ 26.5 µmol/L (≥0.3 mg/dL) or ↑ SCr ≥ 150 to 200% (1.5 to 2X)	<0.5 mL/kg/h (>6 h)	<0.5 mL/kg/h (>6 h)	<0.5 mL/kg/h (>6 h)
Injury/2 *	↑ SCr X 2 or ↓ GFR > 50%	↑ SCr > 200 to 300% (>2 to 3X)	↑ SCr > 200 to 300% (>2 to 3X)	<0.5 mL/kg/h (>12 h)	<0.5 mL/kg/h (>12 h)	<0.5 mL/kg/h (>12 h)
Failure/3*	↑ SCr X 3 or ↓ GFR >75% or if baseline SCr ≥ 353.6 µmol/L (≥4 mg/dL) ↑ SCr > 44.2 µmol/L (>0.5 mg/dL)	↑ SCr >300% (>3X) or if baseline SCr ≥ 353.6 µmol/L (≥4 mg/dL) ↑ SCr ≥ 44.2 µmol/L (≥0.5 mg/dL) or initiation of renal replacement therapy	↑ SCr > 300% (>3X) or ↑ SCr to ≥353.6 µmol/L (≥4 mg/dL) or initiation of renal replacement therapy	<0.3 mL/kg/h (>24 h) or anuria (>12 h)	<0.3 mL /kg/h (24 h) or anuria (12 h)	<0.3 mL/kg/h (24 h) or anuria (12 h) or GFR < 35 mL/min/1.73 m² in patients younger than 18 years

SCr: serum creatinine; GFR: glomerular filtration rate; UO: urine output; RIFLE: Risk, Injury, Failure, Loss of kidney function (dialysis dependence for at least 4 weeks), End-stage kidney disease (dialysis dependence for at least 3 months); AKIN: Acute Kidney Injury Network; KDIGO: Kidney Disease Improving Global Outcomes. * Risk class (RIFLE) corresponds to stage 1 (AKIN and KDIGO), Injury class (RIFLE) corresponds to stage 2 (AKIN and KDIGO), and Failure class (RIFLE) corresponds to stage 3 (AKIN and KDIGO), ↑ increase, ↓ decrease.

Accordingly, AKI is defined as an increase in SCr of at least 0.3 mg/dL within 48 h, or an increase in SCr to more than 1.5 times of baseline level, which is known or presumed to have occurred within the prior 7 days, or a UO decrease to less than 0.5 mL/kg/h for 6 h. AKI stratification according to KDIGO follows the stages of the AKIN criteria, except for a simplification of stage 3 [40].

2.4. RIFLE vs. AKIN vs. KDIGO

The KDIGO classification, theoretically, offers superior diagnostic and prognostic accuracy than the former classifications. Recent studies have conducted evaluations of these classifications to assess differences, advantages, and limitations in their incidence determination and prognostic ability in different settings (Table 2).

Table 2. Incidence of AKI and patient outcomes according to AKI definitions.

Study	Design	Setting	Criteria	AKI Definition	N	AKI Incidence	Mortality
Nisula et al. (2013) [41]	Prospective, multi-centre	ICU	SCr, UO	AKIN, KDIGO	2901	AKIN 39.3%, KDIGO 39.3%	AKIN 26%, KDIGO 26%
Roy et al. (2013) [42]	Prospective	Hospitalized, HF	SCr	RIFLE, AKIN, KDIGO	637	RIFLE 25.6%, AKIN 27.9%, KDIGO 36.7%	RIFLE AUROC 0.76, AKIN AUROC 0.72, KDIGO AUROC 0.74, $p = 0.02$
Bastin et al. (2013) [43]	Retrospective	Cardiac surgery	SCr	RIFLE, AKIN, KDIGO	1881	RIFLE 24.9%, AKIN 25.9%, KDIGO 25.9%	RIFLE AUROC 0.78, AKIN AUROC 0.86, $p < 0.001$
Zeng et al. (2014) [44]	Retrospective	Hospitalized	SCr	RIFLE, AKIN, KDIGO	31,970	RIFLE 16.1%, AKIN 16.6%, KDIGO 18.3%	RIFLE OR 2.9, AKIN OR 2.6, KDIGO OR 2.8
Levi et al. (2013) [45]	Prospective	ICU	SCr, UO	RIFLE, AKIN, KDIGO	190	RIFLE 62.6%, AKIN 63.2%, KDIGO 63.2%	RIFLE OR 0.56, AKIN OR 0.58, KDIGO OR 0.58
Rodrigues et al. (2013) [46]	Prospective	AMI	SCr	RIFLE, KDIGO	1050	RIFLE 14.8%, KDIGO 36.6%	RIFLE HR 3.51 (early) 1.84 (late), KDIGO HR 3.99 (early) 2.43 (late)
Luo et al. (2014) [47]	Prospective	ICU	SCr, UO	RIFLE, AKIN, KDIGO	3107	RIFLE 46.9%, AKIN 38.4%, KDIGO 51%, $p = 0.001$	RIFLE AUROC 0.738, AKIN AUROC 0.746, KDIGO AUROC 0.757, KDIGO vs. RIFLE $p = 0.12$, KDIGO vs. AKIN $p < 0.001$
Fuji et al. (2014) [48]	Retrospective	Hospitalized	SCr	RIFLE, AKIN, KDIGO	49,518	RIFLE 11.0%, AKIN 4.8%, KDIGO 11.8%	RIFLE AUROC 0.77, AKIN AUROC 0.69, KDIGO AUROC 0.78, $p = 0.02$
Neves et al. (2014) [49]	Prospective	Hospitalized	SCr, UO	RIFLE, AKIN, KDIGO	1045	RIFLE 6.2%, AKIN 5.5%, KDIGO 5.5%	N/A
Li et al. (2014) [50]	Retrospective	Hospitalized	SCr	RIFLE, AKIN, KDIGO	1005	RIFLE 32.1%, AKIN 34.7%, KDIGO 38.9%	RIFLE OR 2.56, AKIN OR 2.68, KDIGO OR 4.00, $p < 0.05$
Pereira et al. (2017) [51]	Retrospective	ICU, Sepsis	SCr, UO	RIFLE, AKIN, KDIGO	457	RIFLE 84.2%, AKIN 72.8%, KDIGO 87.5%	RIFLE AUROC 0.652, AKIN AUROC 0.686, KDIGO AUROC 0.658, $p < 0.001$

Table 2. *Cont.*

Study	Design	Setting	Criteria	AKI Definition	N	AKI Incidence	Mortality
Koeze et al. (2017) [52]	Retrospective	ICU	SCr, UO	RIFLE, AKIN, KDIGO	1376	RIFLE 28% (SCr) 35% (SCr + UO) AKIN 12% (SCr) 38% (SCr + UO) KDIGO 11% (SCr) 38% (SCr + UO)	RIFLE 84.2%, AKIN 72.8%, KDIGO 87.5%
Tsai et al. (2017) [53]	Retrospective	ECMO	SCr, UO	RIFLE, AKIN, KDIGO	167	RIFLE 75.4%, AKIN 84.4%, KDIGO 85%	RIFLE AUROC 0.826 AKIN AUROC 0.774 KDIGO AUROC 0.840 $p < 0.001$
Wu et al. (2016) [54]	Retrospective	ICU, Surgical	SCr, UO	AKIN, KDIGO	826	AKIN 31% KDIGO 30%	AKIN 21.8% (1), 20.2% (2), 27.8% (3) KDIGO 16.9% (1), 17.5% (2), 34.1% (3)
Zhou et al. (2016) [55]	Retrospective	ICU	SCr, UO, Cys-C	RIFLE, AKIN, KDIGO	1036	RIFLE 26.4%, AKIN 34.1%, KDIGO 37.8%, Cys-C 36.1%	RIFLE 57.9%, AKIN 54.4%, KDIGO 51.8%, Cys-C 52.1%
Pan et al. (2016) [56]	Retrospective	ICU, Cirrhosis	SCr, UO	RIFLE, AKIN, KDIGO	242	RIFLE, AKIN, KDIGO	RIFLE AUROC 0.774 AKIN AUROC 0.741 KDIGO AUROC 0.781 $p < 0.001$

ICU: Intensive care unit, SCr: Serum creatinine, UO: Urinary output, HF: Heart failure, AMI: acute myocardial infarction, Cys-C: Cystatin C, N/A not applicable, AUROC: area under the receiving operating characteristic curve, HR: hazard ratio, OR: odds ratio.

The Finnaki study demonstrated similar incidence in AKI defined by AKIN and KDIGO in a cohort of 2901 critically patients [41]. Roy et al. also found that the incidence of AKI was similar using the RIFLE, AKIN, and KDIGO criteria in a prospective study of 637 hospitalized patients with acute heart failure, although there were discrete differences in the predictive ability of the 30-day outcomes between RIFLE and KDIGO (area under the receiving operating characteristic curve (AUROC) of 0.76 and 0.74, respectively) [42]. In a retrospective study of 1881 cardiac surgery patients, the RIFLE, AKIN, and KDIGO criteria reported a similar incidence of AKI, although AKIN performed significantly better than RIFLE (AUROC = 0.86 versus 0.78, $p < 0.001$) [43]. Another retrospective cohort study of 31970 hospitalizations reported similar AKI incidence and prognosis using RIFLE, AKIN, and KDIGO [44]. Levi et al. compared the classifications in a study of 190 critical care patients and reported similar incidences [45]. In a prospective study of 1045 hospitalized patients on internal medicine wards conducted by Neves et al., the incidence of AKI was also similar using AKIN and KDIGO criteria, but higher with the RIFLE classification due to the incidence of pre-renal AKI [46].

The KDIGO classification was superior to RIFLE in diagnosing AKI (36.6% versus 14.8%) and predicting early and late mortality (adjusted hazard ratio (HR) for 30-day death of 3.51 by RIFLE and 3.99 by KDIGO; adjusted hazard ratio for 1-year mortality of 1.84 by RIFLE and 2.43 by KDIGO) in a cohort of 1050 patients with acute myocardial infarction [47].

The KDIGO criteria demonstrated a higher incidence of AKI than both RIFLE (51% versus 46.9%, $p = 0.001$) and AKIN (51% versus 38.4%, $p < 0.001$) criteria in a prospective cohort of 3107 critically ill patients [47]. Furthermore, evaluating in-hospital mortality, KDIGO was more predictive than RIFLE ($p < 0.001$), but not AKIN ($p = 0.12$) [48].

AKI was identified in more patients using the RIFLE and KDIGO criteria than AKIN (11% versus 4.8%) in a retrospective analysis of 49518 hospitalizations [49]. In this study, the KDIGO criteria had superior prognostic ability (AUROC: KDIGO 0.78, RIFLE 0.77, AKIN 0.69) [49]. Li et al. also demonstrated the superior performance of KDIGO in diagnosis and outcome prediction compared to RIFLE and AKIN in a retrospective study of 1005 patients with type 1 cardiorenal syndrome (AUROC: KDIGO 4.00, AKIN 2.68, RIFLE 2.56) [50].

We performed a single-center study of 457 critically ill septic patients and demonstrated that RIFLE and KDIGO criteria identified more AKI cases than did AKIN criteria (RIFLE 84.2% vs. KDIGO 87.5% vs. AKIN 72.8%, $p < 0.001$), although there were no differences in AKI incidence comparing RIFLE and KDIGO classifications, and the prediction of in-hospital mortality was similar between the three classifications [51]. Additionally, in this cohort of septic patients, AKI defined only by UO criteria was a better predictor of in-hospital mortality than was AKI defined either by SCr itself or by both SCr and UO (adjusted odds ratio (OR) = 2.7 (95% CI 1.7–4.5), $p < 0.001$), demonstrating the diagnostic and prognostic importance of UO in patients with septic AKI [51].

In a cohort of 1376 critically ill patients by Koeze et al., the AKIN (15%) and KDIGO (14%) criteria identified more AKI patients than the RIFLE criteria (10%). Moreover, by adding UO criteria, patients were detected earlier than when using only SCr criteria (median time of detection using UO 13 h and SCr 24 h) [52].

The KDIGO classification was also superior to AKIN and RIFLE in predicting in-hospital mortality (AUROC: KDIGO 0.840, AKIN 0.836, RIFLE 0.826, $p < 0.001$) in a study of 167 patients on extracorporeal membrane oxygenation (ECMO) support [53].

Wu et al. performed a retrospective analysis of 826 critically ill surgical patients and demonstrated that KDIGO was a better predictor of in-hospital mortality after surgery than AKIN (AUROC: KDIGO 0.678, AKIN 0.670, $p < 0.001$) [54].

In a retrospective multi-center cohort of 1036 critically ill patients, the KDIGO criteria identified more AKI patients than RIFLE and AKIN (37.8%, 26.4%, and 34.1%, respectively) [55]. The KDIGO criteria was also a better predictor of mortality (AUROC: KDIGO 0.7013, AKIN 0.6934, RIFLE 0.7016, $p < 0.001$) [55]. Additionally, this study incorporated the Cystatin-C (Cys-C) criteria, which demonstrated good concordance with the RIFLE, AKIN, and KDIGO criteria, and had better predictive ability of mortality than the three definitions (AUROC 0.7023), validating Cys-C as an important biomarker of AKI [55,56].

In a prospective study of 242 critically ill cirrhotic patients, the incidence of AKI was higher with the KDIGO criteria (67%) than with AKIN (65%) or RIFLE (63%), and KDIGO was a better predictor of in-hospital mortality (AUROC: KDIGO 0.781, AKIN 0.741, RIFLE 0.744, $p < 0.001$) [57].

The KDIGO classification appears to perform better in diagnosis and prognosis determination than AKIN and RIFLE. Nonetheless, future prospective studies with larger populations are still required to better assess the sensitivity and prognostic performance of these definitions.

2.5. Limitations

Despite the importance of these classifications in defining the epidemiology of AKI, it is increasingly recognized that novel biomarkers have to be researched to improve the definition of AKI and its application in predicting outcomes.

The fact that these classifications rely on SCr, eGFR, and UO, which are insensitive and unspecific markers of AKI and do not account for its duration or cause, is a significant caveat [58]. The value of SCr is influenced by factors altering its production (age, gender, diet, muscle mass), elimination (previous renal dysfunction), secretion (medications) and, importantly, concentration according to fluid balance variations. Baseline SCr is frequently unknown and its assessment is complex, with several studies pointing to the use of minimum preadmission SCr or estimated SCr using the Modification of Diet in Renal Disease formula. Furthermore, UO is difficult to assess without a urinary catheter and can be significantly altered by hypovolemic status and diuretics, and UO adjustment to actual versus ideal body weight affects AKI incidence reports [58–64].

2.6. Future Biomarkers

Recently, potential biomarkers of AKI have been identified. Ideally, novel biomarkers should be specific, identify the cause, identify patients at risk, provide an early diagnosis, stratify the severity of the injury, and predict outcomes.

With the enhanced understanding of the pathophysiology of AKI, novel biomarkers were identified, including proteins filtered by the glomerulus, enzymes released by tubular cells after injury, and inflammatory mediators [65]. These include Cys-C, neutrophil gelatinase associated lipocalin (NGAL), N-acetyl-glucosaminidase (NAG), kidney injury molecule 1 (KIM-1), interleukin-6 (IL-6), interleukin-8 (IL-8), interleukin 18 (IL-18), liver-type fatty acid-binding protein (L-FABP), calprotectin, urine angiotensinogen (AGT), urine microRNAs, insulin-like growth factor-binding protein 7 (IGFBP7), and tissue inhibitor of metalloproteinases-2 (TIMP-2), which have been evaluated in multiple settings, primarily on critically ill and surgical patients [66–77].

NGAL was one of the primarily studied biomarkers, which has demonstrated significant prediction of AKI in critically ill, cardiac surgery, sepsis, trauma, and contrast nephropathy patients [65,66,72]. Most recently, the use of IGFBP7 and TIMP-2 has been promising in the critical care setting, demonstrating greater accuracy and stability than former biomarkers [77–82]. However, further studies in different clinical settings are still required.

Most of these biomarkers can be detected in both serum and urine, and have been significantly associated with early AKI prediction. The association of these novel biomarkers with the need for dialysis, renal recovery, progression to CKD, and mortality has also been reported, although further studies are still warranted [65,77].

With recent advances in the understanding of AKI pathogenesis, the role of intrarenal and systemic inflammation leading to multi-organ dysfunction has been emphasized [82,83]. A new marker of systemic inflammation has become available, the neutrophil-lymphocyte ratio (NLR), which has been identified as an AKI prediction tool in multiple settings, being a simple, effective, and low-cost marker [84–86].

Despite the current progress in the development of new biomarkers, important drawbacks have limited their widespread applicability in clinical practice. For instance, they have not been able to reliably distinguish pre-renal and renal AKI; moreover, several patient characteristics and comorbidities, such as age, gender, diabetes mellitus, and chronic inflammation, are associated with range variations that limit their validity. The increased cost associated with testing and the need for multiple assessments to increase accuracy limits the cost-effectiveness. Furthermore, evidence of improvement of outcomes associated with using these biomarkers is still lacking [65,77].

Indeed, AKI is a complex syndrome and perhaps the use of a panel of several biomarkers covering different phases of the syndrome could provide a better understanding of its etiology and pathophysiology, and identify targets for future treatments [87].

Additionally, the use of automated electronic alerts (e-alerts) has received much attention in the past few years [88,89]. These consist of algorithms configured from patients' electronic medical records and clinical information to notify of early or imminent AKI, prompting an earlier clinical evaluation and application of prevention and treatment strategies, potentially improving clinical outcomes [89–92]. Indeed, a UK consensus conference has encouraged the use of these e-alerts for early detection of AKI [93]. Nevertheless, e-alerts are heterogeneous, do not include clear decision-making strategies, and have not been associated with decreased mortality or renal replacement technique (RRT) use [94]. Further development of these alerts is required to assess their impact on clinical outcomes and recommendation of use in clinical practice. We believe that it is essential to incorporate these scientific advances in daily clinical practice in the near future.

3. Conclusions

AKI is a complex syndrome with significant impact on patient outcomes; thus, its prevention, early detection, and prompt treatment are important to minimize the associated morbidity and mortality.

Research has led to an improvement in our understanding of AKI, raising our awareness of its incidence and prognostic impact. The KDIGO classification unified previous definitions and improved the recognition of AKI in clinical practice. The search for the perfect biomarker of AKI is still ongoing. Future studies should focus on early diagnostic measures, outcome predictors, and new treatments.

Author Contributions: Conceptualization, J.G. and J.A.L.; Methodology, J.G. and J.A.L.; Investigation, J.A.F.; Resources, S.J.; Writing-Original Draft Preparation, J.G.; Writing-Review & Editing, S.J. and J.A.L.

References

1. Hoste, E.A.J.; Kellum, J.A.; Selby, N.M.; Zarbock, A.; Palevsky, P.M.; Bagshaw, S.M.; Goldstein, S.L.; Cerdá, J.; Chawla, L.S. Global epidemiology and outcomes of acute kidney injury. *Nat. Rev. Nephrol.* **2018**, *14*, 607–625. [CrossRef] [PubMed]

2. Susantitaphong, P.; Cruz, D.N.; Cerda, J.; Abulfaraj, M.; Alqahtani, F.; Koulouridis, I.; Jaber, B.L. Acute Kidney Injury Advisory Group of the American Society of Nephrology. World incidence of AKI: A meta-analysis. *Clin. J. Am. Soc. Nephrol.* **2013**, *8*, 1482–1493. [CrossRef] [PubMed]

3. Chertow, G.; Burdick, E.; Honour, M.; Bonventre, J.; Bates, D. Acute kidney injury, mortality, length of stay, and costs in hospitalized patients. *J. Am. Soc. Nephrol.* **2005**, *16*, 3365–3370. [CrossRef] [PubMed]

4. Lameire, N.; van Biesen, W.; Vanholder, R. The changing epidemiology of acute renal failure. *Nat. Clin. Nephrol.* **2006**, *2*, 364–377. [CrossRef] [PubMed]

5. Bagshaw, S.M.; George, C.; Bellomo, R.; ANZICS Database Management Committee. Changes in the incidence and outcome for early acute kidney injury in a cohort of Australian intensive care units. *Crit. Care* **2007**, *11*, R68. [CrossRef] [PubMed]

6. Bellomo, R. The epidemiology of acute renal failure: 1975 versus 2005. *Curr. Opin. Crit. Care.* **2006**, *12*, 557–560. [CrossRef] [PubMed]

7.   Feest, T.G.; Round, A.; Hamad, S. Incidence of severe acute renal failure in adults: Results of a community-based study. *BMJ* **1993**, *306*, 481–483. [CrossRef] [PubMed]

8.   Liano, F.; Pascual, J. Epidemiology of acute renal failure: A prospective, multicenter, community-based study. *Kidney Int.* **1996**, *50*, 811–818. [CrossRef] [PubMed]

9.   Amin, A.P.; Salisbury, A.C.; McCullough, P.A.; Gosch, K.; Spertus, J.A.; Venkitachalam, L.; Stolker, J.M.; Parikh, C.R.; Masoudi, F.A.; Jones, P.G.; et al. Trends in the incidence of acute kidney injury in patients hospitalized with acute myocardial infarction. *Arch. Intern. Med.* **2012**, *172*, 246–253. [CrossRef] [PubMed]

10. Ronco, C.; McCullough, P.; Anker, S.D.; Anand, I.; Aspromonte, N.; Bagshaw, S.M.; Bellomo, R.; Berl, T.; Bobek, I.; Cruz, D.N.; et al. Cardio-renal syndromes: Report from the consensus conference of the acute dialysis quality initiative. *Eur. Heart J.* **2010**, *31*, 703–711. [CrossRef] [PubMed]

11. Hsu, R.K.; McCulloch, C.E.; Dudley, R.A.; Lo, L.J.; Hsu, C.Y. Temporal changes in incidence of dialysis-requiring AKI. *J. Am. Soc. Nephrol.* **2013**, *24*, 37–42. [CrossRef] [PubMed]

12. Singbartl, K.; Kellum, J.A. AKI in the ICU: Definition, epidemiology, risk stratification, and outcomes. *Kidney Int.* **2012**, *81*, 819–825. [CrossRef] [PubMed]

13. Uchino, U.S.; Kellum, J.A.; Bellomo, R.; Doig, G.S.; Morimatsu, H.; Morgera, S.; Schetz, M.; Tan, I.; Bouman, C.; Macedo, E.; et al. Acute renal failure in critically ill patients: A multinational, multicenter study. *JAMA* **2005**, *294*, 813–818. [CrossRef] [PubMed]

14. Bellomo, R.; Kellum, J.A.; Ronco, C.; Wald, R.; Martensson, J.; Maiden, M.; Bagshaw, S.M.; Glassford, N.J.; Lankadeva, Y.; Vaara, S.T.; et al. Acute kidney injury in sepsis. *Intensive Care Med.* **2017**, *43*, 816–828. [CrossRef] [PubMed]

15. Bagshaw, S.M.; George, C.; Bellomo, R.; ANZICS Database Management Committee. Early acute kidney injury and sepsis: A multicentre evaluation. *Crit. Care* **2008**, *12*, R47. [CrossRef] [PubMed]

16. Lopes, J.A.; Jorge, S.; Resina, C.; Santos, C.; Pereira, A.; Neves, J.; Antunes, F.; Prata, M.M. Acute kidney injury in patients with sepsis: A contemporary analysis. *Int. J. Infect. Dis.* **2009**, *13*, 176–181. [CrossRef] [PubMed]

17. Thakar, C.V. Perioperative acute kidney injury. *Adv. Chronic Kidney Dis.* **2013**, *20*, 67–75. [CrossRef] [PubMed]

18. Grams, M.E.; Sang, Y.; Coresh, J.; Ballew, S.; Matsushita, K.; Molnar, M.Z.; Szabo, Z.; Kalantar-Zadeh, K.; Kovesdy, C.P. Acute kidney injury after major surgery: A retrospective analysis of veteran's health administration data. *Am. J. Kidney Dis.* **2016**, *67*, 872–880. [CrossRef] [PubMed]

19. Gameiro, J.; Fonseca, J.A.; Neves, M.; Jorge, S.; Lopes, J.A. Acute kidney injury in major abdominal surgery: Incidence, risk factors, pathogenesis and outcomes. *Ann. Intensive Care* **2018**, *8*, 22. [CrossRef] [PubMed]

20. Chawla, L.S.; Bellomo, R.; Bihorac, A.; Goldstein, S.L.; Siew, E.D.; Bagshaw, S.M.; Bittleman, D.; Cruz, D.; Endre, Z.; Fitzgerald, R.L.; et al. Acute kidney disease and renal recovery: Consensus report of the Acute Disease Quality Initiative (ADQI) 16 workgroup. *Nat. Rev. Nephrol.* **2017**, *13*, 241–257. [CrossRef] [PubMed]

21. Husain-Syed, F.; Ronco, C. The odyssey of risk stratification in acute kidney injury. *Nat. Rev. Nephrol.* **2018**. [CrossRef] [PubMed]

22. Bellomo, R.; Ronco, C.; Kellum, J.A.; Mehta, R.L.; Palevsky, P. Acute renal failure—Definition, outcome measures, animal models, fluid therapy and information technology needs: The second international consensus conference of the Acute Dialysis Quality Initiative (ADQI) group. *Crit. Care* **2004**, *8*, R204–R212. [CrossRef] [PubMed]

23. Manjunath, G.; Sarnak, M.J.; Levey, A.S. Prediction equations to estimate glomerular filtration rate: An update. *Curr. Opin. Nephrol. Hypertens.* **2001**, *10*, 785–792. [CrossRef] [PubMed]

24. Brivet, F.G.; Kleinknecht, D.J.; Loirat, P.; Landais, P.J. Acute renal failure in intensive care units—Causes, outcome, and prognostic factors of hospital mortality: A prospective, multicenter study. *Crit. Care Med.* **1996**, *24*, 192–198. [CrossRef] [PubMed]

25. Silvester, W.; Bellomo, R.; Cole, L. Epidemiology, management, and outcome of severe acute renal failure of critical illness in Australia. *Crit. Care Med.* **2001**, *29*, 1910–1915. [CrossRef] [PubMed]

26. Lopes, J.A.; Jorge, S. The RIFLE and AKIN classifications for acute kidney injury: A critical and comprehensive review. *Clin. Kidney J.* **2013**, *6*, 8–14. [CrossRef] [PubMed]

27. Mehta, R.L.; Kellum, J.A.; Shah, S.V.; Molitoris, B.A.; Ronco, C.; Warnock, D.G.; Levin, A. Acute Kidney Injury Network: Report of an initiative to improve outcomes in acute kidney injury. *Crit. Care* **2007**, *11*, R31. [CrossRef] [PubMed]

28. Uchino, S.; Bellomo, R.; Goldsmith, D.; Bates, S.; Ronco, C. An assessment of the RIFLE criteria for acute renal failure in hospitalized patients. *Crit. Care Med.* **2006**, *34*, 1913–1917. [CrossRef] [PubMed]

29. Hoste, E.A.; Clermont, G.; Kersten, A.; Venkataraman, R.; Angus, D.C.; De Bacquer, D.; Kellum, J.A. RIFLE criteria for acute kidney injury are associated with hospital mortality in critically ill patients: A cohort analysis. *Crit. Care* **2006**, *10*, R73. [CrossRef] [PubMed]

30. Lassnigg, A.; Schmidlin, D.; Mouhieddine, M.; Bachmann, L.M.; Druml, W.; Bauer, P.; Hiesmayr, M. Minimal changes of serum creatinine predict prognosis in patients after cardiothoracic surgery: A prospective cohort study. *J. Am. Soc. Nephrol.* **2004**, *15*, 1597–1605. [CrossRef] [PubMed]

31. Lopes, J.A.; Fernandes, P.; Jorge, S.; Gonçalves, S.; Alvarez, A.; Costae, S.Z.; França, C.; Prata, M.M. Acute kidney injury in intensive care unit patients: A comparison between the RIFLE and the Acute Kidney Injury Network classifications. *Crit. Care* **2008**, *12*, R110. [CrossRef] [PubMed]

32. Barrantes, F.; Feng, Y.; Ivanov, O.; Yalamanchili, H.B.; Patel, J.; Buenafe, X.; Cheng, V.; Dijeh, S.; Amoateng-Adjepong, Y.; Manthous, C.A. Acute kidney injury predicts outcomes of non-critically ill patients. *Mayo Clin. Proc.* **2009**, *84*, 410–416. [CrossRef]

33. Barrantes, F.; Tian, J.; Vazquez, R.; Amoateng-Adjepong, Y.; Manthous, C.A. Acute kidney injury criteria predict outcomes of critically ill patients. *Crit. Care Med.* **2008**, *36*, 1397–1403. [CrossRef] [PubMed]

34. Bagshaw, S.M.; George, C.; Bellomo, R. A comparison of the RIFLE and AKIN criteria for acute kidney injury in critically ill patients. *Nephrol. Dial. Transplant.* **2008**, *23*, 1569–1574. [CrossRef] [PubMed]

35. Lassnigg, A.; Schmid, E.R.; Hiesmayr, M.; Falk, C.; Druml, W.; Bauer, P.; Schmidlin, D. Impact of minimal increases in serum creatinine on outcome in patients after cardiothoracic surgery: Do we have to revise current definitions of acute renal failure? *Crit. Care Med.* **2008**, *36*, 1129–1137. [CrossRef] [PubMed]

36. Joannidis, M.; Metnitz, B.; Bauer, P.; Schusterschitz, N.; Moreno, R.; Druml, W.; Metnitz, P.G. Acute kidney injury in critically ill patients classified by AKIN versus RIFLE using the SAPS 3 database. *Intensive Care Med.* **2009**, *35*, 1692–1702. [CrossRef] [PubMed]

37. Ostermann, M.; Chang, R.W. Challenges of defining acute kidney injury. *QJM* **2011**, *104*, 237–243. [CrossRef] [PubMed]

38. Englberger, L.; Suri, R.M.; Li, Z.; Casey, E.T.; Daly, R.C.; Dearani, J.A.; Schaff, H.V. Clinical accuracy of RIFLE and Acute Kidney Injury Network (AKIN) criteria for acute kidney injury in patients undergoing cardiac surgery. *Crit. Care* **2011**, *15*, R16. [CrossRef] [PubMed]

39. Robert, A.M.; Kramer, R.S.; Dacey, L.J.; Charlesworth, D.C.; Leavitt, B.J.; Helm, R.E.; Hernandez, F.; Sardella, G.L.; Frumiento, C.; Likosky, D.S.; et al. Cardiac surgery associated acute kidney injury: A comparison of two consensus criteria. *Ann. Thorac. Surg.* **2010**, *90*, 1939–1943. [CrossRef] [PubMed]

40. Khwaja, A. KDIGO clinical practice guideline for acute kidney injury. *Nephron Clin. Pract.* **2012**, *120*, c179–c184. [CrossRef] [PubMed]

41. Nisula, S.; Kaukonen, K.M.; Vaara, S.T.; Korhonen, A.M.; Poukkanen, M.; Karlsson, S.; Haapio, M.; Inkinen, O.; Parviainen, I.; Suojaranta-Ylinen, R.; et al. Incidence, risk factors and 90-day mortality of patients with acute kidney injury in Finnish intensive care units: The FINNAKI study. *Intensive Care Med.* **2013**, *39*, 420–428. [CrossRef] [PubMed]

42. Roy, A.K.; Mc Gorrian, C.; Treacy, C.; Kavanaugh, E.; Brennan, A.; Mahon, N.G.; Murray, P.T. A comparison of traditional and novel definitions (RIFLE, AKIN, and KDIGO) of acute kidney injury for the prediction of outcomes in acute decompensated heart failure. *Cardiorenal Med.* **2013**, *3*, 26–37. [CrossRef] [PubMed]

43. Bastin, A.J.; Ostermann, M.; Slack, A.J.; Diller, G.P.; Finney, S.J.; Evans, T.W. Acute kidney injury after cardiac surgery according to risk/injury/failure/loss/end-stage, acute kidney injury network, and kidney disease: Improving global outcomes classifications. *J. Crit. Care* **2013**, *28*, 389–396. [CrossRef] [PubMed]

44. Zeng, X.; McMahon, G.M.; Brunelli, S.M.; Bates, D.W.; Waikar, S.S. Incidence, outcomes, and comparisons across definitions of AKI in hospitalized individuals. *Clin. J. Am. Soc. Nephrol.* **2014**, *9*, 12–20. [CrossRef] [PubMed]

45. Levi, T.M.; de Souza, S.P.; de Magalhães, J.G.; de Carvalho, M.S.; Cunha, A.L.; Dantas, J.G.; Cruz, M.G.; Guimarães, Y.L.; Cruz, C.M. Comparison of the RIFLE, AKIN and KDIGO criteria to predict mortality in critically ill patients. *Rev. Bras. Ter. Intensiva* **2013**, *25*, 290–296. [CrossRef] [PubMed]

46. Neves, M.; Fidalgo, P.; Gonçalves, C.; Leitão, S.; Santos, R.M.; Carvalho, A.; Costa, J.M. Acute kidney injury in an internal medicine ward in a Portuguese quaternary hospital. *Eur. J. Intern. Med.* **2014**, *25*, 169–172. [CrossRef] [PubMed]

47. Rodrigues, F.B.; Bruetto, R.G.; Torres, U.S.; Otaviano, A.P.; Zanetta, D.M.; Burdmann, E.A. Incidence and mortality of acute kidney injury after myocardial infarction: A comparison between KDIGO and RIFLE criteria. *PLoS ONE* **2013**, *8*, e69998. [CrossRef] [PubMed]

48. Luo, X.; Jiang, L.; Du, B.; Wen, Y.; Wang, M.; Xi, X. A comparison of different diagnostic criteria in acute kidney injury in critically ill patients. *Crit. Care* **2014**, *18*, R144. [CrossRef] [PubMed]

49. Fujii, T.; Uchino, S.; Takinami, M.; Bellomo, R. Validation of the kidney disease improving global outcomes criteria for AKI and comparison of three criteria in hospitalized patients. *Clin. J. Am. Soc. Nephrol.* **2014**, *9*, 848–854. [CrossRef] [PubMed]

50. Li, Z.; Cai, L.; Liang, X.; Du, Z.; Chen, Y.; An, S.; Tan, N.; Xu, L.; Li, R.; Li, L.; et al. Identification and predicting short-term prognosis of early cardiorenal syndrome type 1: KDIGO is superior to RIFLE or AKIN. *PLoS ONE* **2014**, *9*, e114369. [CrossRef] [PubMed]

51. Pereira, M.; Rodrigues, N.; Godinho, I.; Gameiro, J.; Neves, M.; Gouveia, J.; Costa, E.; Silva, Z.; Lopes, J.A. Acute kidney injury in patients with severe sepsis or septic shock: A comparison between the "Risk, Injury, Failure, Loss of kidney function, End-stage kidney disease" (RIFLE), Acute Kidney Injury Network (AKIN) and Kidney Disease: Improving Global Outcomes (KDIGO) classifications. *Clin. Kidney J.* **2017**, *10*, 332–340. [PubMed]

52. Koeze, J.; Keus, F.; Dieperink, W.; van der Horst, I.C.C.; Zijlstra, J.G.; van Meurs, M. Incidence, timing and outcome of AKI in critically ill patients varies with the definition used and the addition of urine output criteria. *BMC Nephrol.* **2017**, *18*, 70. [CrossRef] [PubMed]

53. Tsai, T.Y.; Chien, H.; Tsai, F.C.; Pan, H.C.; Yang, H.Y.; Lee, S.Y.; Hsu, H.H.; Fang, J.T.; Yang, C.W.; Chen, Y.C. Comparison of RIFLE, AKIN, and KDIGO classifications for assessing prognosis of patients on extracorporeal membrane oxygenation. *J. Formos. Med. Assoc.* **2017**, *116*, 844–851. [CrossRef] [PubMed]

54. Wu, H.C.; Lee, L.C.; Wang, W.J. Incidence and mortality of postoperative acute kidney injury in non-dialysis patients: Comparison between the AKIN and KDIGO criteria. *Ren. Fail.* **2016**, *38*, 330–339. [CrossRef] [PubMed]

55. Zhou, J.; Liu, Y.; Tang, Y.; Liu, F.; Zhang, L.; Zeng, X.; Feng, Y.; Tao, Y.; Yang, L.; Fu, P. A comparison of RIFLE, AKIN, KDIGO, and Cys-C criteria for the definition of acute kidney injury in critically ill patients. *Int. Urol. Nephrol.* **2016**, *48*, 125–132. [CrossRef] [PubMed]

56. Zhang, Z.; Lu, B.; Sheng, X.; Jin, N. Cystatin C in prediction of acute kidney injury: A systemic review and meta-analysis. *Am. J. Kidney Dis.* **2011**, *58*, 356–365. [CrossRef] [PubMed]

57. Pan, H.C.; Chien, Y.S.; Jenq, C.C.; Tsai, M.H.; Fan, P.C.; Chang, C.H. Acute kidney injury classification for critically Ill cirrhotic patients: A comparison of the KDIGO, AKIN, and RIFLE classifications. *Sci. Rep.* **2016**, *6*, 23022. [CrossRef] [PubMed]

58. Thomas, M.E.; Blaine, C.; Dawnay, A.; Devonald, M.A.; Ftouh, S.; Laing, C.; Latchem, S.; Lewington, A.; Milford, D.V.; Ostermann, M. The definition of acute kidney injury and its use in practice. *Kidney Int.* **2015**, *87*, 62–73. [CrossRef] [PubMed]

59. Thongprayoon, C.; Cheungpasitporn, W.; Kittanamongkolchai, W.; Srivali, N.; Ungprasert, P.; Kashani, K. Optimum methodology for estimating baseline serum creatinine for the acute kidney injury classification. *Nephrology (Carlton)* **2015**, *20*, 881–886. [CrossRef] [PubMed]

60. Thongprayoon, C.; Cheungpasitporn, W.; Harrison, A.M.; Kittanamongkolchai, W.; Ungprasert, P.; Srivali, N.; Akhoundi, A.; Kashani, K.B. The comparison of the commonly used surrogates for baseline renal function in acute kidney injury diagnosis and staging. *BMC Nephrol.* **2016**, *17*, 6. [CrossRef] [PubMed]

61. Waikar, S.S.; Betensky, R.A.; Emerson, S.C.; Bonventre, J.V. Imperfect gold standards for kidney injury biomarker evaluation. *J. Am. Soc. Nephrol.* **2012**, *23*, 13–21. [CrossRef] [PubMed]

62. Macedo, E.; Malhotra, R.; Claure-Del Granado, R.; Fedullo, P.; Mehta, R.L. Defining urine output criterion for acute kidney injury in critically ill patients. *Nephrol. Dial. Transplant.* **2011**, *26*, 509–515. [CrossRef] [PubMed]

63. Macedo, E.; Bouchard, J.; Soroko, S.H.; Chertow, G.M.; Himmelfarb, J.; Ikizler, T.A.; Paganini, E.P.; Mehta, R.L. Fluid accumulation, recognition and staging of acute kidney injury in critically-ill patients. *Crit. Care* **2010**, *14*, R82. [CrossRef] [PubMed]

64. Thongprayoon, C.; Cheungpasitporn, W.; Akhoundi, A.; Ahmed, A.H.; Kashani, K.B. Actual versus ideal body weight for acute kidney injury diagnosis and classification in critically ill patients. *BMC Nephrol.* **2014**, *15*, 176. [CrossRef] [PubMed]

65. Ostermann, M.; Philips, B.J.; Forni, L.G. Clinical review: Biomarkers of acute kidney injury: Where are we now? *Crit. Care* **2012**, *16*, 233. [CrossRef] [PubMed]

66. Schinstock, C.A.; Semret, M.H.; Wagner, S.J.; Borland, T.M.; Bryant, S.C.; Kashani, K.B.; Larson, T.S.; Lieske, J.C. Urinalysis is more specific and urinary neutrophil gelatinase-associated lipocalin is more sensitive for early detection of acute kidney injury. *Nephrol. Dial. Transplant.* **2013**, *28*, 1175–1185. [CrossRef] [PubMed]

67. Han, W.K.; Bailly, V.; Abichandani, R.; Thadhani, R.; Bonventre, J.V. Kidney Injury Molecule-1 (KIM-1): A novel biomarker for human renal proximal tubule injury. *Kidney Int.* **2002**, *62*, 237–244. [CrossRef] [PubMed]

68. Parikh, C.R.; Mishra, J.; Thiessen-Philbrook, H.; Dursun, B.; Ma, Q.; Kelly, C.; Dent, C.; Devarajan, P.; Edelstein, C.L. Urinary IL-18 is an early predictive biomarker of acute kidney injury after cardiac surgery. *Kidney Int.* **2006**, *70*, 199–203. [CrossRef] [PubMed]

69. Di Somma, S.; Magrini, L.; De Berardinis, B.; Marino, R.; Ferri, E.; Moscatelli, P.; Ballarino, P.; Carpinteri, G.; Noto, P.; Gliozzo, B.; et al. Additive value of blood neutrophil gelatinase associated lipocalin to clinical judgement in acute kidney injury diagnosis and mortality prediction in patients hospitalized from the emergency department. *Crit. Care* **2013**, *17*, R29–R13. [CrossRef] [PubMed]

70. Bennett, M.; Dent, C.L.; Ma, Q.; Dastrala, S.; Grenier, F.; Workman, R.; Syed, H.; Ali, S.; Barasch, J.; Devarajan, P. Urine NGAL predicts severity of acute kidney injury after cardiac surgery: A prospective study. *Clin. J. Am. Soc. Nephrol.* **2008**, *3*, 665–673. [CrossRef] [PubMed]

71. Hall, I.E.; Yarlagadda, S.G.; Coca, S.G.; Wang, Z.; Doshi, M.; Devarajan, P.; Han, W.K.; Marcus, R.J.; Parikh, C.R. IL-18 and urinary NGAL predict dialysis and graft recovery after kidney transplantation. *J. Am. Soc. Nephrol.* **2010**, *21*, 189–197. [CrossRef] [PubMed]

72. Jia, H.M.; Huang, L.F.; Zheng, Y.; Li, W.X. Diagnostic value of urinary tissue inhibitor of metalloproteinase-2 and insulin-like growth factor binding protein 7 for acute kidney injury: A meta-analysis. *Crit. Care* **2017**, *21*, 77. [CrossRef] [PubMed]

73. Bargnoux, A.S.; Piéroni, L.; Cristol, J.P. Analytical study of a new turbidimetric assay for urinary neutrophil gelatinase-associated lipocalin (NGAL) determination. *Clin. Chem. Lab. Med.* **2013**, *51*, e293–e296. [CrossRef] [PubMed]

74. Westhoff, J.H.; Tönshoff, B.; Waldherr, S.; Pöschl, J.; Teufel, U.; Westhoff, T.H.; Fichtner, A. Urinary tissue inhibitor of metalloproteinase-2 (TIMP-2) insulin-like growth factor-binding protein 7 (IGFBP7) predicts adverse outcome in pediatric acute kidney injury. *PLoS ONE* **2015**, *10*, e0143628. [CrossRef] [PubMed]

75. Lima, C.; Macedo, E. Urinary biochemistry in the diagnosis of acute kidney injury. *Dis. Markers* **2018**. [CrossRef] [PubMed]

76. Vanmassenhove, J.; Vanholder, R.; Nagler, E.; van Biesen, W. Urinary and serum biomarkers for the diagnosis of acute kidney injury: An in-depth review of the literature. *Nephrol. Dial. Transplant.* **2013**, *28*, 254–273. [CrossRef] [PubMed]

77. Kashani, K.; Cheungpasitporn, W.; Ronco, C. Biomarkers of acute kidney injury: The pathway from discovery to clinical adoption. *Clin. Chem. Lab. Med.* **2017**, *55*, 1074–1089. [CrossRef] [PubMed]

78. Fan, W.; Ankawi, G.; Zhang, J.; Digvijay, K.; Giavarina, D.; Yin, Y.; Ronco, C. Current understanding and future directions in the application of TIMP-2 and IGFBP7 in AKI clinical practice. *Clin. Chem. Lab. Med.* **2018**. [CrossRef]

79. Koyner, J.L.; Garg, A.X.; Coca, S.G.; Sint, K.; Thiessen-Philbrook, H.; Patel, U.D.; Shlipak, M.G.; Parikh, C.R. TRIBE-AKI Consortium. Biomarkers predict progression of acute kidney injury after cardiac surgery. *J. Am. Soc. Nephrol.* **2012**, *16*, 905–914. [CrossRef] [PubMed]

80. Bell, M.; Granath, F.; Martensson, J.; Lofberg, E.; Ekbom, A.; Martling, C.R. Cystatin C is correlated with mortality in patients with and without acute kidney injury. *Nephrol. Dial. Transplant.* **2009**, *16*, 3096–3102. [CrossRef] [PubMed]

81. Srisawat, N.; Murugan, R.; Lee, M.; Kong, L.; Carter, M.; Angus, D.C.; Kellum, J.A. Plasma neutrophil gelatinase-associated lipocalin predicts recovery from acute kidney injury following community-acquired pneumonia. *Kidney Int.* **2011**, *16*, 545–552. [CrossRef] [PubMed]

82. Rabb, H.; Griffin, M.D.; McKay, D.B.; Swaminathan, S.; Pickkers, P.; Rosner, M.H.; Kellum, J.A.; Ronco, C. Inflammation in AKI: Current understanding, key questions, and knowledge gaps. *J. Am. Soc. Nephrol.* **2016**, *27*, 371–379. [CrossRef] [PubMed]

83. Gomez, H.; Ince, C.; De Backer, D.; Pickkers, P.; Payen, D.; Hotchkiss, J.; Kellum, J.A. A unified theory of sepsis-induced acute kidney injury: Inflammation, microcirculatory dysfunction, bioenergetics, and the tubular cell adaptation to injury. *Shock* **2014**, *41*, 3–11. [CrossRef] [PubMed]

84. Yilmaz, H.; Cakmak, M.; Inan, O.; Darcin, T.; Akcay, A. Can neutrophil-lymphocyte ratio be independent risk factor for predicting acute kidney injury in patients with severe sepsis? *Ren. Fail.* **2015**, *37*, 225–229. [CrossRef] [PubMed]

85. Kim, W.H.; Park, J.Y.; Ok, S.H.; Shin, I.W.; Sohn, J.T. Association Between the neutrophil/lymphocyte ratio and acute kidney injury after cardiovascular surgery: A retrospective observational study. *Medicine (Baltimore)* **2015**, *94*, e1867. [CrossRef] [PubMed]

86. Abu Alfeilat, M.; Slotki, I.; Shavit, L. Single emergency room measurement of neutrophil/lymphocyte ratio for early detection of acute kidney injury (AKI). *Intern. Emerg. Med.* **2017**. [CrossRef] [PubMed]

87. Marx, D.; Metzger, J.; Pejchinovski, M.; Gil, R.B.; Frantzi, M.; Latosinska, A.; Belczacka, I.; Heinzmann, S.S.; Husi, H.; Zoidakis, J.; et al. Proteomics and Metabolomics for AKI Diagnosis. *Semin. Nephrol.* **2018**, *38*, 63–87. [CrossRef] [PubMed]

88. Hobson, C.E.; Darmon, M.; Mohan, S.; Hudson, D.; Goldstein, S.L.; Ronco, C.; Kellum, J.A.; Bagshaw, S.M. Applications for detection of acute kidney injury using electronic medical records and clinical information systems: Workgroup statements from the 15(th) ADQI Consensus Conference. *Can. J. Kidney Health Dis.* **2016**, *3*, 9.

89. Selby, N.M.; Crowley, L.; Fluck, R.J.; McIntyre, C.W.; Monaghan, J.; Lawson, N.; Kolhe, N.V. Use of electronic results reporting to diagnose and monitor AKI in hospitalized patients. *Clin. J. Am. Soc. Nephrol.* **2012**, *7*, 533–540. [CrossRef] [PubMed]

90. Cheungpasitporn, W.; Kashani, K. Electronic data systems and acute kidney injury. *Contrib. Nephrol.* **2016**, *187*, 73–83. [PubMed]

91. Sutherland, S.M.; Goldstein, S.L.; Bagshaw, S.M. Leveraging big data and electronic health records to enhance novel approaches to acute kidney injury research and care. *Blood Purif.* **2017**, *44*, 68–76. [CrossRef] [PubMed]

92. Prendecki, M.; Blacker, E.; Sadeghi-Alavijeh, O.; Edwards, R.; Montgomery, H.; Gillis, S.; Harber, M. Improving outcomes in patients with acute kidney injury: The impact of hospital based automated AKI alerts. *Postgrad. Med. J.* **2016**, *92*, 9–13. [CrossRef] [PubMed]

93. Feehally, J.; Gilmore, I.; Barasi, S.; Bosomworth, M.; Christie, B.; Davies, A.; Dhesi, J.; Dowdle, R.; Gibbins, C.; Gonzalez, I.; et al. Royal College of Physicians of Edinburgh UK Consensus Conference on Management of acute kidney injury: The role of fluids, e-alerts and biomarkers. *J. R. Coll. Physicians Edinb.* **2013**, *43*, 37–38. [CrossRef] [PubMed]

94. Lachance, P.; Villeneuve, P.M.; Rewa, O.G.; Wilson, F.P.; Selby, N.M.; Featherstone, R.M.; Bagshaw, S.M. Association between e-alert implementation for detection of acute kidney injury and outcomes: A systematic review. *Nephrol. Dial. Transplant.* **2017**, *32*, 265–272. [CrossRef] [PubMed]

6

Continuous Renal Replacement Therapy (CRRT) in Children and the Specialized CRRT Team: A 14-Year Single-Center Study

Keum Hwa Lee [1,2,3], **In Suk Sol** [4,5], **Jung Tak Park** [3,6], **Ji Hong Kim** [1,7], **Jae Won Shin** [1], **Mi Rireu Park** [1], **Jae Hyun Lee** [1], **Yoon Hee Kim** [4,7], **Kyung Won Kim** [4,*] and **Jae Il Shin** [1,2,3,*]

[1] Department of Pediatrics, Yonsei University College of Medicine, Yonsei-ro 50, Seodaemun-gu, C.P.O. Box 8044, Seoul 03722, Korea; AZSAGM@yuhs.ac (K.H.L.); KKKJHD@yuhs.ac (J.H.K.); AGUILERA83@naver.com (J.W.S.); QKRALFM27@yuhs.ac (M.R.P.); LJH89515@yuhs.ac (J.H.L.)
[2] Division of Pediatric Nephrology, Severance Children's Hospital, Seoul 03722, Korea
[3] Institute of Kidney Disease Research, Yonsei University College of Medicine, Seoul 03722, Korea; JTPARK@yuhs.ac
[4] Department of Pediatrics, Severance Hospital, Yonsei University College of Medicine, Seoul 03722, Korea; issolkk0312@gmail.com (I.S.S.); YHKIM@yuhs.ac (Y.H.K.)
[5] Department of Pediatrics, Hallym University Chuncheon Sacred Heart Hospital, Sakju-ro 77, Gangwon-do, Chuncheon 24253, Korea
[6] Department of Internal Medicine, Yonsei University College of Medicine, Seoul 03722, Korea
[7] Department of Pediatrics, Gangnam Severance Hospital, Yonsei University College of Medicine, Eonjuro 211, Gangnam-gu, Seoul 06273, Korea
[*] Correspondence: KWKIM@yuhs.ac (K.W.K.); shinji@yuhs.ac (J.I.S.)

Abstract: Continuous renal replacement therapy (CRRT) has been used as an important intervention in critically ill children. Our center has the only specialized CRRT team (SCT) for children in Korea, which consists of pediatric intensivists, a pediatric nephrologist and CRRT-specialized-nurses. This study was a retrospective single-center analysis, including all pediatric patients admitted to the intensive care unit (ICU) of Severance hospital in Korea and received CRRT between 2003 and 2016, grouped as before SCT (group A, $n = 51$) and after SCT (group B, $n = 212$). We obtained the data for sex, age, weight, diagnosis, blood flow rate or type of CRRT machine used, administration of inotropic agents or anticoagulants, and ICU duration before CRRT (hours). A total of 263 patients were included. The age was significantly younger ($p < 0.001$) and blood flow rate was lower ($p = 0.001$) in group B than group A. Vasopressors ($p < 0.001$), continuous veno-venous hemodiafiltration (CVVHDF) ($p < 0.001$), nafamostat mesilate ($p < 0.001$), and extracorporeal membrane oxygenation (ECMO)-CRRT ($p = 0.004$) were more frequently used in group B. Based on our 14-year experience, we conclude that SCT operation could have played an important role in increasing the amount of CRRT utilization.

Keywords: continuous renal replacement therapy (CRRT); specialized CRRT team (SCT); retrospective study

1. Introduction

Acute kidney injury (AKI) is defined according to the elevated plasma creatinine level and decreased urine output [1–4]. It shows diverse clinical manifestations ranging from asymptomatic, through anuria, to multiple organ dysfunctions [5,6]. The prevalence of AKI has been reported to be about 30%–60% for critically ill patients in an intensive care unit (ICU) [7]. In 2017, Kaddourah et al. reported that AKI developed in 26.9%, and severe AKI (renal replacement therapy required) developed in 11.6% of the children in ICU during the first seven days after ICU admission [8]. They also described that AKI itself may crucial to the associated morbidity and mortality and the mortality rate in severe AKI group could be up to 20% [8].

From this point of view, since continuous renal replacement therapy (CRRT) was first introduced by Kramer et al. in 1977 [9], and pediatric CRRT was first used in 1985 [10]; it has been the most important renal replacement modality in critically ill patients. Although both hemodialysis (HD) and peritoneal dialysis (PD) are established interventions for patients who require renal replacement, CRRT is known to be a more efficient therapy for stabilizing circulatory, acid-base, and electrolyte balance when the patient has unstable vital parameters [11].

As well as technological advances, other attempts in worldwide have been made to drive the success of the CRRT in the critical patient with AKI. In adult patients, Ronco et al. firstly emphasized the importance of a multidisciplinary approach, including collaboration between various clinical teams [12,13]. After then, several centers opened a specialized CRRT team (SCT) to manage CRRT [14], and two recent observational studies showed that patients had improved CRRT outcomes after the SCT approach [15,16].

Despite several studies that have been published demonstrating that CRRT is a very important therapy for critically ill children so far [17–19], there have been no reports about the real efficacy of a SCT in the clinic and managing results. Our center is the biggest tertiary care center in Korea with over 14 years of experience in CRRT and has the only specialized CRRT team (SCT) for children in Korea, which consists of pediatric intensivists, a pediatric nephrologist, and CRRT-specialized nurses. Because the SCT was started in August 2008, the objective of this study was to compare and analyze the factors before and after starting SCT management.

2. Methods

2.1. Search Strategy

Medical records of 291 patients were collected from January 1, 2003 to April 30, 2016. Of these, 28 underwent more than one CRRT treatment run. Final analysis was done by removing duplicates and leaving only the longest CRRT run.

During the study period, patients undergoing CRRT were included and grouped as before SCT (group A) and after SCT (group B). Group A included patients treated from March 2003 to July 2008 and group B those from August 2008 to April 2016. Before SCT, pediatric CRRT was run by occasional operators, but after the SCT began, ICU nurses joined and began to work as the member of SCT. Double-lumen catheters ranging between 6.5 and 13.5 F in diameter (Gambro Healthcare, Lakewood, CO, USA) were inserted into the central veins depending on the child's age and weight. Polyarylethersulfone hollow-fiber hemofilters (PAES; the Prismaflex® HF20, Gambro Lundia AB, Lund, Sweden) and polyacrilonytrile hollow-fiber hemofilters (① AN69® membrane before the year 2010; the Prismaflex® M-10/60/100, Gambro Lundia AB, Lund, Sweden; ② AN69® ST membrane since the year 2010; the Prismaflex® ST-60/100, Gambro Lundia AB, Lund, Sweden) were used in all patients, depending on the patient's weight. HF-20 or M-10 were used in children weighing less than 10 kg; ST-60 or M-60 were used in patients weighing 10–20 kg, and ST-100 or M-100 were used in children weighing more than 20 kg. Commercially prepared bicarbonate-buffered hemofiltration replacement fluid (Hemosol B0; Gambro Healthcare, Seoul, Korea; potassium free), was used as a dialysate and replacement fluid. Potassium chloride (KCl) was added if the patient has a risk of hypokalemia (20 mEq KCl mix in the 5L Hemozol® when serum potassium level ranged from 3.6 to 4.5 mEg/L and 40 mEq KCl mix in the 5L Hemozol® when serum potassium level lowered than 3.6 mEg/L). The blood flow rate was set as 5 mL/kg/min [18]. The predilution replacement fluid rate or dialysate rate was set at a rate of 2000 mL/1.73 m^2/hour [18]. The mode of CRRT was selected from one of the following, depending on the patient's status of solute imbalance: continuous veno-venous hemofiltration (CVVH), continuous veno-venous hemodialysis (CVVHD), and continuous veno-venous hemodiafiltration

(CVVHDF). These were determined by the pediatric nephrologist and pediatric intensivist through in-depth discussion.

The time to initiate CRRT was decided by the pediatric intensivist, depending on each patient's clinical condition, such as anuria, oliguria (<0.5 mL/kg/hour), or positive fluid balance, regardless of administration of high doses of diuretics (furosemide more than 1 mg/kg/hour). Anticoagulation was not administered during CRRT initiation; however, our protocol establishes that if the filter was blocked within 12 hours of CRRT initiation, anticoagulation agents such as continuous heparin or nafamostat mesilate infusion via the pre-blood pump port were used. The percentage of fluid overload at CRRT initiation (%FO) was calculated using the following formula [20]:

$$\%FO = (\text{Fluid In} - \text{Fluid Out})/(\text{ICU admission weight}) \times 100\% \tag{1}$$

At the initiation of CRRT, the following data were obtained for all patients: sex, age, diagnosis, underlying patient conditions, blood flow rate, use of inotropic agents, anticoagulants, and hours to starting CRRT.

2.2. Definition of SCT

The SCT is a specialized team of physicians and nurses who perform pediatric CRRT. It includes a pediatric nephrologist, pediatric intensivists, nephrologists (internal medicine), and five CRRT-specialized nurses. The pediatric intensivist oversees the critical care and overall decisions on critically ill children–related problems. The pediatric nephrologist determines the distribution of CRRT machines depending upon the daily status of adult and pediatric inpatients in the ICU in consultation with the pediatric intensivist and the nephrologists for adults. CRRT-specialized nurses undergo a CRRT-specialized training course, which includes the basic principles, practical operations, alarm control, and troubleshooting of CRRT; checking hemodynamic stability and CRRT kit status; and management of CRRT catheter-related problems. They work three shifts daily, and their role is separate from that of ICU bedside nurses and chronic HD nurses. They regularly monitor the hemodynamic status and CRRT-related problems of children undergoing CRRT. They are in contact with the machine company and monitor periodic inspections to prevent problems of the CRRT machine itself. Every month, the members of the SCT have a conference, where they share their clinical experiences and provide educational feedback on pediatric CRRT.

2.3. Statistical Analysis

Statistical analyses were performed using the SPSS for Windows version 18.0 (IBM Corp., Armonk, NY, USA). An independent t-test was used for continuous variables, and they were expressed as means ± standard deviations. Chi-square test and Fisher's exact test were used to analyze the categorical variables. All differences were considered statistically significant at $p < 0.05$.

3. Results

3.1. Characteristics of Patients

The demographics and characteristics of the patients treated with CRRT are presented in Table 1. Two hundred and sixty-three patients were included, 212 in group A and 51 in group B. The overall mean age was significantly lower in group B than in group A ($p < 0.001$). There were significantly more patients in group B, especially those aged 1 to 11 months, 3 to 5 years, and 11 to 14 years ($p = 0.003$, $p = 0.022$, $p = 0.013$, respectively).

The use of inotropic agents at CRRT initiation was also significantly higher in group B than in group A ($p < 0.001$). The differences in the male-to-female ratio (17/34 versus 87/125) and the mean durations in the ICU before CRRT initiation were not significantly different between the two groups ($p > 0.05$).

Table 1. Characteristics of patients receiving continuous renal replacement therapy (CRRT).

Variables	Number of Patients (%)		p-Value
	Group A (n = 51)	Group B (n = 212)	
Age	5.0 ± 0.0	3.01 ± 0.21	<0.001
<1 month	0 (0.0%)	8 (3.8%)	0.361
1–11 month	1 (2.0%)	37 (17.5%)	0.003
1–2 year	5 (9.8%)	43 (20.3%)	0.082
3–5 year	15 (29.4%)	33 (15.6%)	0.022
6–10 year	12 (23.5%)	38 (17.9%)	0.360
11–14 year	14 (27.5%)	28 (13.2%)	0.013
15–18 year	4 (7.8%)	25 (11.8%)	0.419
Sex			0.312
Male	17 (33.3%)	87 (41.0%)	0.312
Vasopressors at CRRT initiation			<0.001
0	14 (27.5%)	154 (72.6%)	<0.001
>1	37 (72.5%)	58 (27.4%)	<0.001
ICU duration before CRRT (hours)	6.72 ± 6.39	5.78 ± 6.80	0.476

CRRT: continuous renal replacement therapy; ICU: intensive care unit.

The diagnoses of patients who received CRRT were renal disease (e.g., nephrotic syndrome and hemolytic uremic syndrome (HUS)), malignancy and drug intoxication. Cardiac diseases were significantly higher in group B than in group A ($p = 0.001$), and they negatively affect outcome. Malignancy was the most common underlying disease in both groups (70.6% in group A and 36.3% in group B). In contrast to cardiac disease, malignancy was more frequent in group A than in group B, with a statistically significant difference ($p < 0.001$) (Table 2).

Table 2. Underlying diseases of patients receiving CRRT.

Parameter	Number of Patients (%)		p-Value
	Group A (n = 51)	Group B (n = 212)	
Neurologic disease	5 (9.8%)	43 (20.3%)	0.112
Cardiac disease	2 (3.8%)	31 (14.6%)	0.001
Renal disease	3 (5.8%)	16 (7.5%)	1.000
Nephrotic syndrome	1 (1.9%)	2 (0.9%)	1.000
Obstructive uropathy	0 (0.0%)	2 (0.9%)	1.000
HUS	1 (1.9%)	3 (1.4%)	0.580
Rhabdomyolysis	0 (0.0%)	4 (1.9%)	1.000
Denys-Drash syndrome	1 (1.9%)	1 (0.5%)	0.351
AKI on CKD [+]	0 (0.0%)	4 (1.9%)	1.000
Liver disease	1 (2.0%)	20 (9.4%)	0.088
Malignancy	36 (70.6%)	77 (36.3%)	<0.001
No tumor lysis syndrome	35 (68.7%)	72 (34.0%)	<0.001
Tumor lysis syndrome	1 (1.9%)	5 (2.3%)	1.000
Drug intoxication	0 (0.0%)	1 (0.5%)	1.000
Pulmonary disease	1 (2.0%)	11 (5.2%)	0.471
Metabolic disease	1 (2.0%)	1 (0.5%)	0.351
Immune deficiency	0 (0.0%)	1 (0.5%)	1.000
Sepsis	1 (2.0%)	11 (5.2%)	0.471
Other	1 (2.0%)	0 (0.0%)	0.194

CRRT: continuous renal replacement therapy; HUS: hemolytic uremic syndrome; AKI: acute kidney injury; CKD: chronic kidney disease. [+] Patients who are CKD stage 3–5, not depending upon the cause of CKD. These patients received CRRT due to aggravation of AKI.

The indications for initiating CRRT are listed in Table 3. The most common indications for CRRT in both groups were oliguria refractory to diuretic treatment (54.9% in group A and 49.5% in group B). Fluid overload and sepsis were marked significantly higher in group B than in group A ($p = 0.041$, $p = 0.027$, respectively).

Table 3. Indications of initiating CRRT.

Indication	Total Number of Patients (%) *		p-Value
	Group A (n = 51)	Group B (n = 212)	
Oliguria	28(54.9%)	105(49.5%)	0.491
Fluid overload	28(54.9%)	83(39.2%)	0.041
Uremia	27(52.9%)	96(45.3%)	0.325
Metabolic acidosis	3(5.9%)	30(14.2%)	0.156
Electrolyte imbalance	8(15.7%)	20(9.4%)	0.208
Sepsis	9(17.6%)	16(7.5%)	0.027
Others [†]	1(2.0%)	8(3.8%)	1.000

CRRT: continuous renal replacement therapy. * Duplicates are allowed. [†] Other indications contain kidney transplantation, applied immediately after continuous ambulatory peritoneal dialysis catheter insertion, rhabdomyolysis, operation, etc.

Table 4 demonstrates a comparison of the laboratory variables between the group A and B. There were statistically significant differences between the groups in white blood cell counts ($p = 0.022$) and platelet counts ($p < 0.001$). Other parameters, including blood urea nitrogen (BUN) and creatinine, had no significant difference ($p > 0.05$).

Table 4. Laboratory results of patients receiving CRRT.

Parameter	Group A (n = 51)	Group B (n = 212)	p-Value
Complete blood count			
WBC (/mm^3)	6584.78 ± 8331.47	12822.82 ± 12368.29	0.022
Hemoglobin (g/L)	9.32 ± 2.53	9.63 ± 2.31	0.569
Hematocrit (%)	26.83 ± 7.52	29.33 ± 7.53	0.147
Platelet count (×10^3/µL)	81.30 ± 61.36	160.84 ± 149.86	<0.001
Coagulation tests			
Prothrombin Time (s)	30.53 ± 35.66	28.14 ± 29.32	0.737
aPTT (s)	71.00 ± 50.98	72.87 ± 55.14	0.884
ABGA			
pH	7.33 ± 0.17	7.27 ± 0.18	0.147
pCO$_2$ (mmHg)	44.21 ± 26.20	41.98 ± 25.57	0.704
pO$_2$ (mmHg)	92.20 ± 73.53	99.97 ± 67.20	0.619
Lactate (mg/dL)	4.20 ± 0.00	7.03 ± 5.90	0.634
Routine chemistry			
Glucose (mg/dL)	135.32 ± 103.59	144.63 ± 82.83	0.644
Potassium (mg/dL)	4.11 ± 1.18	4.43 ± 1.50	0.342
tCO$_2$ (mg/dL)	20.27 ± 8.09	17.29 ± 7.17	0.081
BUN (mg/dL)	32.60 ± 18.43	39.21 ± 38.54	0.433
Creatinine (mg/dL)	1.53 ± 1.30	1.97 ± 2.95	0.497

WBC: white blood cell; aPTT: activated partial thromboplastin time; ABGA: arterial blood gas analysis; pH: acidity; pCO$_2$: partial pressure of carbon dioxide; pO$_2$: partial pressure of oxygen; tCO$_2$: total carbon dioxide; BUN: blood urea nitrogen.

3.2. Technical Characteristics of CRRT

The details of the technical characteristics of CRRT are shown in Table 5. In the univariate analyses, more children in group B significantly received a combination of diffusion and convection (CVVHDF)

($p < 0.001$) and fewer received the diffusion-only CRRT modality (CVVHD) ($p < 0.001$). In both groups, only one patient received the convective modality (CVVH).

Table 5. Technical characteristics of CRRT.

Characteristics	Number of Patients (%)		p-Value
	Group A (n = 51)	Group B (n = 212)	
Modality			<0.001
CVVH	0 (0.7%)	1 (0.5%)	1.000
CVVHD	47 (92.2%)	17 (8.0%)	<0.001
CVVHDF	4 (7.8%)	194 (91.5%)	<0.001
Anticoagulation			<0.001
No anticoagulation	29 (56.9%)	119 (56.1%)	0.925
Heparin	19 (37.2%)	22 (10.4%)	<0.001
Nafamostat mesilate	2 (3.9%)	60 (28.3%)	<0.001
Nafamostat mesilate → Heparin	0 (0.0%)	6 (2.8%)	0.600
Heparin → Nafamostat mesilate	1 (2.0%)	5 (2.4%)	1.000
Initial catheter position			<0.001
Left femoral	13 (25.5%)	70 (33.0%)	0.299
Right femoral	21 (41.2%)	54 (25.5%)	0.026
Right internal jugular	1 (2.0%)	26 (12.3%)	0.036
Left internal jugular	0 (0.0%)	19 (9.0%)	0.029
Subclavian	7 (13.7%)	16 (7.5%)	0.131
ECMO (PCPS)	0 (0.0%)	27 (12.7%)	0.004
No information *	9 (17.6%)	0 (0.0%)	<0.001
Blood flow rate (mL/min)	89.86 ± 36.13	70.64 ± 29.59	0.001
Range	30–180	15–120	0.001

CRRT: continuous renal replacement therapy; CVVH: continuous veno-venous hemofiltration. CVVHD: continuous veno-venous hemodialysis; CVVHDF: continuous veno-venous hemodiafiltration ECMO: extracorporeal membrane oxygenation; PCPS: percutaneous cardiopulmonary support. * There was no information about catheter position in the patient chart.

A total of 148 (56.3%) patients were initiated on CRRT without anticoagulants. More patients in group B were initiated on CRRT with a single infusion of nafamostat mesilate ($p < 0.001$) and a single dose of heparin ($p < 0.001$) once the hemofilter clotted within 12 hours. When anticoagulation started, six (2.8%) patients in group B were switched from heparin to nafamostat mesylate, and five (2.4%) patients were switched from nafamostat mesilate to heparin, but it was not statistically significant ($p > 0.05$). The mean blood flow rate was lower in group B than in group A ($p = 0.001$).

The most common sites of insertion of the initial hemocatheter are the right and left femoral veins in groups A and B, respectively. Since the administration of extracorporeal membrane oxygenation (ECMO)-CRRT to a patient in January 2, 2012, all 27 (12.7%) patients who underwent simultaneous ECMO and CRRT belonged in group B ($p = 0.004$). In most of such cases, the CRRT pump was cannulated into the ECMO circuit. There were only two cases in 2013, including the first case; however, the number of cases had been increasing dramatically over the years following the increase in the rate of CRRT utilization (Figure 1).

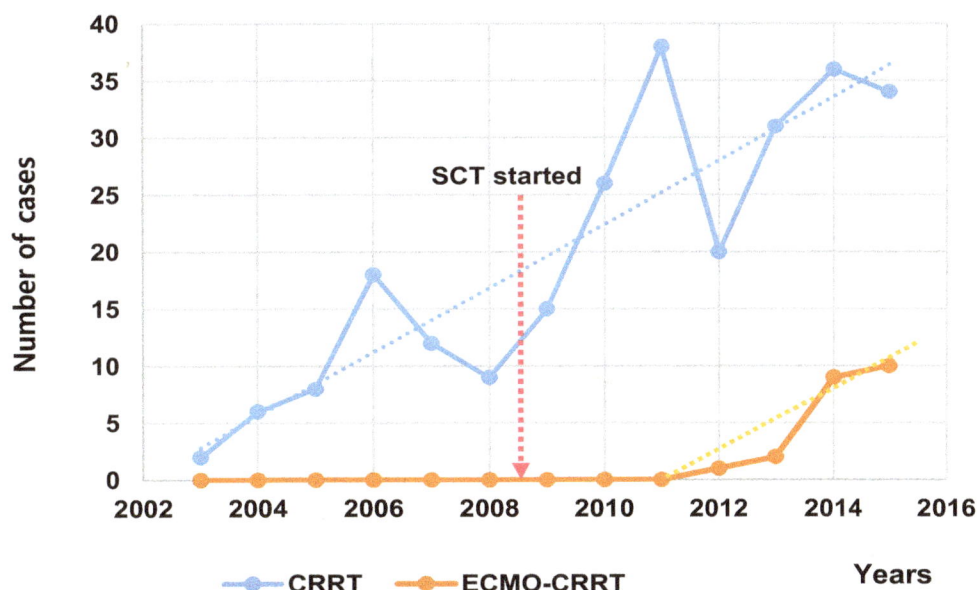

Figure 1. Distribution of CRRT and ECMO-CRRT numbers according to the years. CRRT: continuous renal replacement therapy; ECMO: extracorporeal membrane oxygenation; SCT: specialized CRRT team.

Three different types of CRRT machines were used in pediatric patients: the MultiFiltrate™ CRRT device (FMC), PRISMA® (Gambro Healthcare, Lakewood, CO, USA), and PRISMAFLEX® (Gambro Healthcare). Both PRISMA® and PRISMAFLEX® were more frequently used in group B than in group A, with a statistically significant difference ($p < 0.001$, $p < 0.001$). Only one patient received CRRT with the FMC machine (Table 6).

Table 6. Distribution of CRRT machines which used to patients.

CRRT Machines	Number of Patients (%)		p-Value
	Group A ($n = 51$)	Group B ($n = 212$)	
PRISMA ®	51 (100.0%)	166 (78.3%)	<0.001
PRISMAFLEX ®	0 (0.0%)	45 (21.2%)	<0.001
FMC ®	0 (0.0%)	1 (0.5%)	1.000

CRRT: continuous renal replacement therapy.

Table 7 shows a comparison of the outcomes and parameters between two groups. There were no differences in the duration between CRRT, number of filters used and transfusion during CRRT treatment run, and urine output. Mortality also showed no statistically significance between both groups ($p > 0.05$).

Table 7. Comparison of outcomes and parameters between the groups in patients receiving CRRT.

Valuables	Group A ($n = 51$)	Group B ($n = 212$)	p-Value
Duration of CRRT ± SD (days)	6.72 ± 6.39	5.85 ± 6.83	0.508
Number of filter use during CRRT ± SD (n) [†]	3.67 ± 3.66	4.79 ± 4.39	0.091
Number of TF during CRRT ± SD (n) [†]	0.53 ± 1.50	0.20 ± 0.59	0.133
%FO at CRRT (%)	5.97 ± 7.61	7.35 ± 8.40	0.348
Urine output rate at CRRT (mL/kg/h)	1.24 ± 1.53	1.49 ± 1.80	0.427
CRRT mortality, n (%)	34 (66.7%)	150 (70.8%)	0.863

CRRT: continuous renal replacement therapy; TF: transfusion; %FO: percent of fluid overload; SD: standard deviation.
[†] Number of filters used and TFs during CRRT were counted per patient.

4. Discussion

In our study, the increase in the use of CRRT followed the general world trend. In our center, there are about 10 cases of PD, including acute peritoneal dialysis and continuous ambulatory peritoneal dialysis, and about 10 cases of intermittent HD annually. In the same periods in which CRRT data were compared, from March 2003 to July 2008, patients treated with PD and HD numbered 90. On the other hand, from August 2008 to April 2016, patients treated with PD and HD numbered 160. Confirming the general trend, CRRT increased more in group B than group A. The possible reasons are: (1) Before CRRT was developed, only PD could be applied to children, but PD could be dangerous for children in poor condition when inserting PD catheter through the abdomen by major surgery. Compared to PD surgery, hemo-catheter insertion is easier to insert with short duration. (2) We could further consider applying CRRT in ICU because HD has hemodynamic problems in children lighter than 20 kg with unstable vital signs.

CRRT is an important treatment modality in the field of intensive care. In critically ill children, appropriate treatment has a significant impact on their survival or prognosis. However, research on CRRT has been delayed compared to that on HD or PD worldwide because CRRT must be administered for 24 hours a day, almost all CRRT machines can only be used in the ICU, and a skilled physician is needed to operate these machines. Like elsewhere, in Korea, the numbers of skilled pediatric nephrologists, pediatric intensivists, and well-trained CRRT-specialized nurses are very small, and the number of pediatric patients is much smaller than that of adults. These factors make research on pediatric CRRT difficult.

According to our results, most patients undergoing CRRT were younger than 10 (73.0%), and there were significantly more infants aged 1 to 11 months and children aged 3 to 5 years after initiating SCT ($p = 0.003$, $p = 0.022$). Furthermore, eight neonates were newly started on CRRT. Young patients develop acute kidney injury (AKI) in the early stage, which might progress rapidly, thus requiring renal replacement. If children develop AKI, they should be carefully monitored in the ICU, and early initiation of CRRT should be considered. The intervention of a SCT exclusively dedicated to pediatric CRRT can avoid the dispersion of knowledge by concentrating the expertise in the hands of few, highly specialized operators, thereby maximally exploiting the information coming from a restricted number of patients.

The most common positions for catheter insertion were the left and right femoral veins (60.1%). Probably, as the number of younger patients increases, the femoral site is more easily accessible without ultrasonographic guidance. Besides, as the technique improved, entrance into the right and left internal jugular veins, which was previously difficult, became significantly easier after SCT ($p = 0.036$, $p = 0.029$). Along with the worldwide trend, we increased the number of patients treated with CRRT in recent years (see Figure 1). Before SCT, some patients were initiated on CRRT in the emergency room or in the ward rather than in the ICU. The advent of a SCT allowed us a more specific control over a larger number of patients, standardization of procedures, and catheter related problems. Although not measurable, this may have had a positive impact on patient treatment.

For acceptable number of patients, there were more who started CRRT without vasopressors, and less started on vasopressors in group B, indicating, likely, the early use of CRRT ($p < 0.001$). Our study also showed a significant reduction in blood flow rate significantly after the start of the SCT activity ($p = 0.001$). A possible explanation is the improvement of the machine and filter performance, together with the ability of the SCT to cope with the improvement of technology, in order to obtain adequate results with lesser blood flow rates, and consequently, less hemodynamic stress. SCT may allow for improving diagnose the early AKI, giving early application of CRRT, facilitating decision-making and standardized safe extracorporeal therapy.

Similar to other studies [17,18], the CVVHDF mode was the most common modality used in our study. The initial version of CRRT, which used continuous arteriovenous (AV) filtration modes, is very different from the present one. Because the AV mode is maintained by the patient's own cardiac output, it showed a high access complication rate; thus, it was not widely applied [21]. Since 2000, after the development of external venovenous circuit pumps, the number of cases using CRRT greatly increased, and it is now a standard therapy for AKI. It effectively resolves fluid retention and improves the electrolyte imbalance simultaneously, especially the CVVHDF mode, which is the most recent modality among the external venovenous modes. In a similar context, the use of PRISMAFLEX®, a more specialized CRRT machine for children, also has increased.

There were 27 (10.3%) patients on percutaneous cardiopulmonary support or with ECMO connected to CRRT. In particular, since the first success of ECMO-CRRT in 2012, the rate of ECMO-CRRT utilization has increased rapidly (Figure 1). As mentioned above, this may be due to the fact that the CRRT backup of the SCT has performed well following the development of ECMO technology. The methods of CRRT connection to ECMO, duration of use, and the difference in survival rate were not separately analyzed in this study. Additional studies should be undertaken if plasmapheresis is performed simultaneously with CRRT in patients with liver disease.

The major difference in the use of anticoagulants is that citrate was used in patients with a bleeding tendency in the US study [17], whereas nafamostat mesilate is used in Korea because citrate is not licensed in Korea. In some studies, nafamostat mesilate has been known to have fewer complications, such as hypocalcemia, compared to citrate [22,23]. Because well-trained CRRT-specialized nurses are more efficient in handling nafamostat mesilate, the use of nafamostat mesilate significantly increased after the SCT was established ($p < 0.001$). In Korea, compared with Japan or China, especially in single-group institutions like ours, it is surprising and unusual that nafamostat mesilate has been largely used without notable side effects so far.

Fluid overload or oliguria was an important indication for initiating CRRT in this study. %FO was not significant in the univariate analysis ($p = 0.348$); however, higher %FO indication to CRRT in group B probably reflects an improved sensitization to the %FO importance in outcome determination; i.e., what is expectable in more current times. Although %FO was an important factor to initiate CRRT in the Prospective Pediatric Continuous Renal Replacement Therapy (ppCRRT) Registry study [17], it was not very significant in this study. This could be because the %FO was not accurately measured before and after CRRT.

The limitations of our study are as follows: Since this was a single-center study, it might have had some bias. Moreover, this was a retrospective study. Over this study period, there were significant changes in the development of machines, technique, and proficiency of the SCT, including the pediatric physicians and CRRT-specialized nurses. In addition, although the number of patients with CRRT increased, it could not be associated with SCT because of other factors, such as increased number of beds in ICU, CRRT machines, and critically ill patients in our center compared to other hospitals. Moreover, univariate analysis of both neonates and 1 to 2-year-old infants showed no statistical significance ($p = 0.361$, $p = 0.082$), but no accurate reason for this could be identified. This could be due to a bias in the process of collecting data and selecting patients.

Nevertheless, Severance Hospital is one of the five major hospitals in Korea, and the number of patients who underwent CRRT in this single center is almost similar to the number of patients in 13 major hospitals in the US. In addition, the study period was relatively longer than that of the ppCRRT (14 versus 5 years), reflecting almost all of the cases of pediatric CRRT in Korea. Moreover, since this was a study of Korean children, it also reflects specific ethnic and national characteristics compared with the US studies. The application of SCT to pediatric patients under the collaboration of pediatric nephrologists, pediatric intensivists, and CRRT-specialized nurses has not been reported worldwide and has never been reported in the US.

There have been no multicentric CRRT studies in pediatric patients worldwide, apart from the US ppCRRT. Since 2005, when ppCRRT was implemented, there has been no significant research on pediatric CRRT. Based on this study, an effort should be made in Korea to design an index to predict the mortality and increase the survival of patients.

5. Conclusions

The creation of a homogenous group with common tasks, interests, and devotion is essential in managing pediatric CRRT. This is the first study to have identified that the SCT and the organic collaboration of pediatric nephrologists, pediatric intensivists, and CRRT-specialized nurses could have widened the indication of CRRT for critically ill children with AKI and improved management of our patients.

Although CRRT is used as a first-line treatment for severe AKI in developed countries, it has not yet been introduced in less developed countries. In this global point of view, thorough CRRT training, introduction, and application for physicians are necessary. Further prospective studies will be necessary to evaluate the additional factors for sensitive markers of a SCT efficacy.

Author Contributions: Conceptualization, K.H.L., K.W.K. and J.I.S.; Methodology, K.H.L., I.S.S., J.T.P., J.H.K., K.W.K. and J.I.S.; Software, J.T.P. and J.I.S.; Validation, K.H.L., I.S.S., J.T.P., J.H.K., K.W.K. and J.I.S.; Formal Analysis, K.H.L.; Investigation, J.W.S., M.R.P. and J.H.L.; Resources, Y.H.K., K.W.K. and J.I.S.; Data Curation, K.H.L., I.S.S., K.W.K. and J.I.S.; Writing—Original Draft Preparation, K.H.L.; Writing—Review & Editing, K.H.L., J.T.P., J.H.K., K.W.K. and J.I.S.; Visualization, K.H.L., I.S.S., K.W.K. and J.I.S.; Supervision, I.S.S., J.T.P., J.H.K., K.W.K. and J.I.S. All authors had full access to all of the study data. All authors reviewed, wrote, and approved the final version. The corresponding author was responsible for the final decision to submit the paper for publication. All authors have read and agreed to the published version of the manuscript.

Acknowledgments: The Institutional Review Board and Research Ethics Committee of Yonsei University Severance Hospital approved this study (4-2018-0883). We were given exemption from getting informed consent by the IRB because the study was a retrospective study, personal identifiers were completely removed, and the data were analyzed anonymously. Our study was conducted according to the ethical standards laid down in the 1964 Declaration of Helsinki and its later amendments.

References

1. Kellum, J.A.; Lameire, N.; Aspelin, P.; Barsoum, R.S.; Burdmann, E.A.; Goldstein, S.L.; Herzog, C.A.; Joannidis, M.; Kribben, A.; Levey, A.S.; et al. Kidney Disease: Improving Global Outcomes (KDIGO) Acute Kidney Injury Work Group. KDIGO clinical practice guideline for acute kidney injury. *Kidney Int.* **2012**, 2 (Suppl. S1), 1–138.
2. Hoste, E.A.; Clermont, G.; Kersten, A.; Venkataraman, R.; Angus, D.C.; De Bacquer, D.; Kellum, J.A. RIFLE criteria for acute kidney injury are associated with hospital mortality in critically ill patients: A cohort analysis. *Crit. Care* **2006**, 10, R73. [CrossRef]
3. Selewski, D.T.; Cornell, T.T.; Heung, M.; Troost, J.P.; Ehrmann, B.J.; Lombel, R.M.; Blatt, N.B.; Luckritz, K.; Hieber, S.; Gajarski, R.; et al. Validation of the KDIGO acute kidney injury criteria in a pediatric critical care population. *Intensive Care Med.* **2014**, 40, 1481–1488. [CrossRef]
4. Sutherland, S.M.; Byrnes, J.J.; Kothari, M.; Longhurst, C.A.; Dutta, S.; Garcia, P.; Goldstein, S.L. AKI in hospitalized children: Comparing the pRIFLE, AKIN, and KDIGO definitions. *Clin. J. Am. Soc. Nephrol.* **2015**, 10, 554–561. [CrossRef] [PubMed]
5. Uchino, S.; Kellum, J.A.; Bellomo, R.; Doig, G.S.; Morimatsu, H.; Morg-era, S.; Schetz, M.; Tan, I.; Bouman, C.; Macedo, E.; et al. Acute renal failure in critically ill patients: A multina-tional, multicenter study. *JAMA* **2005**, 294, 813–818. [CrossRef] [PubMed]
6. Mehta, R.L.; Burdmann, E.A.; Cerdá, J.; Feehally, J.; Finkelstein, F.; García-García, G.; Godin, M.; Jha, V.; Lameire, N.H.; Levin, N.W.; et al. Recognition and management of acute kidney injury in the International Society of Nephrology 0by25 Global Snapshot: A multinational cross-sectional study. *Lancet* **2016**, 387, 2017–2025. [CrossRef]
7. Lameire, N.H.; Bagga, A.; Cruz, D.; De Maeseneer, J.; Endre, Z.; Kellum, J.A.; Liu, K.D.; Mehta, R.L.; Pannu, N.; Van Biesen, W.; et al. Acute kidney injury: An increasing global concern. *Lancet* **2013**, 382, 170–179. [CrossRef]

8. Kaddourah, A.; Basu, R.K.; Bagshaw, S.M.; Goldstein, S.L. AWARE Investigators. Epidemiology of Acute Kidney Injury in Critically Ill Children and Young Adults. *N. Engl. J. Med.* **2017**, *376*, 11–20. [CrossRef]

9. Kramer, P.; Wigger, W.; Rieger, J.; Matthaei, D.; Scheler, F. Arteriovenous haemofiltration: A new and simple method for treatment of over-hydrated patients resistant to diuretics. *Klin. Wochenschr.* **1977**, *55*, 1121–1122. [CrossRef]

10. Ronco, C.; Brendolan, A.; Bragantini, L.; Chiaramonte, S.; Fabris, A.; Feriani, M.; Frigiola, A.; La Greca, G. Treatment of acute renal failure in the newborn by continuous arteriovenous hemofiltration. *Trans. Am. Soc. Artif. Intern. Organs* **1985**, *31*, 634–638.

11. Riegel, W.; Habicht, A.; Ulrich, C.; Kohler, H. Hepatoactive substances eliminated by continuous venovenous hemofiltration in acute renal failure patients. *Kidney Int. Suppl.* **1999**, *72*, S67–S70. [CrossRef]

12. Ronco, C.; Bellomo, R. Critical care nephrology: The time has come. *Nephrol. Dial. Transplant.* **1998**, *13*, 264–267. [CrossRef] [PubMed]

13. Endre, Z.H. The role of nephrologist in the intensive care unit. *Blood. Purif.* **2017**, *43*, 78–81. [CrossRef]

14. Gilbert, R.W.; Caruso, D.M.; Foster, K.N.; Canulla, M.V.; Nelson, M.L.; Gilbert, E.A. Development of a continuous renal replacement program in critically ill patients. *Am. J. Surg.* **2002**, *184*, 526–532. [CrossRef]

15. Kee, Y.K.; Kim, E.J.; Park, K.S.; Han, S.G.; Han, I.M.; Yoon, C.Y.; Lee, E.; Joo, Y.S.; Kim, D.Y.; Lee, M.J.; et al. The effect of specialized continuous renal replacement therapy team in acute kidney injury patients treatment. *Yonsei Med. J.* **2015**, *56*, 658–665. [CrossRef]

16. Oh, H.J.; Lee, M.J.; Kim, C.H.; Kim, D.Y.; Lee, H.S.; Park, J.T.; Na, S.; Han, S.H.; Kang, S.-W.; Koh, S.O.; et al. The benefit of specialized team approaches in patients with acute kidney injury undergoing continuous renal replacement therapy: Propensity score matched analysis. *Crit. Care* **2014**, *18*, 454. [CrossRef]

17. Goldstein, S.L.; Somers, M.J.; Brophy, P.D.; Bunchman, T.E.; Baum, M.; Blowey, D.; Mahan, J.D.; Flores, F.X.; Fortenberry, J.D.; Chua, A.; et al. The Prospective Pediatric Continuous Renal Replacement Therapy (ppCRRT) Registry: Design, development and data assessed. *Int. J. Artif. Organs* **2005**, *427*, 9–14. [CrossRef]

18. Symons, J.M.; Chua, A.N.; Somers, M.J.; Baum, M.A.; Bunchman, T.E.; Benfield, M.R.; Brophy, P.D.; Blowey, D.; Fortenberry, J.D.; Chand, D.; et al. Demographic characteristics of pediatric continuous renal replacement therapy: A report of the prospective pediatric continuous renal replacement therapy registry. *Clin. J. Am. Soc. Nephrol.* **2007**, *2*, 732–738. [CrossRef]

19. Goldstein, S.L.; Somers, M.J.; Baum, M.A.; Symons, J.M.; Brophy, P.D.; Blowey, D.; Bunchman, T.E.; Baker, C.; Mottes, T.; Mcafee, N.; et al. Pediatric patients with multi-organ dysfunction syndrome receiving continuous renal replacement therapy. *Kidney Int.* **2005**, *67*, 653–658. [CrossRef]

20. Goldstein, S.L.; Currier, H.; Graf, C.; Cosio, C.C.; Brewer, E.D.; Sachdeva, R. Outcome in children receiving continuous venovenous hemofiltration. *Pediatrics* **2001**, *107*, 1309–1312. [CrossRef]

21. Pannu, N.; Gibney, R.N. Renal replacement therapy in the intensive care unit. *Ther. Clin. Risk Manag.* **2005**, *1*, 141–150. [CrossRef]

22. Chadha, V.; Garg, U.; Warady, B.A.; Alon, U.S. Citrate clearance in children receiving continuous venovenous renal replacement therapy. *Pediatr. Nephrol.* **2002**, *16*, 819–824. [CrossRef]

23. Choi, J.Y.; Kang, Y.J.; Jang, H.M.; Jung, H.Y.; Cho, J.H.; Park, S.H.; Kim, Y.L.; Kim, C.D. Nafamostat Mesilate as an Anticoagulant During Continuous Renal Replacement Therapy in Patients with High Bleeding Risk: A Randomized Clinical Trial. *Medicine* **2015**, *94*, e2392. [CrossRef] [PubMed]

7

Common Inflammation-Related Candidate Gene Variants and Acute Kidney Injury in 2647 Critically Ill Finnish Patients

Laura M. Vilander [1,*], Suvi T. Vaara [1], Mari A. Kaunisto [2], Ville Pettilä [1] and The FINNAKI Study Group [†]

[1] Division of Intensive Care Medicine, Department of Anesthesiology, Intensive Care and Pain Medicine, University of Helsinki and Helsinki University Hospital, 00014 Helsinki, Finland; suvi.vaara@hus.fi (S.T.V.); ville.pettila@hus.fi (V.P.)

[2] Institute for Molecular Medicine Finland (FIMM), HiLIFE, University of Helsinki, 000014 Helsinki, Finland; mari.kaunisto@helsinki.fi

[*] Correspondence: laura.vilander@helsinki.fi

[†] Membership of the The FINNAKI Study Group is provided in the Acknowledgments.

Abstract: Acute kidney injury (AKI) is a syndrome with high incidence among the critically ill. Because the clinical variables and currently used biomarkers have failed to predict the individual susceptibility to AKI, candidate gene variants for the trait have been studied. Studies about genetic predisposition to AKI have been mainly underpowered and of moderate quality. We report the association study of 27 genetic variants in a cohort of Finnish critically ill patients, focusing on the replication of associations detected with variants in genes related to inflammation, cell survival, or circulation. In this prospective, observational Finnish Acute Kidney Injury (FINNAKI) study, 2647 patients without chronic kidney disease were genotyped. We defined AKI according to Kidney Disease: Improving Global Outcomes (KDIGO) criteria. We compared severe AKI (Stages 2 and 3, $n = 625$) to controls (Stage 0, $n = 1582$). For genotyping we used iPLEX^{TM} Assay (Agena Bioscience). We performed the association analyses with PLINK software, using an additive genetic model in logistic regression. Despite the numerous, although contradictory, studies about association between polymorphisms rs1800629 in *TNFA* and rs1800896 in *IL10* and AKI, we found no association (odds ratios 1.06 (95% CI 0.89–1.28, $p = 0.51$) and 0.92 (95% CI 0.80–1.05, $p = 0.20$), respectively). Adjusting for confounders did not change the results. To conclude, we could not confirm the associations reported in previous studies in a cohort of critically ill patients.

Keywords: acute kidney injury; genetic variation; human genetics

1. Introduction

Acute kidney injury (AKI) is a syndrome that often complicates critical illness and is associated with significant mortality and morbidity [1,2]. Thus, efforts to distinguish patients at risk for AKI are justifiable, but despite the advances in the understanding of the pathophysiology of AKI, reliable prediction of developing AKI in different clinical scenarios remains a challenge.

In our systematic review in 2014 we found that evidence about genetic predisposition to AKI was heterogeneous, the studies were of inadequate size and the findings were generally not replicated [3]. Based on these findings, we analyzed 27 common genetic variants that situate in genes previously associated with AKI in a Finnish sample of critically ill patients.

2. Materials and Methods

2.1. Patients

We prospectively recruited patients from 17 Finnish intensive care units (ICUs) in the Finnish acute Kidney Injury (FINNAKI) study. The FINNAKI study took place in the years 2011 and 2012, and the study design has been described previously [1]. We included all patients with an emergency ICU admission of any length and elective surgical patients with an expected duration of ICU stay longer than 24 h. We excluded patients that received maintenance dialysis. The complete exclusion criteria are reported in electronic Supplementary Materials (ESM).

Consent for the study was achieved from the patients or next of kin, at the initiation of the study or deferred. A separate consent for genetic analyses was obtained from all patients or their legal representatives. The Ethics Committee of the Department of Surgery in Helsinki University Hospital gave approval for the study (18/13/03/02/2010).

2.2. Definitions

We defined AKI according to Kidney Disease: Improving Global Outcomes (KDIGO) criteria [4]. We performed analyses using both the severe AKI phenotype (KDIGO Stages 2–3 compared to KDIGO 0) and the all-stage (1–3) AKI phenotype. We classified patients into AKI stages according to daily measurements of plasma creatinine and hourly measurements of urine output. Sepsis was defined according to the American College of Chest Physicians/Society of Critical Care Medicine (ACCP/SCCM) definition [5].

2.3. Data Collection

We collected routine data into Finnish Intensive Care Consortium prospective database (Tieto Ltd., Helsinki, Finland). In addition, we completed a standardized case reporting form (CRF) on admission, as well as daily for 5 days and at discharge from ICU. These study-specific data comprised health status previously and present, medications in use, information about some known AKI risk factors, evaluation of organ dysfunctions such as sepsis, and information about treatments administered.

2.4. DNA Samples and Genotyping

Deoxyribonucleic acid (DNA) was extracted from frozen blood samples collected at enrollment. DNA isolation was performed with Chemagic 360 intrument using Chemagic DNA Blood10k Kit, as instructed by the manufacturer (Perkin Elmer, Baesweiler, Germany). For genotyping, we diluted the sample concentration into 10 ng/μL.

We performed the genotyping in two subsequent assays, in the years 2015 and 2017, at the Genotyping Unit of Institute for Molecular Medicine Finland (FIMM), University of Helsinki. The Agena MassARRAY® system, along with the iPLEXTM Gold Assay (Agena BioscienceTM, San Diego, CA, USA) were used for the genotyping. Here, 20 ng of dried genomic DNA were used for genotyping reactions in 384-well plates using manufacturer's reagents, and according to their recommendations [6]. For designing primer sequences, MassARRAY Assay Design software (Agena BioscienceTM) was used (see ESM). The MassARRAY Compact System (Agena BioscienceTM) was used for data collection and TyperAnalyzer software (Agena BioscienceTM) for genotype calling. The quality control procedure consisted of checking the success rate, duplicate samples, control wells with water and testing for Hardy–Weinberg Equilibrium (HWE). In addition, all of the genotype calls were manually checked. The genotyping personnel were unaware of the clinical status of the patients.

In the year 2015 assay 49 samples (1.7% of 2968 samples) were rejected because of low success rate in the tested polymorphisms, and in the year 2017 assay the corresponding number was five samples (0.2% of 2968 samples).

For rs699 the success rate reached only 48% due to assay failure in half of the runs; however, the remainder of allele calling was possible with new extension primer and the results are thus reported.

2.5. Variant Selection

Variations in or nearby genes related to inflammation, circulation, and cell survival have been suggested in candidate polymorphism studies regarding AKI [7–27]. Additionally, the first hypothesis-free studies in AKI genetic predisposition have been published [28–30], with some replicated associations [31]. We chose to test polymorphisms in *TNFA* (rs1800629 [8,19,21–27]), *IL6* (rs1800796 [24,26] and rs1800795 [19,24,26], rs10499563, rs1474347, rs13306435, rs2069842 and rs2069830), *CXCL8* (rs4073 [27]), *IL10* (rs1800896 [19,21,23,25,26]), *NOS3* (rs2070744 [13,24]), *NFKB1A* (rs1050851 [32]), *AGT* (rs699 and rs2493133 [24]), *VEGFA* (rs2010963 and rs3025039 [27]), *EPO* (rs1617640 [14]), *SUFU* (rs10748825 [9]), *HIF1A* (rs11549465 [15]), *PNMT* (rs876493 [17]), *MPO* (rs7208693 [16]), *COMT* (rs4680 [10–12]), *HSPB1* (rs2868371 [33]), *SFTPD* (rs2243639 and rs721917 [34]), *HAMP* (rs10421768 [35]) and *BBS9* (rs10262995 [30]) genes (see definitions for abbreviations in ESM).

2.6. Statistical Analyses

We used SPSS Statistics version 22 (IBM Corp., Armonk, NY, USA) for analyzing the clinical and demographic variables. The analyses used were the Fisher's exact test in cross tabulation for categorical variables and the Mann–Whitney U for continuous variables. The data are presented as medians (with interquartile range), or absolute count (with percentage).

We performed the association test for genetic variants and AKI phenotype with logistic regression in the PLINK software [36]. We used the additive genetic model. For haplotype analysis, we checked for haploblocks with Haploview [37]. In addition, for polymorphisms in TNFA and IL10 we performed an epistasis test. The haplotype analysis and epistasis test were performed with the PLINK software [36]. In the primary analysis we compared patients with KDIGO stage 2 or 3 AKI to patients without AKI, as the primary outcome of the study. In the secondary analysis we compared all stage AKI (KDIGO 1, 2 or 3) to no AKI. In the tertiary analysis we included patients with chronic kidney disease and compared patients with KDIGO stage 2 or 3 AKI to patients without AKI in an adjusted analysis. We used similar covariates to our previously published article [31] (liver failure, body mass index (BMI), use of nonsteroidal anti-inflammatory drugs (NSAID) or warfarin as permanent medication, use of contrast dye prior to ICU admission, use of colloids prior to ICU admission, use of albumin prior to ICU admission, minimum platelet count, and simplified acute physiology score (SAPS) II without renal and age points), omitting the infection focus for irrelevant information, and maximum leucocyte count and operative admission to avoid multicollinearity, while including cardiac surgery status as well as sepsis status. The missing data within covariates (altogether 2.4%) were addressed by imputing (see ESM for details).

For all analyses, we considered a *p*-value of 0.002 significant after Bonferroni correction for multiple testing (0.05/25 = 0.002).

2.7. Power Calculations

We performed prospective power calculations to determine an appropriate sample size [38]. Assuming an effect size of 1.2 per risk allele (1.4 per homozygote genotype) and a minor allele frequency of 0.2, setting the level of significance to 0.005, there will be 96% (93% for homozygote genotype) power to detect an association in a sample of 1200 cases and 1800 controls.

3. Results

We recruited 2968 patients in the FINNAKI genetic study (Figure 1). We excluded 199 patients (6.7% of 2968 patients) with chronic kidney disease from the primary (green dashed line) and secondary (orange dashed line) analysis. In addition, 122 DNA samples failed at isolation. Of the remaining 2647 patients, 221 (8.3% of 2647) patients had stage 2 AKI, 404 (15.3% of 2647) had stage 3 AKI, and 1582 (59.8% of 2647) patients served as controls without AKI. Overall, 228 (10.9% of 2647) patients received renal replacement therapy (RRT). Moreover, 440 (16.6% of 2647) patients had an ambiguous phenotype

(KDIGO stage 1); we excluded them from the primary and the tertiary (blue dashed line) analysis. Table 1 presents patient demographics.

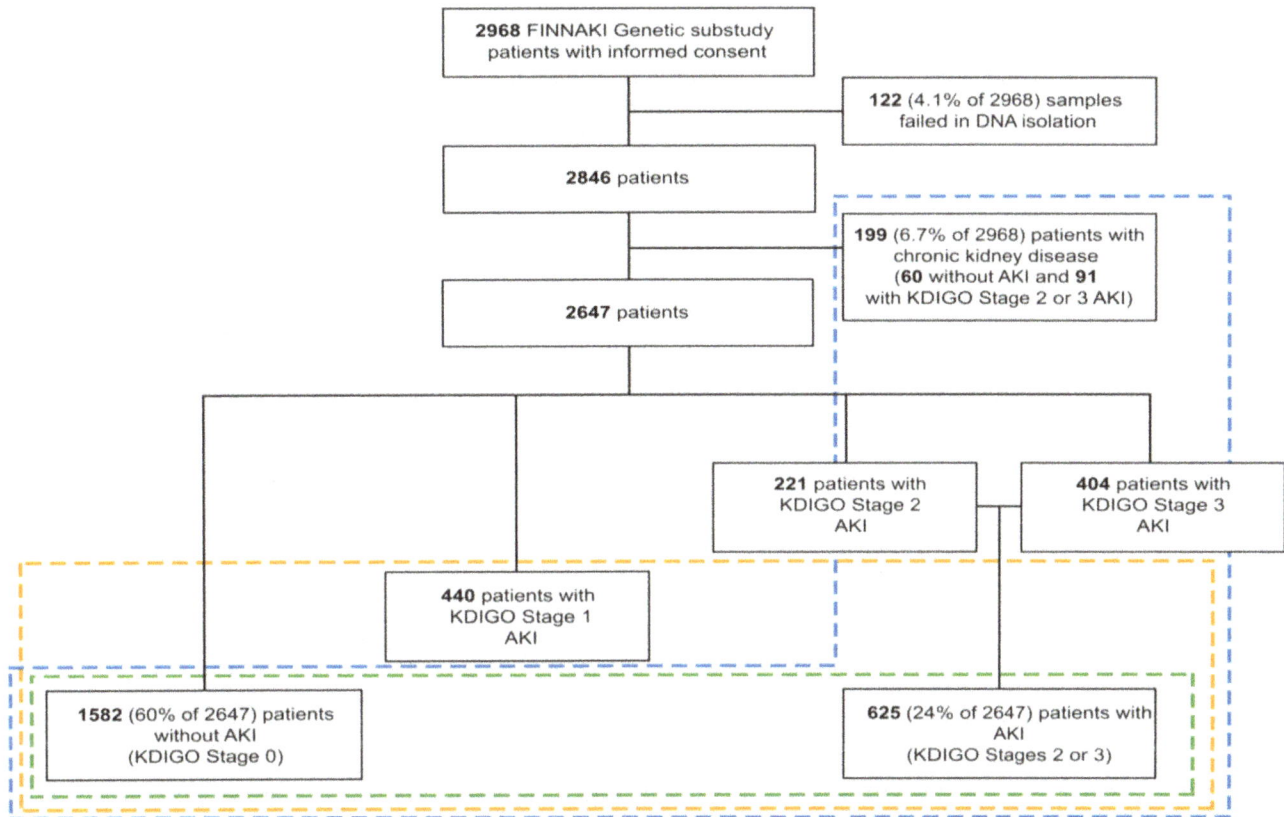

Figure 1. Study flowchart. Abbreviations: FINNAKI; Finnish Acute Kidney Injury; DNA, deoxyribonucleic acid; AKI, acute kidney injury; KDIGO, Kidney Disease: Improving Global Outcomes

Table 1. Demographics of altogether 2647 patients in the FINNAKI genetic substudy after excluding patients with maintenance dialysis. Data are presented according to presence of severe AKI (KDIGO stage 2 or 3, $n = 625$), presence of all stage AKI (KDIGO stage 1, 2, 3, $n = 1065$), or absence of AKI (KDIGO stage 0, $n = 1582$).

Characteristics	Data Available	AKI		No AKI	p *
		KDIGO stage 2 or 3	KDIGO stage 1, 2, 3		
Age (years)	2647	65 (54–74)	65 (54–75)	62 (48–72)	<0.001
Gender (male)	2647	409 (65.4)	700 (65.7)	980 (61.9)	0.130
BMI (kg/m^2)	2627	27.5 (24.5–31.3)	27.5 (24.2–31.2)	25.7 (23.1–28.7)	<0.001
Co-morbidities					
Arterial hypertension	2633	333 (53.3)	561 (52.9)	641 (40.8)	<0.001
Diabetes	2643	169 (27.0)	263 (24.7)	280 (17.7)	<0.001
Arteriosclerosis	2623	94 (15.1)	159 (15.0)	160 (10.2)	0.002
Chronic obstructive pulmonary disease	2630	43 (6.9)	81 (7.7)	136 (8.6)	0.195
Chronic liver disease	2617	46 (7.4)	59 (5.6)	51 (3.3)	<0.001
Systolic heart failure	2628	79 (12.7)	129 (12.2)	139 (8.8)	0.009
Baseline plasma creatinine (μmol/L)	2643	81.0 (68.9–94.0)	81.0 (69.0–94.0)	79.0 (68.0–94.0)	0.210
Pre ICU daily medication					
ACE inhibitor or ARB	2585	263 (42.8)	428 (41.1)	475 (30.8)	<0.001
NSAID	2538	73 (12.1)	112 (10.9)	118 (7.8)	0.002
Diuretic	2596	185 (29.8)	324 (30.8)	323 (20.9)	<0.001

Table 1. *Cont.*

Characteristics	Data Available	AKI	No AKI	*p* *
Metformin	2606	109 (17.6)	163 (15.5)	164 (10.6)	<0.001
Statin	2603	196 (31.6)	320 (30.5)	397 (25.6)	0.005
Corticosteroids	2614	56 (9.0)	94 (8.9)	105 (6.7)	0.070
Warfarin	2608	107 (17.2)	166 (15.8)	179 (11.5)	0.001
		KDIGO stage 2 or 3	**KDIGO stage 1, 2, 3**		
Treatments administered 48 h before admission					
Contrast medium	2632	120 (19.3)	223 (21.1)	417 (26.5)	<0.001
ACE inhibitor or ARB	2601	167 (27.3)	287 (27.5)	329 (21.1)	0.002
Diuretics	2570	217 (35.8)	353 (34.3)	360 (23.4)	<0.001
Colloids (gelatin or starch)	2479	229 (38.3)	395 (39.0)	394 (26.9)	<0.001
Albumin	2584	14 (2.3)	18 (1.7)	14 (0.9)	0.018
Type of admission					
Operative	2646	180 (28.8)	343 (32.2)	557 (35.2)	0.004
Cardiac surgery	2647	35 (5.6)	80 (7.5)	147 (9.3)	0.004
Emergency	2621	575 (92.6)	962 (91.1)	1386 (88.6)	0.005
SAPS II score 24 h without renal or age components	2614	24.0 (16.0–34.0)	24.0 (16.0–32.0)	20.0 (13.0–29.3)	<0.001
Mechanical ventilation	2647	432 (69.1)	776 (72.9)	1031 (65.2)	0.080
Sepsis	2647	309 (49.4)	500 (46.9)	362 (22.9)	<0.001
White blood cell count at admission, max (10^9/L)	2186	12.0 (8.3–17.4)	11.7 (8.2–16.8)	10.9 (7.8–15.3)	<0.001
Platelet count at admission, min (10^9/L)	2419	190.0 (116.5–263.5)	194.0 (127.0–265.0)	205.0 (153.0–268.0)	<0.001

* Comparison of No AKI to KDIGO stages 2 or 3 AKI. The *p*-values are calculated with Fisher's exact test for categorical variables and with Mann–Whitney U test for continuous variables. Data presented as medians and interquartile ranges for continuous variables, and absolute counts and percentages for categorical variables. Abbreviations: FINNAKI; Finnish Acute Kidney Injury; AKI, acute kidney injury; KDIGO, Kidney Disease: Improving Global Outcomes; BMI, body mass index; ICU, intensive care unit; ACE, angiotensin-converting enzyme; ARB, angiotensin II receptor blocker; NSAID, nonsteroidal anti-inflammatory drug; SAPS II, simplified acute physiology score II.

In the primary analysis, none of the previously reported associations replicated in our sample (Figure 2). Of note, the A-allele of rs1800629 in TNFA was not associated with AKI (odds ratio, OR 1.06, 95% confidence interval, CI 0.89–1.28, *p* = 0.51). In addition, the G-allele of rs1800896 in IL10 was not associated with AKI (OR 0.92, 95% CI 0.80–1.05, *p* = 0.20) (Table 2). In the epistasis test between A-allele of rs1800629 and G-allele of rs1800896 we detected no evidence of interaction (OR 1.10, *p* = 0.40). Frequencies of genotype combinations of these two variants are presented in Table 3, grouped according to their reported effect on protein production [25].

We tested IL6 for altogether seven variants and found no association with either endpoint. We found no variation in single nucleotide polymorphisms (SNPs) rs2069842 and rs2069830 in IL6; rs10499563 in IL6 was not in HWE (*p* = 0.034). The haplotypes of the two tested haploblocks were not associated with AKI (data shown in ESM).

The T-allele of rs3025039 in VEGFA had an odds ratio (OR) of 1.20 (95% CI 1.01–1.44, *p* = 0.044) for development of stage 2 or 3 AKI. This finding prevailed in the tertiary analysis (adjusted model, OR 1.21, 95% CI 1.00–1.45, *p* = 0.047; ESM, Table S1).

In the tertiary analysis the G-allele of rs10421768 in HAMP had an OR of 0.81 (95% CI 0.69–0.95, *p* = 0.0090) for development of stage 2 or 3 AKI; however, none of the variants had a statistically significant association in this adjusted model with CKD patients included (Table S1, ESM).

In the secondary analysis with all stage AKI as the endpoint the results did not change (ESM, Table S2).

The variants we investigated had minor allele frequencies ranging from 0.03 to 0.47 and the retrospectively calculated variant-specific power varied accordingly from 13.0% to 91.2% (ESM, Table S3).

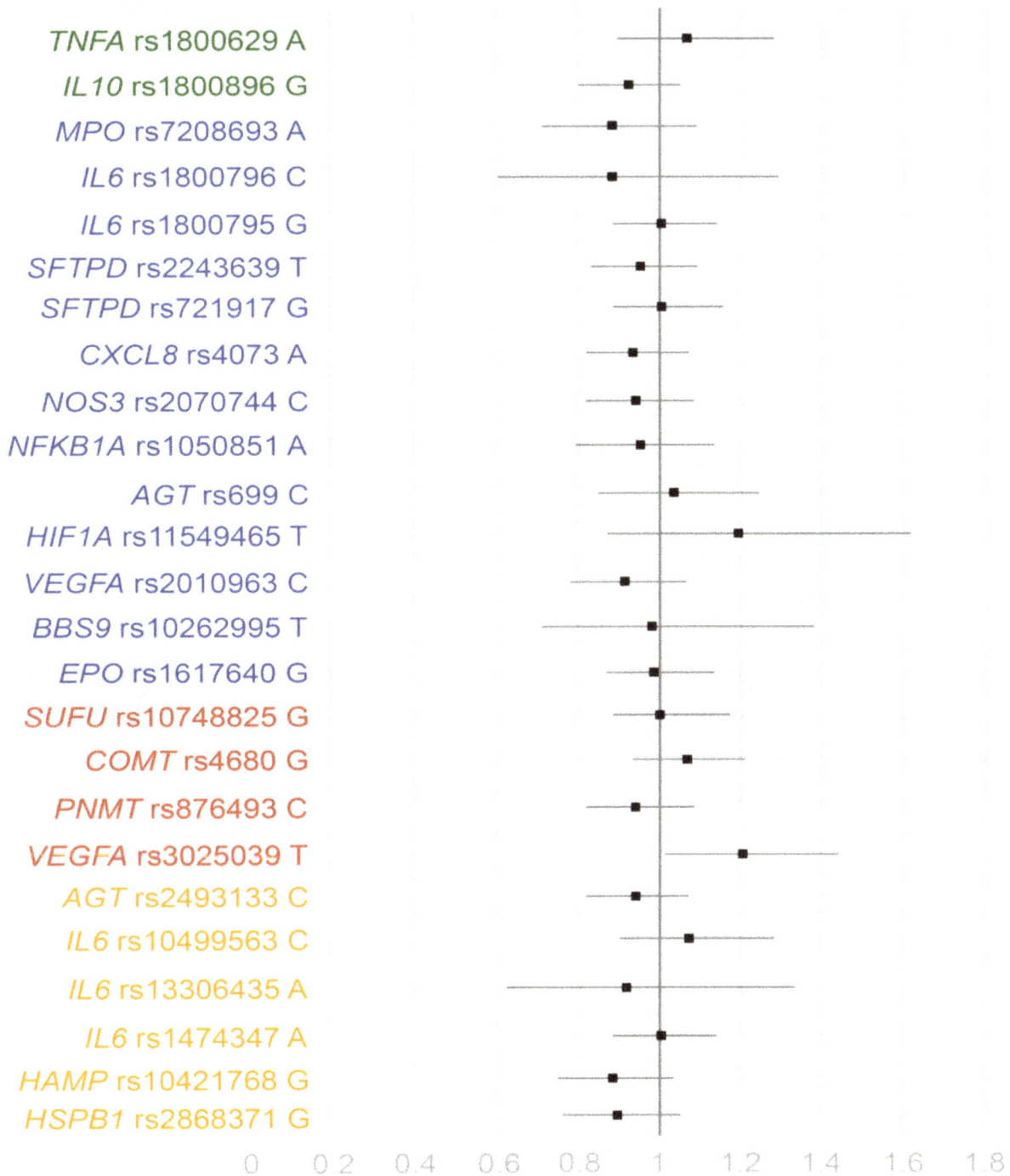

Figure 2. Odds ratios (OR) and confidence intervals (95% CI) for the minor allele for all the studied polymorphisms. For variants in green, there are several previous studies and both alleles have been reported to associate with AKI, variants in blue have been reported with same risk allele, variants in red have been reported with opposite risk allele, and variants in orange have not been previously reported in association to AKI.

Table 2. Association of genetic variants with acute kidney injury (AKI) KDIGO stages 2 and 3 compared to stage 0. Odds ratios (OR) and confidence intervals (95% CI) are reported for each copy of minor allele.

Gene	SNP	Patients	Minor Allele	MAF (Cases/Controls)	Additive Logistic OR	95% CI	p
TNFA	rs1800629	2174	A	0.15/0.14	1.06	0.89–1.28	0.51
IL10	rs1800896	2173	G	0.44/0.46	0.92	0.80–1.05	0.20
IL6	rs10499563	2192	C	0.15/0.14	1.07	0.90–1.28	0.45
	rs1800796	2197	C	0.03/0.03	0.88	0.60–1.29	0.51
	rs1800795	2189	G	0.47/0.47	1.00	0.88–1.14	0.97
	rs1474347	2187	A	0.47/0.47	1.00	0.88–1.14	1.00
	rs13306435	2199	A	0.03/0.03	0.91	0.62–1.33	0.62
CXCL8	rs4073	2193	A	0.42/0.42	0.93	0.82–1.07	0.31
NOS3	rs2070744	2174	C	0.34/0.36	0.94	0.82–1.08	0.37
NFKB1A	rs1050851	2196	A	0.16/0.17	0.95	0.79–1.13	0.54
AGT	rs699	1047	C	0.43/0.42	1.03	0.85–1.24	0.78
	rs2493133	2196	C	0.41/0.42	0.94	0.82–1.07	0.36
VEGFA	rs2010963	2170	C	0.22/0.24	0.91	0.78–1.06	0.22
	rs3025039	2195	T	0.16/0.14	1.20	1.01–1.44	0.044
EPO	rs1617640	2173	G	0.44/0.45	0.99	0.87–1.13	0.91
SUFU	rs10748825	2174	G	0.37/0.37	1.02	0.88–1.17	0.83
HIF1A	rs11549465	2173	T	0.05/0.04	1.19	0.87–1.62	0.28
PNMT	rs876493	2173	C	0.36/0.38	0.94	0.82–1.08	0.37
MPO	rs7208693	2174	A	0.10/0.12	0.88	0.71–1.09	0.23
COMT	rs4680	2173	G	0.47/0.45	1.06	0.93–1.21	0.39
HSPB1	rs2868371	2194	G	0.19/0.21	0.89	0.76–1.05	0.18
SFTPD	rs2243639	2199	T	0.39/0.40	0.95	0.83–1.09	0.47
	rs721917	2193	G	0.39/0.39	1.00	0.88–1.15	0.97
HAMP	rs10421768	2199	G	0.23/0.25	0.88	0.75–1.03	0.11
BBS9	rs10262995	2200	T	0.04/0.04	0.98	0.71–1.38	0.93

Abbreviations: AKI, acute kidney injury; KDIGO, Kidney Disease: Improving Global Outcomes; SNP, single nucleotide polymorphism; MAF, minor allele frequency; OR, odds ratio; CI, confidence interval; *TNFA*, tumor necrosis factor alpha; *IL10*, interleukin 10; *IL6*, interleukin 6; *CXCL8*, interleukin 8; *NOS3*, nitric oxide synthase 3; *NFKB1A*, nuclear factor of kappa light polypeptide gene enhancer in B-cells inhibitor, alpha; *AGT*, angiotensinogen; *VEGFA*, vascular endothelial growth factor; *EPO*, erythropoietin; *SUFU*, suppressor of fused homolog; *HIF1A*, hypoxia-inducible factor 1-alpha; *PNMT*, phenylethanolamine N-methyltransferase; *MPO*, myeloperoxidase; *COMT*, catechol-O-methyltransferase; *HSPB1*, heat shock protein family B (small) member 1; *SFTPD*, surfactant protein D; *HAMP*, hepcidin antimicrobial peptide; *BBS9*, Bardet–Biedl syndrome 9.

Table 3. Number of patients (percentage) with *TNFA* rs1800629 and *IL10* rs1800896 genotype combinations. Genotypes are grouped according to the reported effect in protein production. Acute kidney injury (AKI) KDIGO stages 2 and 3 (cases) compared to stage 0 (controls).

Genotype Combination	AKI (*n* = 615)	No AKI (*n* = 1558)
TNFA GG + *IL10* AA	138 (22%)	340 (22%)
TNFA GG + *IL10* GA + GG	311 (51%)	814 (52%)
TNFA GA + AA + *IL10* AA	52 (8%)	116 (8%)
TNFA GA + AA + *IL10* GA + GG	114 (19%)	288 (18%)

Abbreviations: TNFA, tumor necrosis factor alpha; IL10, interleukin 10; AKI, acute kidney injury; KDIGO, Kidney Disease: Improving Global Outcomes; OR, odds ratio. TNFA GG: TNF-α low producer; IL10 AA: IL-10 low producer; IL10 GA + GG: IL-10 intermediate + high producer; TNFA GA + AA: TNF-α high producer.

4. Discussion

In this study involving nearly 3000 critically ill adult patients, we were unable to replicate the previously reported associations between selected inflammation-related gene variants and AKI. The 27 tested polymorphisms are within 18 candidate genes, the majority of which relate to inflammation, cell survival, or circulation. Despite the suggestive findings in VEGFA and HAMP, we did not achieve the pre-set statistical significance after correcting for multiple comparisons.

The original studies reporting genetic associations have been generally underpowered, and of moderate quality only [3]. Majority of these studies investigated candidate polymorphisms with unknown biological function. Heterogeneity in reporting has hampered conduction of meta-analyses of reported associations [3,39]. In addition, the few replication attempts have given contradicting results. Moreover, most reports are from cardiac surgery patients, whereas septic and mixed ICU patients have been studied less [3]. In our prospective power calculation we determined that a sample of 1200 cases and 1800 controls would suffice to give a 96% power to detect an association, with realistic assumptions of minor allele frequency and effect size considering complex disease origin. However, the true effects of associations are known to be smaller than the ones reported by first authors [40,41]. In addition, false positive associations are numerous in genetic association studies to identify common variants [41]. This, along with population diversity is a possible explanation as to the failure in replication attempt [42]. Because of multiple variants tested, we used a more stringent level of significance. By using Bonferroni method we determined the acceptable level of type 1 error rate to 0.002.

The first results of hypothesis-free study designs in genetic predisposition to AKI have been published in septic [28] and cardiac surgery-associated AKI [29,30]. In their genome wide association study (GWAS), Stafford-Smith and coworkers [30] reported an association of polymorphism rs10262995 in BBS9 with cardiac surgery-associated AKI. However, in our cohort this association was not found.

One of the most studied polymorphisms is the rs1800629 in TNFA: the low producing genotype (GG) has been associated with more frequent and more severe AKI [7,8]. In addition, low producing genotype AA of variant rs1800896 in IL10 has been associated with AKI [7], along with combined genotype of rs1800629 GG + rs1800896 AA [19]. However, contradicting findings have been presented [22–26]. Additionally, TNFA and IL10 variations have been associated with sepsis development [43–45]. Of note, we were unable to detect any significant association between these polymorphisms or their combination in the epistasis test.

Vascular endothelial growth factor (VEGF) is a protein with shown effects in angiogenesis, cell survival and differentiation, as well as vascular permeability [46,47]. In our study, the T-allele in rs3025039 in VEGFA resulted in an OR of 1.20 for AKI (95% CI 1.01–1.44, $p = 0.044$); however, previously the C-allele has been reported to increase AKI risk [27]. In carriers of T-allele, the plasma VEGF levels are lower [48]. The T-allele has been suggested to relate to susceptibility to ARDS and mortality in ARDS [49,50]. Additionally, variation in VEGFA has been associated with diabetic nephropathy [51].

As the IL-6 cytokine has been associated with AKI development [52,53], we aimed to investigate the IL6 gene variation more broadly. We genotyped seven SNPs, five in addition to the two replication variants. However, two of these SNPs did not have any variation in our sample. The remaining five did not associate with AKI, even when studied as a haplotype. In sepsis, the SNP rs1800795 is not associated with susceptibility or mortality [54]. Consistently, rs1800795 does not correlate with the risk of end-stage renal disease [55]. Nevertheless, in patients with CKD, the SNP rs1800796 is suggested to predispose to sepsis and mortality [56]. However, due to multiple differing etiologies the predisposing genetic variants are generally unique to CKD [57–59].

The rs4680 in catechol-O-methyltransferase gene (COMT) causes an amino acid transition (Val158Met), which leads to lower (L) in comparison to higher (H) enzyme activity [60]. The COMT enzyme degrades catecholamines [61], and thus has been thought to contribute in vasodilatory shock and AKI [11]. The LL genotype is associated in cardiac surgery associated AKI (CSA-AKI) in two studies of modest size [11,12], yet in a larger study this association was ruled out [10]. Furthermore, endothelial NO synthase gene (NOS3) variant rs2070744 was studied in association to CSA-AKI with conflicting results [13,24]. The rs2070744 has been investigated in association with diabetic nephropathy, however, results have contradicted [62]. We did not find any association between these variants and AKI.

To our knowledge, this is the first replication of polymorphisms in CXCL8 [27], NFKB1A [32], AGT [24], EPO [14], SUFU [9], HIF1A [15], PNMT [17], MPO [16], and SFTPD [34] in association to

AKI phenotype. None of the investigated variants rendered verification for the initial hypotheses.

In addition to the candidate polymorphism replication, we tested two SNPs due to interesting biological hypotheses. Li and colleagues [33] presented in their in vitro septic AKI model that heat shock protein 27 (Hsp27) overexpression caused the renal epithelial cells to outlive. The C-allele of a functional SNP rs2868371 in the HSPB1 gene associates with decreased expression of Hsp27 [63,64]. However, in our sample this SNP was not associated with AKI in any of the analyses. Another intriguing suggestion regarding the pathophysiology of septic AKI was presented by Schaalan and colleagues [35]: the hepcidin levels were elevated in patients with septic AKI. Hepcidin is encoded by HAMP gene, and the promoter SNP rs10421768 is suggested to affect the gene expression [65,66]. We found G-allele to be protective (OR 0.81, 95% CI 0.69–0.95, p = 0.0090) in the adjusted model; however, this was not a replication of an association to a human AKI model, but a pilot study on this association.

We acknowledge that our study has some limitations. First, we were unable to extract the DNA of 122 (4.1%) patients. However, this random selection is unlikely to cause bias in our remaining data.

Second, our cohort of critically ill patients consists of patients with multiple possible etiologies for AKI, rather than tightly defined phenotypes, such as cardiac surgery or sepsis. However, we did adjust for these confounders in our tertiary analysis.

Third, the actual sample size was somewhat smaller than the estimated sample size we prospectively estimated to be needed for an adequate power. However, even with samples of 2207 patients in primary analysis, 2647 patients in the secondary analysis, and 2358 patients in the tertiary analysis, the retrospectively calculated power of the study, holding to the presumptions about allele frequency and effect size, remained adequate (80.6%, 93.6% and 85.5%, respectively). The minor allele frequency was, however, lower for some of the studied SNPs, affecting the power of these specific analyses. Most SNPs had frequencies exceeding the 0.2 we anticipated. A larger sample of patients with a sub-phenotype such as septic AKI is an interesting challenge for the future.

5. Conclusions

In conclusion, we were unable to replicate previous associations between genetic variants and AKI in critically ill patients. Even if short of significance, an interesting previously unpublished variant in the HAMP gene offers possible insight into mechanism of AKI, although future studies are needed to confirm this finding. In the future, the efforts to decipher "the AKI gene" should be targeted on more carefully assigned AKI sub-phenotypes.

Author Contributions: V.P. is the principal investigator for the FINNAKI study. V.P., M.A.K., and L.M.V. designed the study. S.T.V. contributed to the data acquisition and database access. L.M.V. and M.A.K. analyzed the data. L.M.V. made the manuscript draft and the figures. All authors edited the manuscript. All authors revised the article critically for important intellectual content, giving their approval.

Acknowledgments: We thank the FINNAKI Study Group: Central Finland Central Hospital: Raili Laru-Sompa, Anni Pulkkinen, Minna Saarelainen, Mikko Reilama, Sinikka Tolmunen, Ulla Rantalainen, Marja Miettinen; East Savo Central Hospital: Markku Suvela, Katrine Pesola, Pekka Saastamoinen, Sirpa Kauppinen; Helsinki University Central Hospital: Ville Pettilä, Kirsi-Maija Kaukonen, Anna-Maija Korhonen, Sara Nisula, Suvi Vaara, Raili Suojaranta-Ylinen, Leena Mildh, Mikko Haapio, Laura Nurminen, Sari Sutinen, Leena Pettilä, Helinä Laitinen, Heidi Syrjä, Kirsi Henttonen, Elina Lappi, Hillevi Boman; Jorvi Central Hospital: Tero Varpula, Päivi Porkka, Mirka Sivula, Mira Rahkonen, Anne Tsurkka, Taina Nieminen, Niina Prittinen; KantaHäme Central Hospital: Ari Alaspää, Ville Salanto, Hanna Juntunen, Teija Sanisalo; Kuopio University Hospital: Ilkka Parviainen, Ari Uusaro, Esko Ruokonen, Stepani Bendel, Niina Rissanen, Maarit Lång, Sari Rahikainen, Saija Rissanen, Merja Ahonen, Elina Halonen, Eija Vaskelainen; Lapland Central Hospital: Meri Poukkanen, Esa Lintula, Sirpa Suominen; Länsi Pohja Central Hospital: Jorma Heikkinen, Timo Lavander, Kirsi Heinonen, Anne-Mari Juopperi; Middle Ostrobothnia Central Hospital: Tadeusz Kaminski, Fiia Gäddnäs, Tuija Kuusela, Jane Roiko; North Karelia

Central Hospital: Sari Karlsson, Matti Reinikainen, Tero Surakka, Helena Jyrkönen, Tanja Eiserbeck, Jaana Kallinen; Satakunta Hospital District: Vesa Lund, Päivi Tuominen, Pauliina Perkola, Riikka Tuominen, Marika Hietaranta, Satu Johansson; South Karelia Central Hospital: Seppo Hovilehto, Anne Kirsi, Pekka Tiainen, Tuija Myllärinen, Pirjo Leino, Anne Toropainen; Tampere University Hospital: Anne Kuitunen, Ilona Leppänen, Markus Levoranta, Sanna Hoppu, Jukka Sauranen, Jyrki Tenhunen, Atte Kukkurainen, Samuli Kortelainen, Simo Varila; Turku University Hospital: Outi Inkinen, Niina Koivuviita, Jutta Kotamäki, Anu Laine; Oulu University Hospital: Tero Ala-Kokko, Jouko Laurila, Sinikka Sälkiö; Vaasa Central Hospital: Simo-Pekka Koivisto, Raku Hautamäki, Maria Skinnar. In addition, we thank the Genotyping Unit of the FIMM technology Center (Institute for molecular Medicine Finland, University of Helsinki, Finland) for the genotyping. We thank DeCode (Reykjavik, Iceland) for extracting the DNA. L.M.V. has received grants from Munuaissäätiö fund and The Finnish Society of Anaesthesiologists. In addition V.P. has received funding by grants TYH 2013343, 2016243, 2017241, and Y102011091 from the Helsinki University Hospital research funding, and a grant from the Sigrid Juselius Foundation. S.T.V. has received funding for Clinical Researchers (317061) from the Academy of Finland. The consent given by the study participants and ethical approval for the study limit the individual-level data availability. Summary-level data are presented in ESM.

References

1. Nisula, S.; Kaukonen, K.-M.M.; Vaara, S.T.; Korhonen, A.-M.M.; Poukkanen, M.; Karlsson, S.; Haapio, M.; Inkinen, O.; Parviainen, I.; Suojaranta-Ylinen, R.; et al. Incidence, risk factors and 90-day mortality of patients with acute kidney injury in Finnish intensive care units: The FINNAKI study. *Intensive Care Med.* **2013**, *39*, 420–428. [CrossRef] [PubMed]

2. Hoste, E.A.J.; Bagshaw, S.M.; Bellomo, R.; Cely, C.M.; Colman, R.; Cruz, D.N.; Edipidis, K.; Forni, L.G.; Gomersall, C.D.; Govil, D.; et al. Epidemiology of acute kidney injury in critically ill patients: The multinational AKI-EPI study. *Intensive Care Med.* **2015**, *41*, 1411–1423. [CrossRef] [PubMed]

3. Vilander, L.M.; Kaunisto, M.A.; Pettilä, V. Genetic predisposition to acute kidney injury—A systematic review. *BMC Nephrol.* **2015**, *16*, 197. [CrossRef] [PubMed]

4. Kidney Disease: Improving Global Outcomes (KDIGO) Acute Kidney Injury Work Group. KDIGO Clinical Practice Guideline for Acute Kidney Injury. *Kidney Int. Suppl.* **2012**, *2*, 1–138.

5. Bone, R.C.; Balk, R.A.; Cerra, F.B.; Dellinger, R.P.; Fein, A.M.; Knaus, W.A.; Schein, R.M.; Sibbald, W.J. Definitions for sepsis and organ failure and guidelines for the use of innovative therapies in sepsis. The ACCP/SCCM consensus conference. *Chest J.* **1992**, *101*, 1644–1655. [CrossRef]

6. Jurinke, C.; van den Boom, D.; Cantor, C.R.; Koster, H. Automated genotyping using the DNA MassArray technology. *Methods Mol. Biol.* **2002**, *187*, 179–192. [PubMed]

7. Hashad, D.I.; Elsayed, E.T.; Helmy, T.A.; Elawady, S.M. Study of the role of tumor necrosis factor-α (−308 G/A) and interleukin-10 (−1082 G/A) polymorphisms as potential risk factors to acute kidney injury in patients with severe sepsis using high-resolution melting curve analysis. *Ren. Fail.* **2017**, *39*, 77–82. [CrossRef] [PubMed]

8. Susantitaphong, P.; Perianayagam, M.C.; Tighiouart, H.; Liangos, O.; Bonventre, J.V.; Jaber, B.L. Tumor necrosis factor alpha promoter polymorphism and severity of acute kidney injury. *Nephron* **2013**, *123*, 67–73. [CrossRef] [PubMed]

9. Henao-Martinez, A.; Agler, A.H.; LaFlamme, D.; Schwartz, D.A.; Yang, I. V Polymorphisms in the SUFU gene are associated with organ injury protection and sepsis severity in patients with Enterobacteriacea bacteremia. *Infect. Genet. Evol.* **2013**, *16*, 386–391. [CrossRef] [PubMed]

10. Kornek, M.; Deutsch, M.A.; Eichhorn, S.; Lahm, H.; Wagenpfeil, S.; Krane, M. COMT-Val158Met-polymorphism is not a risk factor for acute kidney injury after cardiac surgery. *Dis. Mark.* **2013**, *35*, 129–134. [CrossRef] [PubMed]

11. Haase-Fielitz, A.; Haase, M.; Bellomo, R.; Lambert, G.; Matalanis, G.; Story, D.; Doolan, L.; Buxton, B.; Gutteridge, G.; Luft, F.C.; et al. Decreased catecholamine degradation associates with shock and kidney injury after cardiac surgery. *J. Am. Soc. Nephrol.* **2009**, *20*, 1393–1403. [CrossRef] [PubMed]

12. Albert, C.; Kube, J.; Haase-Fielitz, A.; Dittrich, A.; Schanze, D.; Zenker, M.; Kuppe, H.; Hetzer, R.; Bellomo, R.; Mertens, P.R.; et al. Pilot study of association of catechol-O-methyl transferase rs4680 genotypes with acute kidney injury and tubular stress after open heart surgery. *Biomark. Med.* **2014**, *8*, 1227–1238. [CrossRef] [PubMed]

13. Popov, A.F.; Hinz, J.; Schulz, E.G.; Schmitto, J.D.; Wiese, C.H.; Quintel, M.; Seipelt, R.; Schoendube, F.A. The eNOS 786C/T polymorphism in cardiac surgical patients with cardiopulmonary bypass is associated with renal dysfunction. *Eur. J. Cardio-Thoracic Surg.* **2009**, *36*, 651–656. [CrossRef] [PubMed]

14. Popov, A.F.; Schulz, E.G.; Schmitto, J.D.; Coskun, K.O.; Tzvetkov, M.V.; Kazmaier, S.; Zimmermann, J.; Schondube, F.A.; Quintel, M.; Hinz, J. Relation between renal dysfunction requiring renal replacement therapy and promoter polymorphism of the erythropoietin gene in cardiac surgery. *Artif. Organs* **2010**, *34*, 961–968. [CrossRef] [PubMed]

15. Kolyada, A.Y.; Tighiouart, H.; Perianayagam, M.C.; Liangos, O.; Madias, N.E.; Jaber, B.L. A genetic variant of hypoxia-inducible factor-1alpha is associated with adverse outcomes in acute kidney injury. *Kidney Int.* **2009**, *75*, 1322–1329. [CrossRef] [PubMed]

16. Perianayagam, M.; Tighiouart, H.; Liangos, O.; Kouznetsov, D.; Wald, R.; Rao, F.; O'Connor, D.; Jaber, B. Polymorphisms in the myeloperoxidase gene locus are associated with acute kidney injuryrelated outcomes. *Kidney Int.* **2012**, *82*, 909–919. [CrossRef] [PubMed]

17. Alam, A.; O'Connor, D.T.; Perianayagam, M.C.; Kolyada, A.Y.; Chen, Y.; Rao, F.; Mahata, M.; Mahata, S.; Liangos, O.; Jaber, B.L. Phenylethanolamine N-methyltransferase gene polymorphisms and adverse outcomes in acute kidney injury. *Nephron* **2010**, *114*, 253–259. [CrossRef] [PubMed]

18. Gaudino, M.; Di Castelnuovo, A.; Zamparelli, R.; Andreotti, F.; Burzotta, F.; Iacoviello, L.; Glieca, F.; Alessandrini, F.; Nasso, G.; Donati, M.B.; et al. Genetic control of postoperative systemic inflammatory reaction and pulmonary and renal complications after coronary artery surgery. *J. Thorac. Cardiovasc. Surg.* **2003**, *126*, 1107–1112. [CrossRef]

19. Dalboni, M.A.; Quinto, B.M.; Grabulosa, C.C.; Narciso, R.; Monte, J.C.; Durao, M. Tumour necrosis factor-alpha plus interleukin-10 low producer phenotype predicts acute kidney injury and death in intensive care unit patients. *Clin. Exp. Immunol.* **2013**, *173*, 242–249. [CrossRef] [PubMed]

20. Wattanathum, A.; Manocha, S.; Groshaus, H.; Russell, J.A.; Walley, K.R. Interleukin-10 Haplotype Associated with Increased Mortality in Critically Ill Patients with Sepsis From Pneumonia But Not in Patients With Extrapulmonary Sepsis. *Chest* **2005**, *128*, 1690–1698. [CrossRef] [PubMed]

21. Chang, C.F.; Lu, T.M.; Yang, W.C.; Lin, S.J.; Lin, C.C.; Chung, M.Y. Gene polymorphisms of interleukin-10 and tumor necrosis factor-alpha are associated with contrast-induced nephropathy. *Am. J. Nephrol.* **2013**, *37*, 110–117. [CrossRef] [PubMed]

22. Boehm, J.; Eichhorn, S.; Kornek, M.; Hauner, K.; Prinzing, A.; Grammer, J. Apolipoprotein E genotype, TNF-alpha 308G/A and risk for cardiac surgery associated-acute kidney injury in Caucasians. *Ren. Fail.* **2014**, *36*, 237–243. [CrossRef] [PubMed]

23. McBride, W.T.; Prasad, P.S.; Armstrong, M.; Patterson, C.; Gilliland, H.; Drain, A. Cytokine phenotype, genotype, and renal outcomes at cardiac surgery. *Cytokine* **2013**, *61*, 275–284. [CrossRef] [PubMed]

24. Stafford-Smith, M.; Podgoreanu, M.; Swaminathan, M.; Phillips-Bute, B.; Mathew, J.P.; Hauser, E.H. Association of genetic polymorphisms with risk of renal injury after coronary bypass graft surgery. *Am. J. Kidney Dis.* **2005**, *45*, 519–530. [CrossRef] [PubMed]

25. Jaber, B.L.; Rao, M.; Guo, D.; Balakrishnan, V.S.; Perianayagam, M.C.; Freeman, R.B.; Pereira, B.J. Cytokine gene promoter polymorphisms and mortality in acute renal failure. *Cytokine* **2004**, *25*, 212–219. [CrossRef] [PubMed]

26. Jouan, J.; Golmard, L.; Benhamouda, N.; Durrleman, N.; Golmard, J.L.; Ceccaldi, R.; Trinquart, L.; Fabiani, J.N.; Tartour, E.; Jeunemaitre, X.; et al. Gene polymorphisms and cytokine plasma levels as predictive factors of complications after cardiopulmonary bypass. *J. Thorac. Cardiovasc. Surg.* **2012**, *144*, 467–473.e2. [CrossRef] [PubMed]

27. Cardinal-Fernandez, P.; Ferruelo, A.; El-Assar, M.; Santiago, C.; Gomez-Gallego, F.; Martin-Pellicer, A. Genetic predisposition to acute kidney injury induced by severe sepsis. *J. Crit. Care* **2013**, *28*, 365–370. [CrossRef] [PubMed]

28. Frank, A.J.; Sheu, C.C.; Zhao, Y.; Chen, F.; Su, L.; Gong, M.N.; Bajwa, E.; Thompson, B.T.; Christiani, D.C. BCL2 genetic variants are associated with acute kidney injury in septic shock. *Crit. Care Med.* **2012**, *40*, 2116–2123. [CrossRef] [PubMed]

29. Zhao, B.; Lu, Q.; Cheng, Y.; Belcher, J.M.; Siew, E.D.; Leaf, D.E.; Body, S.C.; Fox, A.A.; Waikar, S.S.; Collard, C.D.; et al. A Genome-Wide Association Study to Identify Single-Nucleotide Polymorphisms for Acute Kidney Injury. *Am. J. Respir. Crit. Care Med.* **2017**, *195*, 482–490. [CrossRef] [PubMed]

30. Stafford-Smith, M.; Li, Y.-J.; Mathew, J.P.; Li, Y.-W.; Ji, Y.; Phillips-Bute, B.G.; Milano, C.A.; Newman, M.F.; Kraus, W.E.; Kertai, M.D.; et al. Genome-wide association study of acute kidney injury after coronary bypass graft surgery identifies susceptibility loci. *Kidney Int.* **2015**, *88*, 823–832. [CrossRef] [PubMed]

31. Vilander, L.M.; Kaunisto, M.A.; Vaara, S.T.; Pettilä, V.; FINNAKI Study Group. Genetic variants in SERPINA4 and SERPINA5, but not BCL2 and SIK3 are associated with acute kidney injury in critically ill patients with septic shock. *Crit. Care* **2017**, *21*, 47. [CrossRef] [PubMed]

32. Bhatraju, P.; Hsu, C.; Mukherjee, P.; Glavan, B.J.; Burt, A.; Mikacenic, C.; Himmelfarb, J.; Wurfel, M. Associations between single nucleotide polymorphisms in the FAS pathway and acute kidney injury. *Crit. Care* **2015**, *19*, 368. [CrossRef] [PubMed]

33. Li, C.; Wu, J.; Li, Y.; Xing, G. Cytoprotective Effect of Heat Shock Protein 27 Against Lipopolysaccharide-Induced Apoptosis of Renal Epithelial HK-2 Cells. *Cell. Physiol. Biochem.* **2017**, *41*, 2211–2220. [CrossRef] [PubMed]

34. Liu, J.; Li, G.; Li, L.; Liu, Z.; Zhou, Q.; Wang, G.; Chen, D. Surfactant protein-D (SP-D) gene polymorphisms and serum level as predictors of susceptibility and prognosis of acute kidney injury in the Chinese population. *BMC Nephrol.* **2017**, *18*, 67. [CrossRef]

35. Schaalan, M.F.; Mohamed, W.A. Determinants of hepcidin levels in sepsis-associated acute kidney injury: Impact on pAKT/PTEN pathways? *J. Immunotoxicol.* **2016**, *13*, 751–757. [CrossRef] [PubMed]

36. Purcell, S.; Neale, B.; Todd-Brown, K.; Thomas, L.; Ferreira, M.A.; Bender, D.; Maller, J.; Sklar, P.; de Bakker, P.I.; Daly, M.J.; et al. PLINK: A tool set for whole-genome association and population-based linkage analyses. *Am. J. Hum. Genet.* **2007**, *81*, 559–575. [CrossRef] [PubMed]

37. Barrett, J.C.; Fry, B.; Maller, J.; Daly, M.J. Haploview: Analysis and visualization of LD and haplotype maps. *Bioinformatics* **2005**, *21*, 263–265. [CrossRef] [PubMed]

38. Purcell, S.; Cherny, S.S.; Sham, P.C. Genetic Power Calculator: Design of linkage and association genetic mapping studies of complex traits. *Bioinformatics* **2003**, *19*, 149–150. [CrossRef] [PubMed]

39. Larach, D.B.; Engoren, M.C.; Schmidt, E.M.; Heung, M. Genetic variants and acute kidney injury: A review of the literature. *J. Crit. Care* **2018**, *44*, 203–211. [CrossRef] [PubMed]

40. Ioannidis, J.P. Why most discovered true associations are inflated. *Epidemiology* **2008**, *19*, 640–648. [CrossRef] [PubMed]

41. Lohmueller, K.E.; Pearce, C.L.; Pike, M.; Lander, E.S.; Hirschhorn, J.N. Meta-analysis of genetic association studies supports a contribution of common variants to susceptibility to common disease. *Nat. Genet.* **2003**, *33*, 177–182. [CrossRef] [PubMed]

42. Kraft, P.; Zeggini, E.; Ioannidis, J.P.A. Replication in genome-wide association studies. *Stat. Sci.* **2009**, *24*, 561–573. [CrossRef] [PubMed]

43. Teuffel, O.; Ethier, M.C.; Beyene, J.; Sung, L. Association between tumor necrosis factor-α promoter −308 A/g polymorphism and susceptibility to sepsis and sepsis mortality: A systematic review and meta-analysis. *Crit. Care Med.* **2010**, *38*, 276–282. [CrossRef] [PubMed]

44. Christaki, E.; Giamarellos-Bourboulis, E.J. The beginning of personalized medicine in sepsis: Small steps to a bright future. *Clin. Genet.* **2014**, *86*, 56–61. [CrossRef] [PubMed]

45. Pan, W.; Zhang, A.Q.; Yue, C.L.; Gao, J.W.; Zeng, L.; Gu, W.; Jiang, J.X. Association between interleukin-10 polymorphisms and sepsis: A meta-analysis. *Epidemiol. Infect.* **2015**, *143*, 366–375. [CrossRef] [PubMed]

46. Ferrara, N.; Gerber, H.-P.; LeCouter, J. The biology of VEGF and its receptors. *Nat. Med.* **2003**, *9*, 669–676. [CrossRef] [PubMed]

47. Bates, D.O. Vascular endothelial growth factors and vascular permeability. *Cardiovasc. Res.* **2010**, *87*, 262–271. [CrossRef] [PubMed]

48. Renner, W.; Kotschan, S.; Hoffmann, C.; Obermayer-Pietsch, B.; Pilger, E. A common 936 C/T mutation in the gene for vascular endothelial growth factor is associated with vascular endothelial growth factor plasma levels. *J. Vasc. Res.* **2000**, *37*, 443–448. [CrossRef] [PubMed]

49. Medford, A.R.L.; Keen, L.J.; Bidwell, J.L.; Millar, A.B. Vascular endothelial growth factor gene polymorphism and acute respiratory distress syndrome. *Thorax* **2005**, *60*, 244–248. [CrossRef] [PubMed]

50. Zhai, R.; Gong, M.N.; Zhou, W.; Thompson, T.B.; Kraft, P.; Su, L.; Christiani, D.C. Genotypes and haplotypes of the VEGF gene are associated with higher mortality and lower VEGF plasma levels in patients with ARDS. *Thorax* **2007**, *62*, 718–722. [CrossRef] [PubMed]

51. Nazir, N.; Siddiqui, K.; Al-Qasim, S.; Al-Naqeb, D. Meta-analysis of diabetic nephropathy associated genetic variants in inflammation and angiogenesis involved in different biochemical pathways. *BMC Med. Genet.* **2014**, *15*, 103. [CrossRef] [PubMed]

52. Nechemia-Arbely, Y.; Barkan, D.; Pizov, G.; Shriki, A.; Rose-John, S.; Galun, E.; Axelrod, J.H. IL-6/IL-6R axis plays a critical role in acute kidney injury. *J. Am. Soc. Nephrol.* **2008**, *19*, 1106–1115. [CrossRef] [PubMed]

53. Simmons, E.M.; Himmelfarb, J.; Sezer, M.T.; Chertow, G.M.; Mehta, R.L.; Paganini, E.P.; Soroko, S.; Freedman, S.; Becker, K.; Spratt, D.; et al. Plasma cytokine levels predict mortality in patients with acute renal failure. *Kidney Int.* **2004**, *65*, 1357–1365. [CrossRef] [PubMed]

54. Gao, J.; Zhang, A.; Pan, W.; Yue, C.; Zeng, L.; Gu, W.; Jiang, J. Association between IL-6-174G/C polymorphism and the risk of sepsis and mortality: A systematic review and meta-analysis. *PLoS ONE* **2015**, *10*, e0118843. [CrossRef] [PubMed]

55. Feng, Y.; Tang, Y.; Zhou, H.; Xie, K. A meta-analysis on correlation between interleukin-6 -174G/C polymorphism and end-stage renal disease. *Ren. Fail.* **2017**, *39*, 350–356. [CrossRef] [PubMed]

56. Panayides, A.; Ioakeimidou, A.; Karamouzos, V.; Antonakos, N.; Koutelidakis, I.; Giannikopoulos, G.; Makaritsis, K.; Voloudakis, N.; Toutouzas, K.; Rovina, N.; et al. -572 G/C single nucleotide polymorphism of interleukin-6 and sepsis predisposition in chronic renal disease. *Eur. J. Clin. Microbiol. Infect. Dis.* **2015**, *34*, 2439–2446. [CrossRef] [PubMed]

57. Agrawal, S.; Agarwal, S.; Naik, S. Genetic contribution and associated pathophysiology in end-stage renal disease. *Appl. Clin. Genet.* **2010**, *3*, 65–84. [CrossRef] [PubMed]

58. Wuttke, M.; Köttgen, A. Insights into kidney diseases from genome-wide association studies. *Nat. Rev. Nephrol.* **2016**, *12*, 549–562. [CrossRef] [PubMed]

59. O'Seaghdha, C.M.; Fox, C.S. Genome-wide association studies of chronic kidney disease: What have we learned? *Nat. Rev. Nephrol.* **2011**, *8*, 89–99. [CrossRef] [PubMed]

60. Chen, J.; Lipska, B.K.; Halim, N.; Ma, Q.D.; Matsumoto, M.; Melhem, S.; Kolachana, B.S.; Hyde, T.M.; Herman, M.M.; Apud, J.; et al. Functional Analysis of Genetic Variation in Catechol-O-Methyltransferase (COMT): Effects on mRNA, Protein, and Enzyme Activity in Postmortem Human Brain. *Am. J. Hum. Genet.* **2004**, *75*, 807–821. [CrossRef] [PubMed]

61. Axelrod, J. O-Methylation of Epinephrine and Other Catechols in vitro and in vivo. *Science* **1957**, *126*, 400–401. [CrossRef] [PubMed]

62. Dellamea, B.; Leitão, C.; Friedman, R.; Canani, L. Nitric oxide system and diabetic nephropathy. *Diabetol. Metab. Syndr.* **2014**, *6*, 17. [CrossRef] [PubMed]

63. Guo, H.; Bai, Y.; Xu, P.; Hu, Z.; Liu, L.; Wang, F.; Jin, G.; Wang, F.; Deng, Q.; Tu, Y.; et al. Functional promoter -1271G/C variant of HSPB1 predicts lung cancer risk and survival. *J. Clin. Oncol.* **2010**, *28*, 1928–1935. [CrossRef] [PubMed]

64. Pang, Q.; Wei, Q.; Xu, T.; Yuan, X.; Lopez Guerra, J.L.; Levy, L.B.; Liu, Z.; Gomez, D.R.; Zhuang, Y.; Wang, L.-E.; et al. Functional Promoter Variant rs2868371 of HSPB1 Is Associated with Risk of Radiation Pneumonitis After Chemoradiation for Non-Small Cell Lung Cancer. *Int. J. Radiat. Oncol.* **2013**, *85*, 1332–1339. [CrossRef] [PubMed]

65. Liang, L.; Liu, H.; Yue, J.; Liu, L.; Han, M.; Luo, L.; Zhao, Y.; Xiao, H. Association of Single-Nucleotide Polymorphism in the Hepcidin Promoter Gene with Susceptibility to Extrapulmonary Tuberculosis. *Genet. Test. Mol. Biomark.* **2017**, *21*, 351–356. [CrossRef] [PubMed]

66. Parajes, S.; González-Quintela, A.; Campos, J.; Quinteiro, C.; Domínguez, F.; Loidi, L. Genetic study of the hepcidin gene (HAMP) promoter and functional analysis of the c.-582A > G variant. *BMC Genet.* **2010**, *11*, 110. [CrossRef] [PubMed]

8

Diagnostic Performance of Cyclophilin A in Cardiac Surgery-Associated Acute Kidney Injury

Cheng-Chia Lee [1,2,†], **Chih-Hsiang Chang** [1,2,†], **Ya-Lien Cheng** [1], **George Kuo** [1],
Shao-Wei Chen [2,3], **Yi-Jung Li** [1,2], **Yi-Ting Chen** [4] **and Ya-Chung Tian** [1,*]

[1] Kidney Research Center, Department of Nephrology, Chang Gung Memorial Hospital, College of Medicine,
Chang Gung University, Taoyuan 333, Taiwan; chia7181@gmail.com (C.-C.L.);
franwisandsun@gmail.com (C.-H.C.); yolien0205@gmail.com (Y.-L.C.); b92401107@gmail.com (G.K.);
r5259@cgmh.org.tw (Y.-J.L.)

[2] Graduate Institute of Clinical Medical Sciences, College of Medicine, Chang Gung University, Taoyuan 333,
Taiwan; josephchen0939@gmail.com

[3] Department of Cardiothoracic and Vascular Surgery, Chang Gung Memorial Hospital, Linkou branch,
College of Medicine, Chang Gung University, Taoyuan 333, Taiwan

[4] Department of Biomedical Sciences, College of Medicine, Chang Gung University, Taoyuan 333, Taiwan;
ytchen@mail.cgu.edu.tw

* Correspondence: dryctian@adm.cgmh.org.tw

† These authors contributed equally to this manuscript.

Abstract: Acute kidney injury (AKI) is associated with increased morbidity and mortality and is frequently encountered in cardiovascular surgical intensive care units (CVS-ICU). In this study, we aimed at investigating the utility of cyclophilin A (CypA) for the early detection of postoperative AKI in patients undergoing cardiac surgery. This was a prospective observational study conducted in a CVS-ICU of a tertiary care university hospital. All prospective clinical and laboratory data were evaluated as predictors of AKI. Serum and urine CypA, as well as urine neutrophil gelatinase-associated lipocalin (uNGAL), were examined within 6 h after cardiac surgery. The discriminative power for the prediction of AKI was evaluated using the area under the receiver operator characteristic curve (AUROC). We found that both serum CypA and urine CypA were significantly higher in the AKI group than in the non-AKI group. For discriminating AKI and dialysis-requiring AKI, serum CypA demonstrated acceptable AUROC values (0.689 and 0.738, respectively). The discrimination ability of urine CypA for predicting AKI was modest, but it was acceptable for predicting dialysis-requiring AKI (AUROC = 0.762). uNGAL best predicted the development of AKI, but its sensitivity was not good. A combination of serum CypA and uNGAL enhanced the overall performance for predicting the future development of AKI and dialysis-requiring AKI. Our results suggest that CypA is suitable as a biomarker for the early detection of postoperative AKI in CVS–ICU. However, it has better discriminating ability when combined with uNGAL for predicting AKI in CVS-ICU patients.

Keywords: cardiovascular surgical intensive care units; cardiac surgery; acute kidney injury; cyclophilin A; neutrophil gelatinase-associated lipocalin

1. Introduction

Acute kidney injury (AKI) is a severe complication after cardiac surgery and significantly affects morbidity and mortality [1,2]. Up to 15–40% of patients undergoing cardiac surgery develop AKI, with 1–6% requiring renal replacement therapy (RRT) [1–4]. The mortality rate in cardiac surgery patients with a severe, RRT-requiring AKI can be as high as 60% [3,4]. Even minor increases in serum creatinine (SCr) levels (that is, 20–25% from preoperative baseline) following cardiac surgery are associated with increased mortality [5,6]. AKI is associated with not only postoperative mortality but long-term complications, such as increased risks of myocardial infarction, heart failure, mediastinitis, and stroke [2,7–9]. Therefore, novel biomarkers that can predict the development and severity of AKI earlier after cardiac surgery are important tools in clinical practice.

Recently, a secreted molecule, cyclophilin A (CypA), was found to have a physiological and pathological role in cardiovascular diseases, including atherosclerosis, acute coronary syndrome, and aortic aneurysm [10–14]. Extracellular CypA has been found to promote either the development of atherosclerosis or the vulnerability of atherosclerotic plaques by enhancing vascular oxidative stress and inflammation [14]. CypA has also been shown to be a damage-associated molecular pattern molecule that can initiate and perpetuate the inflammatory response [15]. It can stimulate inflammatory cell recruitment and subsequent tissue injury through binding to membrane receptor CD147 [16]. Critically, Dear et al., by using a mouse model of sepsis based on cecal ligation and puncture, found that inhibition of CypA receptor CD147 attenuates sepsis-induced acute renal failure [17]. Furthermore, the increased secretion of CypA from human proximal tubular cells has been demonstrated after exposure to harmful insults, such as free radical treatment [18]. Thus, it is conceivable that urine CypA might be a potential early marker of kidney injury.

Our hypothesis was that serum CypA can be a crucial mediator leading to adverse outcomes in patients after cardiac surgery. Therefore, this study aimed to evaluate whether serum or urine CypA could be a potential marker to predict AKI after cardiac surgery.

2. Materials and Methods

2.1. Study Design

We conducted a prospective, observational study in the CVS-ICU at a tertiary care referral center in Taiwan between September 2015 and December 2016. Patients who received cardiac surgery were enrolled in this investigation. A total of 186 patients were included and divided into the AKI and non-AKI groups. Patients who had an estimated glomerular filtration rate (eGFR) < 30 mL/min/1.73 m^2, were receiving dialysis, were aged < 18 years, or reported any prior organ transplantation were excluded. To ensure early detection, only those who underwent cardiac surgery and were admitted to the CVS-ICU within 72 h were enrolled. Demographic data, clinical characteristics, and echocardiographic data were collected. Routine biochemistry test results, such as white blood cell, hemoglobin, creatinine (Cr), and alanine aminotransferase levels were measured by the central laboratory of Chang Gung Memorial Hospital. Based on the Kidney Disease Improving Global Outcomes (KDIGO) Clinical Practice Guidelines for Acute Kidney Injury, AKI was defined under either of the following criteria: increase in SCr by ≥0.3mg/dL within 48 h or increase in SCr to ≥1.5 times the baseline within 7 days. In addition, the severity of AKI was staged according to the KDIGO guidelines [19]. The study protocol was approved by the local Institutional Review Board (number 103-1993B).

2.2. Clinical Assessment

All the patients received standard medical therapy after cardiac surgery. The cardiac surgical details included coronary artery bypass grafting (CABG), valve surgery, and aortic surgery. Surgical risk was assessed using the European System for Cardiac Operative Risk Evaluation (EuroSCORE) II score [20]. To determine the predictive value of potential biomarkers for AKI, the primary outcome was the development of AKI within 7 days after cardiac surgery. To assess the prognostic utility of potential biomarkers, new-onset dialysis-requiring AKI and 90-day mortality were considered secondary outcomes. After hospital discharge, a 6-month follow-up examination was performed by reviewing the electronic medical records or using telephone interviews as needed.

2.3. Sampling and Quantifying Urine Neutrophil Gelatinase-Associated Lipocalin (uNGAL) and Cyclophilin A (CypA)

Urine samples were collected in sterile non-heparinized tubes immediately after cardiac surgery and then centrifuged at 5000× g for 30 min at 4 °C to remove cells and debris. The clarified supernatants were stored at −80 °C until analysis. CypA and uNGAL were measured by an enzyme-linked immunosorbent assay using kits purchased from Cusabio Biotech (Carlsbad, CA, USA) and R&D Systems (DLCN20; Minneapolis, MN, USA), respectively, according to the manufacturers' specifications.

2.4. Statistical Analysis

Continuous data, such as preoperative laboratory value, were expressed as means ± standard deviations. Since most biomarkers did not fit a normal distribution, we expressed them as median and interquartile range. Data of continuous variables for the AKI and non-AKI groups were compared using the Student's t-test or Mann–Whitney U test. Fisher's exact test was used to compare the categorical variables. The trends of uNGAL/Cr and serum CypA across chronic kidney disease (CKD) stages was assessed by the Jonckheere–Terpstra trend test. Pairwise comparisons among the CKD stages were made by the Kruskal–Wallis test with Bonferroni adjustment. The discrimination abilities of several markers (i.e., serum CypA, uNGAL/Cr, serum CypA + uNGAL/Cr, and urine CypA/Cr) in diagnosing outcomes (including AKI, hemodialysis, and 90-day mortality) were assessed using the area under the receiver operating characteristic curve (AUROC). Subsequently, optimal cut-off points and the corresponding sensitivities/specificities were obtained according to the Youden index. The areas under the curve (AUCs) of different markers were compared by the DeLong test. All tests were two-tailed, and $p < 0.05$ was considered statistically significant. No adjustment for multiple testing (multiplicity) was made in this study. Data analyses were conducted using SPSS 22 (IBM SPSS Inc, Chicago, IL, USA).

3. Results

3.1. Study Population Characteristics

Overall, 186 adult patients (116 men and 70 women) with a mean age of 60 years were investigated. AKI was diagnosed in 92 (49.5%) patients. The patient characteristics, including age, sex, preoperative laboratory data, and surgical details, are listed in Table 1. Diabetes mellitus and congestive heart failure were recorded in 32.8% and 19.9% of the patients, respectively, during recruitment. The AKI patients exhibited significantly higher EuroSCORE II than the non-AKI patients ($p = 0.018$). Furthermore, the AKI patients exhibited lower platelet and albumin levels and higher Cr levels at baseline than the non-AKI patients ($p < 0.05$; Table 1). No significant differences were seen in other clinical and biochemical parameters between the AKI and non-AKI groups after the cardiac surgeries.

Table 1. Baseline characteristics of the patients with and without AKI after cardiac surgeries.

Characteristics	All Patients	AKI	Non-AKI	p
Patient number	186	92	94	-
Age, year	60.0 ± 14.6	60.7 ± 14.8	59.3 ± 14.5	0.504
Male gender, n (%)	116 (62.4)	55 (59.8)	61 (64.9)	0.545
Diabetes mellitus, n (%)	61 (32.8)	33 (35.9)	28 (29.8)	0.436
CHF NYHA III/IV, n (%)	37 (19.9)	22 (23.9)	15 (16.0)	0.201
Mean arterial pressure, mmHg	90.3 ± 14.4	89.5 ± 15.4	91.0 ± 13.3	0.475
LVEF, %	60.9 ± 15.5	59.9 ± 15.9	61.8 ± 15.3	0.394

Table 1. *Cont.*

Characteristics	All Patients	AKI	Non-AKI	*p*
Preoperative laboratory data				
Leukocyte count, 1000/mL	7.8 ± 3.4	7.7 ± 3.6	7.9 ± 3.2	0.730
Hemoglobin, g/dL	12.6 ± 2.4	12.3 ± 2.7	12.9 ± 2.0	0.083
Platelet count, 1000/mL	201 ± 75	189 ± 81	212 ± 66	0.038
ALT, u/L	30.2 ± 34.8	31.2 ± 43.3	29.1 ± 24.0	0.691
Serum creatinine, mg/dL	1.1 ± 1.0	1.3 ± 1.3	0.9 ± 0.4	0.013
Albumin, mg/dL	3.9 ± 0.5	3.9 ± 0.6	4.0 ± 0.4	0.044
EuroSCORE II	6.7 (6.1)	8.0 (7.2)	5.5 (4.5)	0.018
Surgical detail, *n* (%)				0.162
CABG	61 (32.8)	24 (26.1)	37 (39.4)	
Valve surgery	64 (34.4)	33 (35.9)	31 (33.0)	
CABG + valve surgery	17 (9.1)	12 (13.0)	5 (5.3)	
Aorta	34 (18.3)	19 (20.7)	15 (16.0)	
Others	10 (5.4)	4 (4.3)	6 (6.4)	

Continuous data are presented as means ± SDs or medians (interquartile range); AKI, acute kidney injury; CHF, congestive heart failure; NYHA, New York Heart Association; ALT, alanine aminotransferase; CABG, coronary artery bypass grafting.

Table 2 summarizes the postoperative biomarkers and clinical outcomes of the patients with and without AKI in this study. In the AKI and non-AKI groups, the median serum CypA levels were 5.8 ng/mL and 4.0 ng/mL ($p < 0.001$), respectively; the median uNGAL levels were 91 ng/mL and 31 ng/mL ($p < 0.001$), respectively; and the median urine CypA levels were 0.24 ng/mL and 0.17 ng/mL ($p = 0.035$), respectively. To compensate for perioperative variation in urine dilution, urine CypA and uNGAL were adjusted according to urine Cr. The median urine CypA/Cr levels in the AKI and non-AKI groups were 0.004 ng/mL and 0.002 ng/mL ($p = 0.003$), respectively, and the median uNGAL/Cr levels in the two groups were 1.73 ng/mL and 0.43 ng/mL ($p < 0.001$), respectively. Eventually, eleven (12%) of the AKI patients underwent hemodialysis. There were seven (7.6%) and five (5.4%) patients in the AKI group suffered from post-operative bleeding and sepsis respectively. Overall, 12 (6.5%) patients died within 90 days. Patients in the AKI group had a longer hospital stay and a higher incidence of postoperative bleeding and mortality than did those in the non-AKI group.

Table 2. Postoperative biomarkers and outcomes of the patients with and without AKI after cardiac surgeries.

Characteristics	All Patients	AKI	Non-AKI	*p*
Patient number	186	92	94	-
Postoperative biomarkers				
Urine NGAL, ng/mL	44 (104)	91 (141)	31 (39)	<0.001
Urine NGAL/urine creatinine	0.73 (1.9)	1.73 (6.51)	0.43 (0.65)	<0.001
CypA, ng/mL	5.2 (3.3)	5.8 (3.9)	4.0 (4.3)	<0.001
Urine CypA, ng/mL	0.19 (0.29)	0.24 (0.40)	0.17 (0.24)	0.035
Urine CypA/urine creatinine	0.003 (0.007)	0.004 (0.013)	0.002 (0.005)	0.003
Peak serum creatinine, mg/dL	1.6 ± 1.3	2.3 ± 1.8	1.0 ± 0.4	<0.001
Outcome				
AKI stage 1/2/3	-	48/23/21	-	-
Renal replacement therapy, *n* (%)	12 (6.5)	11 (12.0)	1 (1.1)	0.002
Postoperative bleeding, *n* (%)	8 (4.3)	7 (7.6)	1 (1.1)	0.034
Postoperative sepsis, *n* (%)	6 (3.2)	5 (5.4)	1 (1.1)	0.116
Stay of hospital, days	21.4 (15.0)	28.0 (18.5)	14.9 (11.0)	<0.001
Mortality in 90 days, *n* (%)	12 (6.5)	10 (10.9)	2 (2.1)	0.018

Continuous data are presented as means ± SDs or medians (interquartile range); AKI, acute kidney injury; NGAL, neutrophil gelatinase-associated lipocalin; CypA, cyclophilin A.

The patients in the AKI group exhibited significantly higher serum CypA and normalized uNGAL levels than those in the non-AKI group. The level of normalized uNGAL increased along with the more severe AKI stage, but there was no significant difference between the KDIGO 1 and KDIGO 2 stages (Figure 1A). The level of serum CypA was significantly different between the AKI and non-AKI groups, but there was no significant difference among the KDIGO stages 1–3 (Figure 1B).

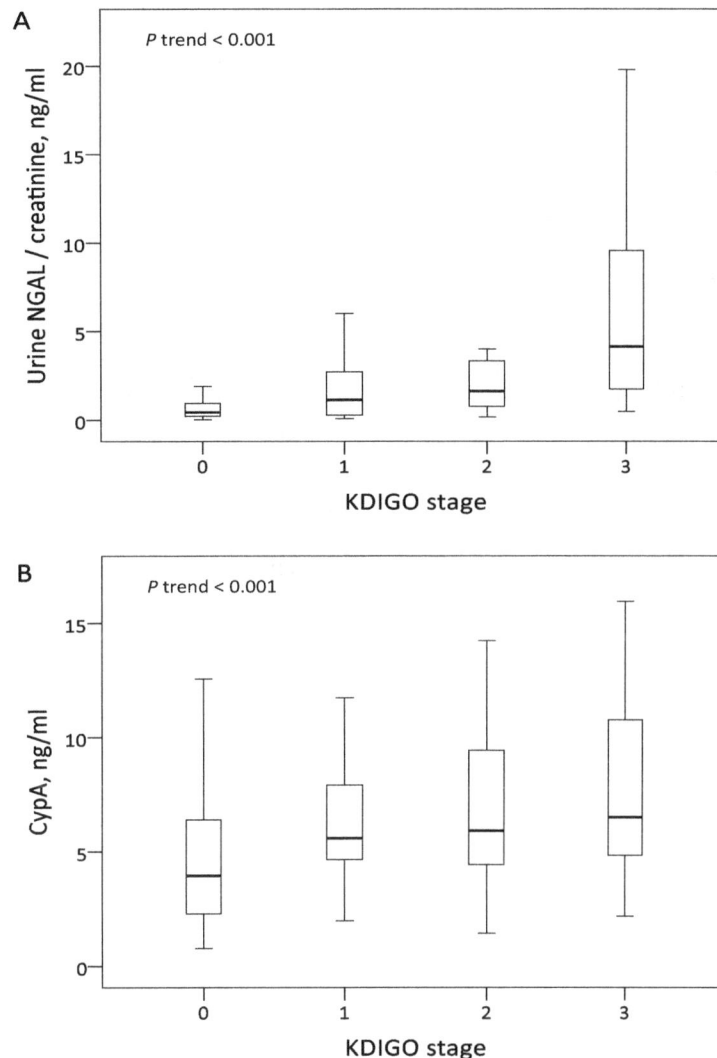

Figure 1. Levels of urine NGAL normalized by urine creatinine (**A**) and serum CypA (**B**) across KDIGO stages. Abbreviations: CypA, cyclophilin A; NGAL, neutrophil gelatinase-associated lipocalin; KDIGO, Kidney Disease Improving Global Outcomes.

3.2. Discrimination Abilities of Serum CypA and Normalized uNGAL in Detecting AKI, Dialysis-Requiring AKI, and 90-Day Mortality

The performances of serum CypA and normalized uNGAL in the detection of outcomes were assessed through AUROC analysis, as shown in Figure 2A–C. The ROC analysis of serum CypA and normalized uNGAL revealed AUROC values of 0.689 (95% confidence interval [CI], 0.618–0.755) and 0.752 (95% CI, 0.684–0.812), respectively, for predicting the future development of AKI. The combination of serum CypA and normalized uNGAL showed the highest AUC of 0.787 (95% CI, 0.721–0.843) in diagnosing AKI. In terms of using a single marker to predict dialysis-requiring AKI, serum CypA and normalized uNGAL had AUROCs of 0.738 (95% CI, 0.668–0.799) and 0.835 (95% CI, 0.773–0.885), respectively. Normalized urine CypA had an AUROC of 0.762 and exhibited a good specificity of 83.9%

for a cutoff value of 0.012. The combination of CypA and normalized uNGAL showed the highest AUC of 0.848 (95% CI, 0.788–0.896).

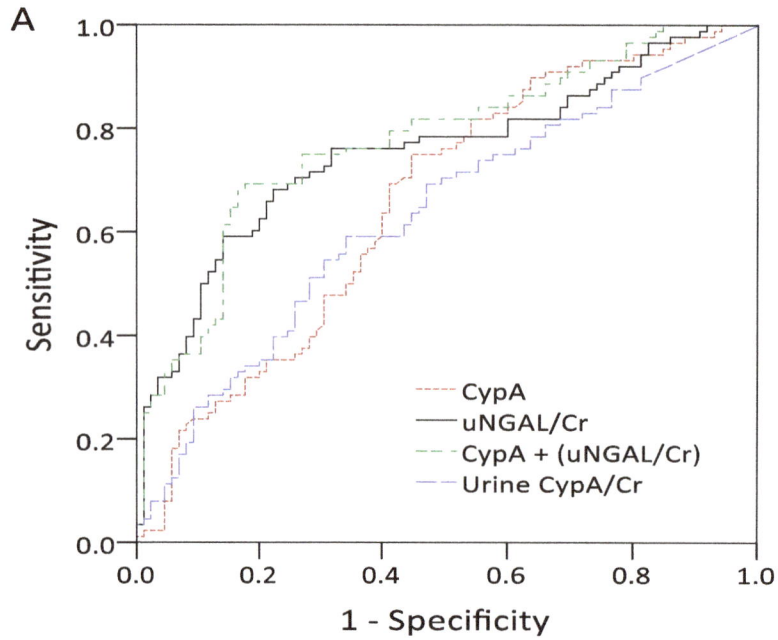

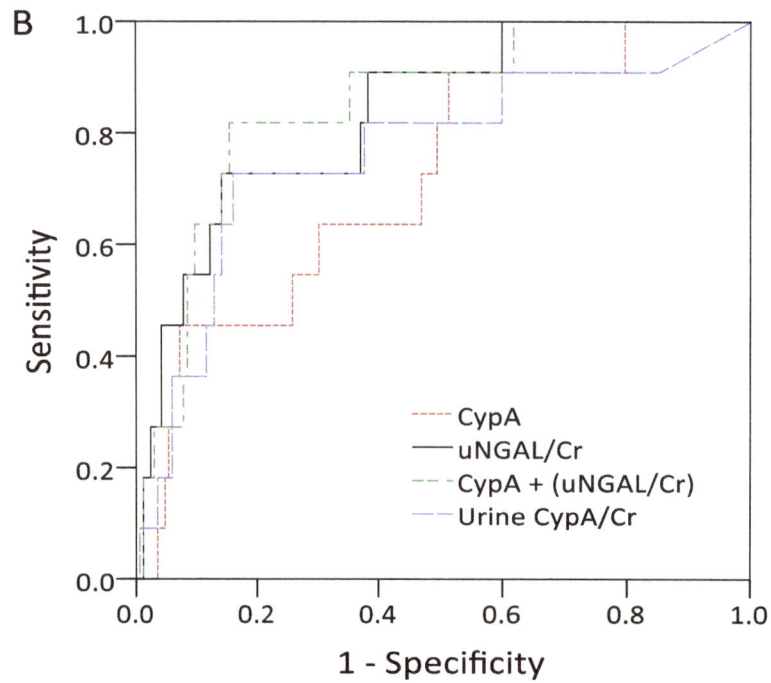

Figure 2. *Cont.*

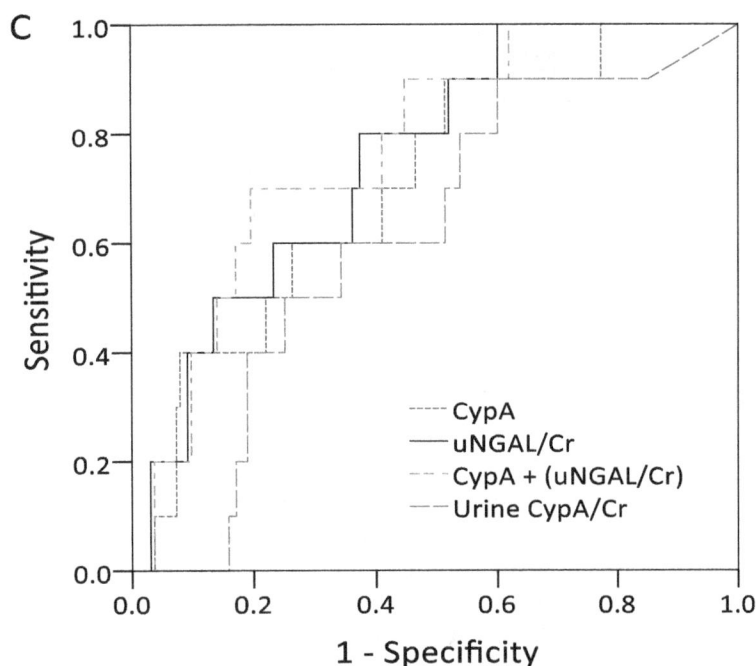

Figure 2. Area under the curves for serum CypA, urine NGAL normalized by urine Cr, serum CypA plus urine NGAL normalized by urine Cr, and urine CypA normalized by urine Cr in discriminating acute kidney injury (**A**), dialysis-requiring acute kidney injury (**B**), and 90-day mortality (**C**). Abbreviations: CypA, cyclophilin A; NGAL, neutrophil gelatinase-associated lipocalin; Cr, creatinine.

As for the detection of AKI, CypA exhibited a sensitivity of 76.1% and a specificity of 58.5% for a threshold value of 4.36 ng/mL, whereas normalized uNGAL exhibited a poor sensitivity of 68.5% and a specificity of 76.6% for a cut-off value of 0.85 (Table 3). However, there was no significant difference in the 90-day survival rates between the subgroups of high/low serum CypA and normalized uNGAL.

Table 3. Diagnostic property of markers in discriminating outcomes.

Outcome/Marker	AUC (95% CI)	Cut-Off #	Sensitivity (95% CI)	Specificity (95% CI)
Acute kidney injury				
CypA	68.9 (61.8–75.5)	>4.36	76.1 (66.1–84.4)	58.5 (47.9–68.6)
Urine NGAL/Cr	75.2 (68.4–81.2)	>0.85	68.5 (58.0–77.8)	76.6 (66.7–84.7)
CypA + (urine NGAL/Cr)	78.7 (72.1–84.3)	NA	NA	NA
Urine CypA/Cr	63.0 (55.3–70.2)	>0.003	59.1 (48.1–69.5)	65.9 (54.8–75.8)
Dialysis-requiring AKI				
CypA	73.8 (66.8–79.9)	>4.84	91.7 (61.5–99.8)	50.0 (42.3–57.7)
Urine NGAL/Cr	83.5 (77.3–88.5)	>3.09	75.0 (42.8–94.5)	85.1 (78.9–90.0)
CypA + (urine NGAL/Cr)	84.8 (78.8–89.6)	NA	NA	NA
Urine CypA/Cr	76.2 (69.2–82.3)	>0.012	72.7 (39.0–94.0)	83.9 (77.4–89.2)
90-day mortality				
CypA	67.0 (59.7–73.7)	>4.84	83.3 (51.6–97.9)	49.4 (41.8–57.1)
Urine NGAL/Cr	75.4 (68.5–81.4)	>1.12	83.3 (51.6–97.9)	62.6 (55.0–69.8)
CypA + (urine NGAL/Cr)	73.1 (66.2–79.4)	NA	NA	NA
Urine CypA/Cr	61.1 (53.4–68.4)	>0.0016	90.0 (55.5–99.7)	39.9 (32.3–47.8)

AUC, area under the curve; CI, confidence interval; CypA, cyclophilin A; NGAL, neutrophil gelatinase-associated lipocalin; Cr, creatinine; AKI, acute kidney injury; NA, not applicable; #, number by Youden index.

4. Discussion

The development of AKI is associated with unfavorable outcomes and high mortality in patients undergoing cardiac surgery. Because renal dysfunction is known as a well-established predictor of all-cause mortality in cardiac surgery, biomarkers for the early detection of AKI after cardiac surgery would be valuable for clinical practices, such as decision making, patient counseling, and optimization of post-operative care [21]. NGAL has been the most popular biomarker for the early identification of AKI following cardiac surgery. However, compared with the excellent discrimination reported in pediatric patients, studies of urinary NGAL in adult patients reported only moderate discrimination, with an AUROC of 0.72 (95% confidence interval, 0.66–0.79) [22]. Thus, new biomarkers with better performance are urgently needed. Strategies combining biomarkers with different types of pathophysiological relevance may also be beneficial in risk stratification. In this study, we found that both serum CypA and normalized urine CypA were elevated in the patients who developed AKI after sample collection. As we have shown, serum CypA is suitable for the early detection of AKI in patients undergoing cardiac surgery, with a good sensitivity and acceptable discriminative power comparable to those of normalized uNGAL. A combination of serum CypA and normalized uNGAL enhanced the overall performance for predicting the development of AKI and dialysis-requiring AKI, with AUROC values of 0.787 and 0.848, respectively.

Cyclophilins are a family of ubiquitous proteins that are evolutionarily well conserved and present in all prokaryotes and eukaryotes [23]. The most abundant member of this family is CypA, which accounts for about 0.1–0.6% of total cytosolic proteins [24]. Although CypA is present intracellularly and was originally identified as the primary cytosolic binding protein of the immunosuppressive drug cyclosporin A, it has been found to be secreted from cells in response to inflammatory stimuli, such as hypoxia, infection, and oxidative stress [25–28]. Secreted CypA has been demonstrated to be a damage-associated molecular pattern molecule that has a potent chemotactic effect on leukocytes, and, in turn, perpetuates the inflammatory response [15,27]. Moreover, high levels of extracellular CypA have also been detected in several different human inflammatory diseases, such as rheumatoid arthritis [29,30] and sepsis [17,31], and found to be correlated with the severity of those diseases. Our data are in accordance with these findings. The distinctive characteristics of cardiac surgery, including aortic clamping and cardiopulmonary bypass, which induce a systemic inflammatory response lead to the development of AKI [32]. Notably, our study also revealed that urine CypA is elevated in patients with AKI. Because CypA is an 18-kDa protein that theoretically can be freely filtered by renal glomeruli, higher levels of urine CypA in patients with AKI may just reflect an increase in serum CypA levels. An alternative explanation is that the actual source of urine CypA may be the injured renal tubular cells. Studies have demonstrated that CypA is highly expressed in the kidney, especially in the proximal tubular epithelial cells [33]. Tsai et al. also demonstrated that CypA is released by human proximal tubular cells in a dose-dependent manner after exposure to free radical treatment [18]. However, our study showed that normalized urine CypA only exhibited modest discrimination ability for predicting AKI, with an AUROC of 0.63. In addition, although normalized urine CypA exhibited a good specificity of 83.9% in predicting dialysis-requiring AKI for a cutoff value of 0.012, its overall performance was not better than that of the well-known marker normalized urine NGAL. Intriguingly, previous studies reported that not only urine soluble components, but human urine exosomes, contain CypA [15]. Whether the exosomal part of urine CypA can exhibit better discrimination power than soluble part of urine CypA alone in stratifying AKI risk needs further investigation.

Our study found that serum CypA levels were higher in the patients who subsequently developed AKI than in those who did not, but the levels were not significantly different among the AKI KDIGO stages 1–3. This might be explained by the notion that the AKI severity is more associated with changes in the serum CypA level over time than with the level at a single time. Indeed, some of the elevation in serum CypA levels in our patients might just reflect their underlying cardiac diseases. Extracellular CypA was previously found to contribute to cardiovascular diseases as a novel player not only through its proinflammatory actions but through its proatherogenic properties [10,11,34]. Yan et al. reported that serum CypA concentrations in patients with unstable angina and acute myocardial infarction were significantly higher than those in patients with stable angina and controls [12]. Serum CypA levels were also previously found to be associated with the clinical outcomes of coronary artery disease [35], ST-elevated myocardial infarction [36], and heart failure [37]. In addition to coronary artery disease, extracellular CypA was identified as a mediator in abdominal aortic aneurysm (AAA) progression. In human AAA lesions, CypA was highly expressed, especially in the area that expresses active metalloproteinase 2 (MMP-2) [14]. Using human AAA-derived vascular smooth muscle cells, angiotensin II induces the release of CypA and enhances vascular inflammation by activating MMP activity, which was significantly reduced by treatment with the CypA inhibitor. Based on these evidences, we hypothesized that increased serum CypA levels may partly be a consequence of underlying cardiovascular diseases, and that patients with more severe cardiovascular diseases might have hemodynamic instability, leading to higher baseline renal dysfunction. Further studies using preoperative serum CypA levels or serum CypA dynamics are needed to help clarify the relationship between CypA and the outcomes of cardiac surgery.

Our study showed that normalized uNGAL best predicted the development of AKI, and the level of normalized uNGAL increased along with the more severe AKI stage. This finding is consistent with previous reports that uNGAL is an early predictive biomarker of AKI following cardiac surgery [38,39]. NGAL was originally identified from neutrophils as a shuttle for iron transport, and its upregulation has been demonstrated in the proximal renal tubule after exposure to harmful insults, such as ischemia [40]. Consequently, increased level of NGAL is rapidly detectable in the urine before SCr is elevated, presumably resulting from acute tubular damage. Although the discrimination ability of CypA levels regarding the development of AKI was not superior to that of normalized uNGAL levels, our study found that normalized uNGAL had only modest sensitivity in predicting AKI and dialysis-requiring AKI. Meanwhile, we further found that the combination of these two biomarkers provides the most accurate predictive ability in these patients, suggesting that their combination is a reasonable strategy to improve the diagnostic performance of biomarkers. Our study also found a moderate discrimination ability of normalized urine CypA when predicting dialysis-requiring AKI, with comparable sensitivity and specificity ability when compared to the well-known marker normalized uNGAL. However, this study only considered AKI identified within a 7-day period; thus, studies focusing on longer-term outcomes, such as acute kidney disease [41], are warranted to clarify the potential pathogenic role of serum CypA or urine CypA in cardiac surgery-related kidney injury.

This study has several limitations. First, only one measurement of the CypA and NGAL levels was used in this cross-sectional study to predict the development of AKI. Repeated measurements to detect persistent or secondary kidney damage may improve the predictive ability. Second, the roles and expression of CypA in AKI require further investigation. Using animal models to evaluate the origin of CypA in urine may help determine the pathogenic role of urine CypA. Third, this research was conducted on a heterogeneous population with different cardiovascular diseases, and no subgroup analysis was conducted to explore the relationships between a specific disease type and the biomarkers. We also did not analyze the relationships between CypA levels and medications that may interfere with CypA levels. Finally, given the small sample size and observational design, additional prospective trials are warranted to explore the role of CypA in different etiologies of AKI.

In summary, both serum CypA and normalized uNGAL are suitable for the early detection of AKI in patients undergoing cardiac surgery, as both have acceptable discriminative power. Moreover, the combination of these two markers provides the highest AUROC and could serve as a new non-invasive test for use in clinical applications to differentiate AKI and RRT, potentially shortening the time to the initiation of appropriate therapy. Relatedly, the careful consideration of the appropriate medication, choice of therapy, and early intervention in patients exhibiting increased biomarker levels may improve AKI outcomes.

Author Contributions: C.-C.L. and C.-H.C. made substantial contribution to conception and design of the study. Y.-L.C., G.K. and S.-W.C. assisted in analysis and interpretation of the data. Y.-J.L. and Y.-T.C. assisted in laboratory analysis and interpretation of results. C.-C.L. and C.-H.C. wrote the manuscript and prepared the figures. C.-H.C., Y.-J.L. and Y.-C.T. supervised the study. All authors have read and agreed to the published version of the manuscript.

Acknowledgments: The authors thank all participants from the Kidney Research Center of Chang Gung Memorial Hospital, Linkou, Taiwan. The authors also thank Alfred Hsing-Fen Lin for his assistance in statistical analysis.

References

1. Hobson, C.E.; Yavas, S.; Segal, M.S.; Schold, J.D.; Tribble, C.G.; Layon, A.J.; Bihorac, A. Acute Kidney Injury Is Associated With Increased Long-Term Mortality After Cardiothoracic Surgery. *Circulation* **2009**, *119*, 2444–2453. [CrossRef] [PubMed]

2. Rydén, L.; Ahnve, S.; Bell, M.; Hammar, N.; Ivert, T.; Holzmann, M.J. Acute kidney injury following coronary artery bypass grafting: Early mortality and postoperative complications. *Scand. Cardiovasc. J.* **2012**, *46*, 114–120. [CrossRef] [PubMed]

3. Chertow, G.M.; Levy, E.M.; Hammermeister, K.E.; Grover, F.; Daley, J. Independent Association between Acute Renal Failure and Mortality following Cardiac Surgery. *Am. J. Med.* **1998**, *104*, 343–348. [CrossRef]

4. Zanardo, G.; Michielon, P.; Paccagnella, A.; Rosi, P.; Caló, M.; Salandin, V.; Da Ros, A.; Michieletto, F.; Simini, G. Acute renal failure in the patient undergoing cardiac operation. Prevalence, mortality rate, and main risk factors. *J. Thorac. Cardiovasc. Surg.* **1994**, *107*, 1489–1495. [CrossRef]

5. Mangano, C.M.; Diamondstone, L.S.; Ramsay, J.G.; Aggarwal, A.; Herskowitz, A.; Mangano, D.T. Renal dysfunction after myocardial revascularization: Risk factors, adverse outcomes, and hospital resource utilization. The Multicenter Study of Perioperative Ischemia Research Group. *Ann. Intern. Med.* **1998**, *128*, 194–203. [CrossRef] [PubMed]

6. Liotta, M.; Olsson, D.; Sartipy, U.; Holzmann, M.J. Minimal changes in postoperative creatinine values and early and late mortality and cardiovascular events after coronary artery bypass grafting. *Am. J. Cardiol.* **2014**, *113*, 70–75. [CrossRef]

7. Olsson, D.; Sartipy, U.; Braunschweig, F.; Holzmann, M.J. Acute Kidney Injury Following Coronary Artery Bypass Surgery and Long-term Risk of Heart Failure. *Circ. Heart Fail.* **2013**, *6*, 83–90. [CrossRef]

8. Rydén, L.; Ahnve, S.; Bell, M.; Hammar, N.; Ivert, T.; Sartipy, U.; Holzmann, M.J. Acute kidney injury after coronary artery bypass grafting and long-term risk of myocardial infarction and death. *Int. J. Cardiol.* **2014**, *172*, 190–195. [CrossRef]

9. Pickering, J.W.; James, M.T.; Palmer, S.C. Acute Kidney Injury and Prognosis After Cardiopulmonary Bypass: A Meta-analysis of Cohort Studies. *Am. J. Kidney Dis.* **2015**, *65*, 283–293. [CrossRef]

10. Nigro, P.; Satoh, K.; O'Dell, M.R.; Soe, N.N.; Cui, Z.; Mohan, A.; Abe, J.-I.; Alexis, J.D.; Sparks, J.D.; Berk, B.C. Cyclophilin A is an inflammatory mediator that promotes atherosclerosis in apolipoprotein E–deficient mice. *J. Exp. Med.* **2011**, *208*, 53–66. [CrossRef]

11. Rezzani, R.; Favero, G.; Stacchiotti, A.; Rodella, L.F. Endothelial and vascular smooth muscle cell dysfunction mediated by cyclophylin A and the atheroprotective effects of melatonin. *Life Sci.* **2013**, *92*, 875–882. [CrossRef] [PubMed]

12. Yan, J.; Zang, X.; Chen, R.; Yuan, W.; Gong, J.; Wang, C.; Li, Y. The clinical implications of increased cyclophilin A levels in patients with acute coronary syndromes. *Clin. Chim. Acta* **2012**, *413*, 691–695. [CrossRef] [PubMed]

13. Satoh, K.; Fukumoto, Y.; Sugimura, K.; Miura, Y.; Aoki, T.; Nochioka, K.; Tatebe, S.; Miyamichi-Yamamoto, S.; Shimizu, T.; Osaki, S.; et al. Plasma Cyclophilin A Is a Novel Biomarker for Coronary Artery Disease. *Circ. J.* **2013**, *77*, 447–455. [CrossRef] [PubMed]

14. Satoh, K.; Nigro, P.; Matoba, T.; O'Dell, M.R.; Cui, Z.; Shi, X.; Mohan, A.; Yan, C.; Abe, J.; Illig, K.A.; et al. Cyclophilin A enhances vascular oxidative stress and the development of angiotensin II-induced aortic aneurysms. *Nat. Med.* **2009**, *15*, 649–656. [CrossRef] [PubMed]

15. Dear, J.W.; Simpson, K.J.; Nicolai, M.P.; Catterson, J.H.; Street, J.; Huizinga, T.; Craig, D.G.; Dhaliwal, K.; Webb, S.; Bateman, D.N.; et al. Cyclophilin A is a damage-associated molecular pattern molecule that mediates acetaminophen-induced liver injury. *J. Immunol.* **2011**, *187*, 3347–3352. [CrossRef]

16. Seizer, P.; Geisler, T.; Bigalke, B.; Schneider, M.; Klingel, K.; Kandolf, R.; Stellos, K.; Schreieck, J.; Gawaz, M.; May, A.E. EMMPRIN and its ligand cyclophilin A as novel diagnostic markers in inflammatory cardiomyopathy. *Int. J. Cardiol.* **2013**, *163*, 299–304. [CrossRef]

17. Dear, J.W.; Leelahavanichkul, A.; Aponte, A.; Hu, X.; Constant, S.L.; Hewitt, S.M.; Yuen, P.S.; Star, R.A. Liver proteomics for therapeutic drug discovery: Inhibition of the cyclophilin receptor CD147 attenuates sepsis-induced acute renal failure. *Crit. Care Med.* **2007**, *35*, 2319–2328. [CrossRef]

18. Tsai, S.F.; Su, C.W.; Wu, M.J.; Chen, C.H.; Fu, C.P.; Liu, C.S.; Hsieh, M. Urinary Cyclophilin A as a New Marker for Diabetic Nephropathy: A Cross-Sectional Analysis of Diabetes Mellitus. *Medicine* **2015**, *94*, e1802. [CrossRef]

19. Palevsky, P.M.; Liu, K.D.; Brophy, P.D.; Chawla, L.S.; Parikh, C.R.; Thakar, C.V.; Tolwani, A.J.; Waikar, S.S.; Weisbord, S.D. KDOQI US Commentary on the 2012 KDIGO Clinical Practice Guideline for Acute Kidney Injury. *Am. J. Kidney Dis.* **2013**, *61*, 649–672. [CrossRef]

20. Nashef, S.A.M.; Roques, F.; Sharples, L.D.; Nilsson, J.; Smith, C.; Goldstone, A.R.; Lockowandt, U. EuroSCORE II. *Eur. J. Cardio-Thorac. Surg.* **2012**, *41*, 734–745. [CrossRef]

21. Lee, C.C.; Chang, C.H.; Chen, S.W.; Fan, P.C.; Chang, S.W.; Chen, Y.T.; Nan, Y.Y.; Lin, P.J.; Tsai, F.C. Preoperative risk assessment improves biomarker detection for predicting acute kidney injury after cardiac surgery. *PLoS ONE* **2018**, *13*, e0203447. [CrossRef] [PubMed]

22. Ho, J.; Tangri, N.; Komenda, P.; Kaushal, A.; Sood, M.; Brar, R.; Gill, K.; Walker, S.; MacDonald, K.; Hiebert, B.M.; et al. Urinary, Plasma, and Serum Biomarkers' Utility for Predicting Acute Kidney Injury Associated With Cardiac Surgery in Adults: A Meta-analysis. *Am. J. Kidney Dis.* **2015**, *66*, 993–1005. [CrossRef] [PubMed]

23. Wang, P.; Heitman, J. The cyclophilins. *Genome Biol.* **2005**, *6*. [CrossRef]

24. Dornan, J.; Taylor, P.; Walkinshaw, M.D. Structures of immunophilins and their ligand complexes. *Curr. Top. Med. Chem.* **2003**, *3*, 1392–1409. [CrossRef] [PubMed]

25. Handschumacher, R.E.; Harding, M.W.; Rice, J.; Drugge, R.J.; Speicher, D.W. Cyclophilin: A specific cytosolic binding protein for cyclosporin A. *Science* **1984**, *226*, 544–547. [CrossRef] [PubMed]

26. Jin, Z.-G.; Melaragno, M.G.; Liao, D.-F.; Yan, C.; Haendeler, J.; Suh, Y.-A.; Lambeth, J.D.; Berk, B.C. Cyclophilin A Is a Secreted Growth Factor Induced by Oxidative Stress. *Circ. Res.* **2000**, *87*, 789–796. [CrossRef]

27. Sherry, B.; Yarlett, N.; Strupp, A.; Cerami, A. Identification of cyclophilin as a proinflammatory secretory product of lipopolysaccharide-activated macrophages. 1992, 89, 3511–3515. *Proc. Natl. Acad. Sci. USA.*

28. Suzuki, J.; Jin, Z.-G.; Meoli, D.F.; Matoba, T.; Berk, B.C. Cyclophilin A Is Secreted by a Vesicular Pathway in Vascular Smooth Muscle Cells. *Circ. Res.* **2006**, *98*, 811–817. [CrossRef]

29. Billich, A.; Winkler, G.; Aschauer, H.; Rot, A.; Peichl, P. Presence of cyclophilin A in synovial fluids of patients with rheumatoid arthritis. *J. Exp. Med.* **1997**, *185*, 975–980. [CrossRef]

30. Wang, L.; Wang, C.H.; Jia, J.F.; Ma, X.K.; Li, Y.; Zhu, H.B.; Tang, H.; Chen, Z.N.; Zhu, P. Contribution of cyclophilin A to the regulation of inflammatory processes in rheumatoid arthritis. *J. Clin. Immunol.* **2010**, *30*, 24–33. [CrossRef]

31. Tegeder, I.; Schumacher, A.; John, S.; Geiger, H.; Geisslinger, G.; Bang, H.; Brune, K. Elevated serum cyclophilin levels in patients with severe sepsis. *J. Clin. Immunol.* **1997**, *17*, 380–386. [CrossRef] [PubMed]

32. O'Neal, J.B.; Shaw, A.D.; Billings, F.T. Acute kidney injury following cardiac surgery: Current understanding and future directions. *Crit. Care* **2016**, *20*, 187. [CrossRef] [PubMed]

33. Demeule, M.; Laplante, A.; Sepehr-Arae, A.; Murphy, G.M.; Wenger, R.M.; Beliveau, R. Association of cyclophilin A with renal brush border membranes: Redistribution by cyclosporine A. *Kidney Int.* **2000**, *57*, 1590–1598. [CrossRef] [PubMed]

34. Seizer, P.; Schönberger, T.; Schött, M.; Lang, M.R.; Langer, H.F.; Bigalke, B.; Krämer, B.F.; Borst, O.; Daub, K.; Heidenreich, O.; et al. EMMPRIN and its ligand cyclophilin A regulate MT1-MMP, MMP-9 and M-CSF during foam cell formation. *Atherosclerosis* **2010**, *209*, 51–57. [CrossRef] [PubMed]

35. Ohtsuki, T.; Satoh, K.; Omura, J.; Kikuchi, N.; Satoh, T.; Kurosawa, R.; Nogi, M.; Sunamura, S.; Yaoita, N.; Aoki, T.; et al. Prognostic Impacts of Plasma Levels of Cyclophilin A in Patients with Coronary Artery Disease. *Arter. Thromb. Vasc. Biol.* **2017**, *37*, 685–693. [CrossRef]

36. Huang, C.-H.; Chang, C.-C.; Kuo, C.-L.; Huang, C.-S.; Lin, C.-S.; Liu, C.-S. Decrease in Plasma Cyclophilin A Concentration at 1 Month after Myocardial Infarction Predicts Better Left Ventricular Performance and Synchronicity at 6 Months: A Pilot Study in Patients with ST Elevation Myocardial Infarction. *Int. J. Biol. Sci.* **2015**, *11*, 38–47. [CrossRef]

37. Zuern, C.S.; Müller, K.A.L.; Seizer, P.; Geisler, T.; Banya, W.; Klingel, K.; Kandolf, R.; Bauer, A.; Gawaz, M.; May, A.E. Cyclophilin A predicts clinical outcome in patients with congestive heart failure undergoing endomyocardial biopsy. *Eur. J. Heart Fail.* **2013**, *15*, 176–184. [CrossRef]

38. Bennett, M.; Dent, C.L.; Ma, Q.; Dastrala, S.; Grenier, F.; Workman, R.; Syed, H.; Ali, S.; Barasch, J.; Devarajan, P. Urine NGAL predicts severity of acute kidney injury after cardiac surgery: A prospective study. *Clin. J. Am. Soc. Nephrol.* **2008**, *3*, 665–673. [CrossRef]

39. Parikh, C.R.; Coca, S.G.; Thiessen-Philbrook, H.; Shlipak, M.G.; Koyner, J.L.; Wang, Z.; Edelstein, C.L.; Devarajan, P.; Patel, U.D.; Zappitelli, M.; et al. Postoperative biomarkers predict acute kidney injury and poor outcomes after adult cardiac surgery. *J. Am. Soc. Nephrol.* **2011**, *22*, 1748–1757. [CrossRef]

40. Paragas, N.; Qiu, A.; Zhang, Q.; Samstein, B.; Deng, S.X.; Schmidt-Ott, K.M.; Viltard, M.; Yu, W.; Forster, C.S.; Gong, G.; et al. The Ngal reporter mouse detects the response of the kidney to injury in real time. *Nat. Med.* **2011**, *17*, 216–222. [CrossRef]

41. Chawla, L.S.; Bellomo, R.; Bihorac, A.; Goldstein, S.L.; Siew, E.D.; Bagshaw, S.M.; Bittleman, D.; Cruz, D.; Endre, Z.; Fitzgerald, R.L.; et al. Acute kidney disease and renal recovery: Consensus report of the Acute Disease Quality Initiative (ADQI) 16 Workgroup. *Nat. Rev. Nephrol.* **2017**, *13*, 241–257. [CrossRef] [PubMed]

9

Plasma Oxalate as a Predictor of Kidney Function Decline in a Primary Hyperoxaluria Cohort

Ronak Jagdeep Shah [1], Lisa E. Vaughan [2], Felicity T. Enders [2], Dawn S. Milliner [1,3] and John C. Lieske [1,4,*]

[1] Division of Nephrology and Hypertension, Mayo Clinic, Rochester, MN 55905, USA;
dr.ronakjagshah@gmail.com (R.J.S.); Milliner.Dawn@mayo.edu (D.S.M.)
[2] Division of Biomedical Statistics and Informatics, Mayo Clinic, Rochester, MN 55905, USA;
Vaughan.Lisa@mayo.edu (L.E.V.); Enders.Felicity@mayo.edu (F.T.E.)
[3] Division of Pediatric Nephrology, Mayo Clinic, Rochester, MN 55905, USA
[4] Division of Laboratory Medicine and Pathology, Mayo Clinic, Rochester, MN 55905, USA
* Correspondence: lieske.john@mayo.edu

Abstract: This retrospective analysis investigated plasma oxalate (POx) as a potential predictor of end-stage kidney disease (ESKD) among primary hyperoxaluria (PH) patients. PH patients with type 1, 2, and 3, age 2 or older, were identified in the Rare Kidney Stone Consortium (RKSC) PH Registry. Since POx increased with falling estimated glomerular filtration rate (eGFR), patients were stratified by chronic kidney disease (CKD) subgroups (stages 1, 2, 3a, and 3b). POx values were categorized into quartiles for analysis. Hazard ratios (HRs) and 95% confidence intervals (95% CIs) for risk of ESKD were estimated using the Cox proportional hazards model with a time-dependent covariate. There were 118 patients in the CKD1 group (nine ESKD events during follow-up), 135 in the CKD 2 (29 events), 72 in CKD3a (34 events), and 45 patients in CKD 3b (31 events). During follow-up, POx Q4 was a significant predictor of ESKD compared to Q1 across CKD2 (HR 14.2, 95% CI 1.8–115), 3a (HR 13.7, 95% CI 3.0–62), and 3b stages (HR 5.2, 95% CI 1.1–25), $p < 0.05$ for all. Within each POx quartile, the ESKD rate was higher in Q4 compared to Q1–Q3. In conclusion, among patients with PH, higher POx concentration was a risk factor for ESKD, particularly in advanced CKD stages.

Keywords: plasma oxalate; primary hyperoxaluria; estimated glomerular filtration rate; chronic kidney disease; Urine Oxalate; end-stage renal disease

1. Introduction

Primary hyperoxaluria (PH) is a rare inherited autosomal recessive genetic disease caused by defects in genes that encode proteins important for glyoxylate metabolism [1]. Currently, three distinct forms are known—PH1 results from mutations in the enzyme alanine-glyoxylate aminotransferase (AGT) which is encoded the *AGXT* gene, PH2 is caused by a deficiency of the glyoxylate reductase/hydroxypyruvate reductase (GRHPR) enzyme encoded by *GRHPR*, and PH3 occurs when the mitochondrial enzyme, 4-hydroxy-2-oxoglutarate aldolase (HOGA) is deficient due to mutations in the *HOGA1* gene. Based upon current numbers in the Rare Kidney Stone Consortium (RKSC) PH registry, approximately 70% of diagnosed patients are PH1, 10% are PH2, 10% PH3, and 10% do not have an identified genetic cause [2].

The metabolic consequence of each of these enzyme deficiencies is a marked increase in hepatic oxalate production. Since oxalate cannot be metabolized by humans, the excess released into the plasma must be excreted by the kidneys, with less than 10% eliminated through the gastronintestinal tract. Calcium oxalate stones and nephrocalcinosis can result from high urinary oxalate (UOx) excretion; the latter can be associated with interstitial inflammation and fibrosis and may contribute to progressive chronic kidney disease (CKD) and end-stage kidney disease (ESKD) [3]. Once patients approach ESKD, excess oxalate can no longer be eliminated by the kidneys, and it accumulates in the body, potentially leading to systemic oxalosis. Among PH patients, there is wide variability in clinical course, with some progressing to ESKD in early childhood, while other PH patients retain kidney function into their fifth or sixth decade. Prediction of long-term outcomes using biomarkers is an important tool for clinical management, particularly now that novel treatment strategies with the potential to reduce hepatic oxalate production in PH are ready for clinical trials [4]. Patients with PH typically excrete >0.7 mmol/1.73 m^2/day [5], and we previously reported that higher UOx predicts future ESKD risk within the PH patient group [2]. We also recently reported that plasma oxalate (POx) concentration correlates with UOx excretion [6].

Since 24 h urine collections can be difficult to obtain, especially on a repeated basis or in younger children, a blood biomarker that predicts UOx and other clinical features of PH could be clinically valuable. Furthermore, in patients with advanced CKD, UOx may no longer reflect systemic oxalate burden; in such cases, POx may represent a more accurate biomarker [7]. Therefore, we examined data in the RKSC PH registry in order to determine whether POx represents a viable biomarker that predicts the future loss of kidney function among patients with confirmed PH and at varying CKD stages.

2. Results

2.1. Baseline Characteristics

There were 227 patients who met the criteria for this study (Figure 1). During follow-up, ESKD developed in nine of the 118 patients (7.6%) in the CKD 1 group, 29 of 135 (21.5%) of the CKD 2 patients, 34 of 72 (47.2%) in the CKD3a, and 31 of 45 (68.8%) in the CKD 3b. There was one death in the CKD 1 group, nine deaths each in the CKD 2 and 3a groups, and 10 deaths in the CKD 3b group. The proportion of patients with PH1 increased by CKD stage (Table 1), representing 56.8% with CKD1, 73.3% with CKD2, 86.1% with CKD3a, and 84.4% with CKD3b. Due to the analysis plan, the median age at PH diagnosis also differed according to which patients experienced each CKD stage, from 5.4 years (CKD1) to 16.0 years (CKD3b). Median follow-up time was 5.3, 8.8, 6.6, and 1.8 years for CKD stages 1–3b, respectively.

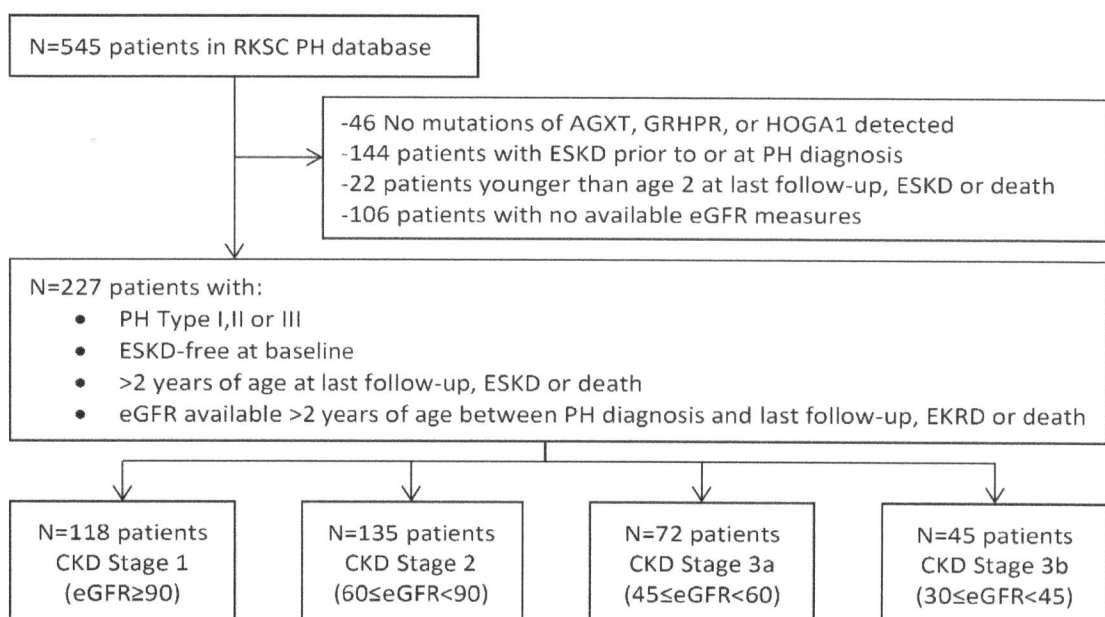

Figure 1. Flowchart of inclusion criteria for analysis cohort. From a total of 545 PH1 patients in the Registry, 227 were eligible for this analysis.

Table 1. Clinical characteristics of patients with primary hyperoxaluria who did not have ESKD at or before diagnosis.

	CKD Stage			
	Stage 1 (≥90)	Stage 2 (60–89)	Stage 3a (45–59)	Stage 3b (30–44)
Characteristics	*n* = 118	*n* = 135	*n* = 72	*n* = 45
Type of PH, % (*n*)				
PH1	67 (56.8%)	99 (73.3%)	62 (86.1%)	38 (84.4%)
PH2	23 (19.5%)	16 (11.9%)	6 (8.3%)	5 (11.1%)
PH3	28 (23.7%)	20 (14.8%)	4 (5.6%)	2 (4.4%)
Sex, % (*n*)				
Male	68 (57.6%)	76 (56.3%)	39 (54.2%)	23 (51.1%)
Female	50 (42.4%)	59 (43.7%)	33 (45.8%)	22 (48.9%)
Age at diagnosis, y	5.4 (2.7, 11.1)	7.9 (4.0, 23.9)	10.7 (4.6, 26.4)	16.0 (7.0, 41.7)
Follow-up time, y	5.3 (2.9, 10.0)	8.8 (3.1, 15.2)	6.6 (3.4, 12.8)	1.8 (1.0, 3.8)
Patients with follow-up Pox labs	*n* = 50	*n* = 69	*n* = 37	*n* = 17
No. follow-up labs	2.5 (1,5)	3 (1,6)	3 (1,5)	1 (1,3)

Continuous variables are expressed as median with 25th, 75th percentiles. *n*, number; PH, primary hyperoxaluria; PH1, primary hyperoxaluria type 1; PH2, primary hyperoxaluria type 2; PH3, primary hyperoxaluria type 3; y, years.

Baseline POx increased by CKD stage from (3.1 (2.1, 5.7) μmol/L in CKD1 (*n* = 38) to 14.4 (10.5, 20.0) μmol/L in CKD3b (*n* = 17) (Table 2). The results were similar within the PH1 subset, increasing from 3.9 [2.4, 6.8] μmol/L in CKD1 (*n* = 24) to 14.9 (11.6, 21.5) μmol/L in CKD3b (*n* = 16). The numbers were not sufficient for a similar sub-analysis in PH2 and PH3. The risk of incident ESKD was higher in patients with PH1 compared to PH2 and PH3 in CKD2 and CKD3b; the results were similar albeit non-significant in CKD1 (HR 7.45; 95% CI 0.92–60.2; p = 0.06) and CKD3a (HR 5.74; 95% CI 0.78–42.1; p = 0.085) (Table 3).

Table 2. Baseline and follow-up POx quartiles, by CKD stage.

Oxalate Measure	*n*	Q1	Median	Q3
Baseline				
POx, umol/L				
CKD stage 1	38	2.1	3.1	5.7
CKD stage 2	44	1.9	4.1	7.2
CKD stage 3a	25	2.9	4.8	8.2
CKD stage 3b	17	10.5	14.4	20.0
Follow-up				
POx, umol/L				
CKD stage 1	171	1.9	3.0	4.8
CKD stage 2	288	2.1	4.1	7.1
CKD stage 3a	165	4.2	7.0	12.9
CKD stage 3b	38	9.9	15.2	18.0

2.2. POx and ESKD

When treated as a continuous predictor, higher baseline POx values were significantly associated with a higher risk of ESKD in CKD2 (HR 1.17; 95% CI 1.01–1.35; p = 0.033), CKD3a (HR 1.29; 95% CI 1.09–1.53; p = 0.004) and CKD3b (HR 1.24; 95% CI 1.08–1.42; p = 0.003) (Table 3). Baseline POx values in Q4 compared to POx in Q1 were also associated with a higher risk of ESKD in CKD3a (HR 13.88; 95% CI 1.41–137; p = 0.024) and CKD3b (HR 42.1; 95% CI 3.29–539; p = 0.004) (Table 3).

During follow-up (Table 4), POx was significantly associated with ESKD risk across all CKD stages: CKD1 (HR 1.12; 95% CI 1.02–1.24, p = 0.018), CKD2 (HR 1.17; 95% CI 1.08–1.25; p < 0.001), CKD3a (HR 1.19; 95% CI 1.11–1.27; p < 0.001), and CKD3b (HR 1.12; 95% CI 1.04–1.21; p = 0.003). When POx was considered by quartile, Q4 was a significant predictor of ESKD compared to Q1 across the CKD stages as well: CKD 2 (HR 14.2; 95% CI 1.76–115; $p = 0.013$), CKD3a (HR 13.7; 95% CI 3.02–62; $p < 0.001$), and CKD3b (HR 5.19; 95% CI 1.10–24.5; $p = 0.038$). Within each POx quartile, the ESKD rate was higher for the later CKD stages. Within each CKD stage, the ESKD rate was also higher in the fourth POx quartile compared to the first three (Table S1 and Figure 2). Thus, the greatest ESKD rate was for the CKD 3b subjects in the highest POx quartile (Figure 2).

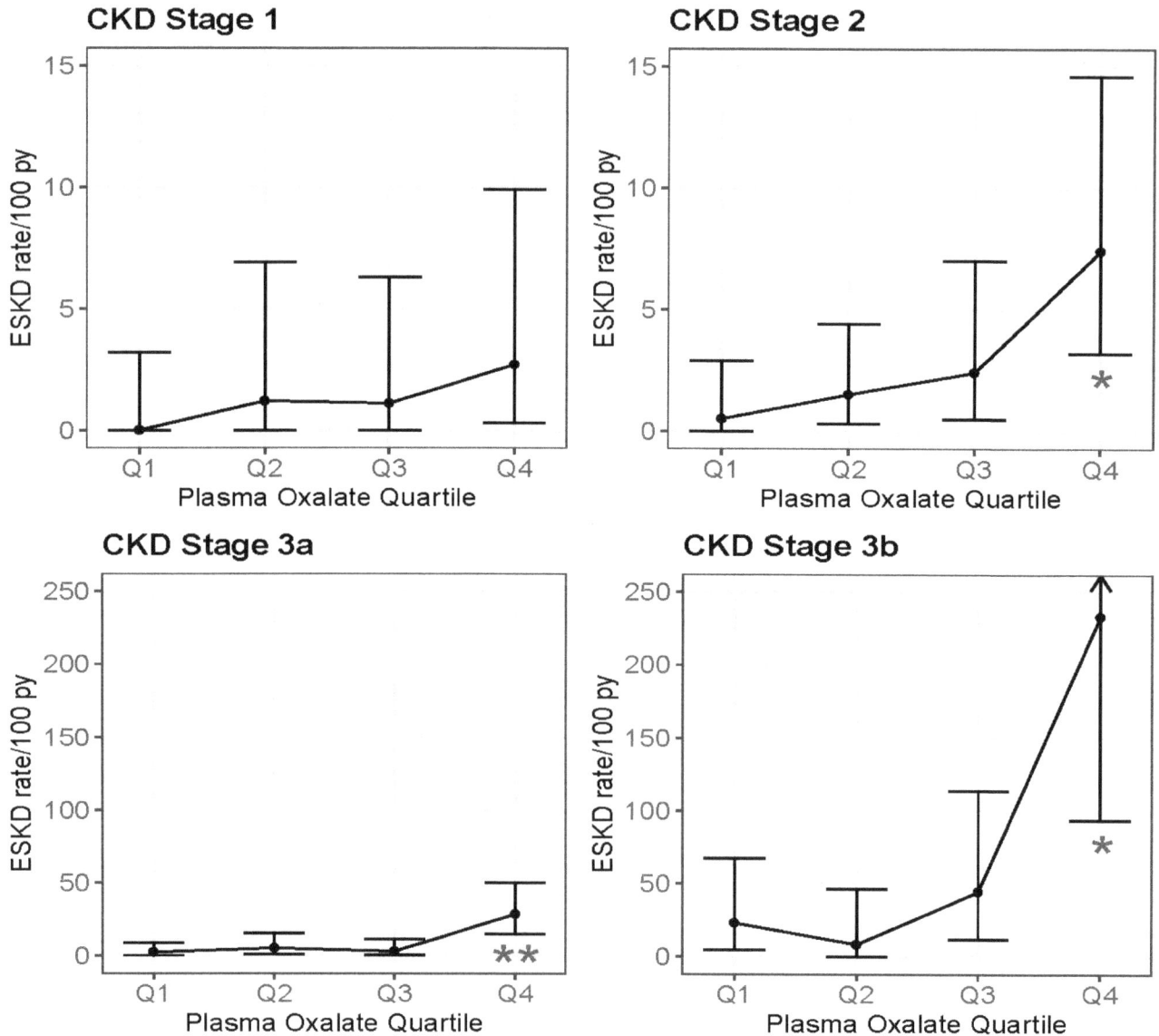

Figure 2. ESKD rate by POx quartile during follow-up by CKD stage. ESKD rates were estimated for each CKD stage group by dividing individual patient follow-up times into intervals based on the time between the POx measures or last follow-up. Person-time and ESKD events were summed within POx quartiles with the rate = [100 × (events/person-time)]; error bars represent 95% CI of the ESKD rate (see Supplemental Table S1 for numerical values). ESKD rates were similar for the lower three quartiles (Q) but increased for the highest POx quartile across CKD stages 2–3b (Q4 vs. Q1 HR 14.21; 95% CI 1.76–114.7; * $p < 0.05$ for CKD stage 2, HR 13.66; 95% CI 3.02–61.91; ** $p < 0.001$ for CKD stage 3a, and HR 5.19; 95% CI 1.10–24.5; * $p < 0.05$ for CKD stage 3b).

Table 3. Factors univariately associated with incident ESKD among patients with primary hyperoxaluria without ESKD at baseline.

| | CKD Stage | | | | | | | | | | | | | | | |
| | Stage 1 (≥90) | | | | Stage 2 (60–89) | | | | Stage 3a (45–59) | | | | Stage 3b (30–44) | | | |
Variable	n; E	HR (95% CI)	p	C-Index	n; E	HR (95% CI)	p	C-Index	n; E	HR (95% CI)	p	C-Index	n; E	HR (95% CI)	p	C-Index
Demographics																
PH1	118; 9	7.45 (0.92–60.2)	0.06	0.677	135; 29	23.9 (3.06–186)	**0.003**	0.630	72; 34	5.74 (0.78–42.1)	0.085	0.544	45; 31	9.45 (1.28–69.8)	**0.028**	0.607
Male	118; 9	1.31 (0.32–5.34)	0.71	0.535	135; 29	1.73 (0.80–3.74)	0.17	0.577	72; 34	1.10 (0.56–2.18)	0.78	0.517	45; 31	1.07 (0.51–2.23)	0.86	0.520
Age at diagnosis	118; 9	0.98 (0.90–1.08)	0.69	0.500	135; 29	1.00 (0.98–1.03)	0.78	0.577	72; 34	1.01 (0.98–1.03)	0.70	0.550	45; 31	0.98 (0.96–1.01)	0.13	0.612
Plasma Oxalate																
POx, umol/L	38; 2	NE†	NE†	NE†	44; 9	1.17 (1.01–1.35)	**0.033**	0.623	25; 10	1.29 (1.09–1.53)	**0.004**	0.727	17; 14	1.24 (1.08–1.42)	**0.003**	0.810
POx, quartile	38; 2	-	-	NE†	44; 9	-	-	0.610	25; 10	-	-	0.698	17; 14	-	-	0.791
Q1	-	REF	REF	-	-	REF	REF	-	-	REF	REF	-	-	REF	REF	-
Q2	-	NE†	NE†	-	-	0.41 (0.04–4.52)	0.47	-	-	2.40 (0.14–40.0)	0.54	-	-	7.85 (0.82–75.0)	0.074	-
Q3	-	NE†	NE†	-	-	1.68 (0.27–10.52)	0.58	-	-	4.39 (0.49–39.5)	0.19	-	-	10.1 (1.11–91.5)	**0.040**	-
Q4	-	NE†	NE†	-	-	1.57 (0.25–9.75)	0.63	-	-	13.88 (1.41–136.5)	**0.024**	-	-	42.1 (3.29–539)	**0.004**	-

PH1, primary hyperoxaluria type 1; n: number available for analysis; E: = ESKD events; 95% CI, 95% confidence interval. p-values in bold denote significance at the 0.05 level. Harrell's c index is provided. † Not estimable, sample size, and no. of events too small for a variable with four levels. The proportional hazards assumption was met for all models with reported HRs.

Table 4. Plasma oxalate excretion on follow-up (>6 months after entry into the CKD group) and risk of ESKD.

| | CKD Stage | | | | | | | | | | | | | | | |
| | Stage 1 (≥90) | | | | Stage 2 (60–89) | | | | Stage 3a (45–59) | | | | Stage 3b (30–44) | | | |
Follow-up Plasma Oxalate	n; E	HR (95% CI)	p	C-Index	n; E	HR (95% CI)	p	C-Index	n; E	HR (95% CI)	p	C-Index	n; E	HR (95% CI)	p	C-Index
POx, umol/L	171; 4	1.12 (1.02–1.24)	**0.018**	0.854	288; 15	1.17 (1.08–1.25)	**<0.001**	0.806	165; 19	1.19 (1.11–1.27)	**<0.001**	0.795	38; 15	1.12 (1.04–1.21)	**0.003**	0.729
POx, quartile	171; 4	-	-	0.818	288; 15	-	-	0.772	165; 19	-	-	0.757	38; 15	-	-	0.752
Q1	-	REF	REF	-	-	REF	REF	-	-	REF	REF	-	-	REF	REF	-
Q2	-	NE†	NE†	-	-	2.70 (0.28–26.03)	0.39	-	-	2.10 (0.35–12.65)	0.42	-	-	0.39 (0.04–4.40)	0.45	-
Q3	-	NE†	NE†	-	-	3.98 (0.41–38.82)	0.24	-	-	1.28 (0.18–9.17)	0.80	-	-	0.98 (0.19–5.04)	0.98	-
Q4	-	NE†	NE†	-	-	14.21 (1.76–114.7)	**0.013**	-	-	13.66 (3.02–61.91)	**<0.001**	-	-	5.19 (1.10–24.5)	**0.038**	-

† Not estimable, sample size, and no. events, too small for a variable with four levels. p-values in bold denote significance at the 0.05 level. Harrell's c index is provided. n = Follow-up intervals; E = ESKD events.

2.3. UOX and ESKD

Risk of ESKD increased at higher UOx levels when follow-up UOx was employed as a continuous time-dependent covariate, yielding an HR of 1.8 (95% CI 1.35–2.5) per each UOx increased of 1 mmol/1.73 m^2/24 h ($p < 0.001$). When examined by follow-up UOx quartile (cut-off points of 0.77, 1.21, and 1.84 mmol/1.73 m^2/24 h), UOx Q4 had a higher ESKD risk than Q1 (HR, 3.7; 95% CI 1.5–9.55) ($p < 0.01$).

2.4. ESKD or 40% Sustained Reduction in eGFR

Results were similar when the combined endpoint of ESKD and a 40% sustained eGFR reduction in eGFR were used for CKD progression. A higher baseline POx remained a significant predictor of incident CKD progression at CKD3b (HR 1.27; 95% CI 1.09–1.48; $p = 0.002$). Higher POx values during follow-up also remained a significant predictor of CKD progression in CKD2 (HR 1.15, 95% CI 1.07–1.23; $p < 0.001$) and CKD3a (HR 1.17, 95% CI 1.08–1.27; $p < 0.001$) when treated both as a continuous predictor and when comparing POx Q4 to POx Q1 (HR 10.71; 95% CI 1.34–85.4; $p = 0.025$ and HR 8.15; 95% CI 1.74–38.2; $p = 0.008$; respectively). Follow-up time was shorter, and there were fewer laboratory parameters available when considering this composite endpoint.

2.5. eGFR Slope

There were 59 patients with a total of 369 POx and eGFR laboratory measures obtained within three months of each other throughout follow-up. The number of lab values per patient ranged from 1 to 20. After adjusting for follow-up time, eGFR was significantly lower among those with higher POx (eGFR reduced by 1.27 mL/min/1.73 m^2 per 1 μmol/L increase in POx; ($p < 0.001$).

3. Discussion

In the current study, we analyzed the predictive value of POx for the subsequent decline in eGFR in PH patients, stratified by CKD stage. These data suggest that POx is a useful predictor of ESKD risk across CKD stages 2–3b (Figure 2), with the effect most pronounced in CKD3b. These data and our previous study [2] suggest that the use of POx and UOx could be complimentary, with UOx being particularly informative across CKD stages 1–3b, and POx particularly informative in CKD stages 3a and 3b.

The clinical management of PH is challenging due to the lifelong nature of the disease and the risk for ESKD observed in a vast majority of PH1 patients, although this can occur at markedly variable ages. The ability to predict long term outcomes using biomarkers facilitates the most effective use of current treatments and also has the potential to provide an important outcome measure for clinical trials of novel therapeutics. Newer treatment options, including the potential use of small inhibitory RNA (siRNA) therapeutics to impact oxalate generating pathways in the liver are under current development [8]. These newer approaches make it important to better understand the prognostic features of PH, which could both identify patients who could be eligible candidates for clinical trials and also potentially be used as surrogate endpoints in future studies.

In the current study, we examined whether POx is a useful prognostic marker for the future of loss of kidney function. The data demonstrate that higher POx levels both at baseline and during follow-up were significantly associated with loss of kidney function over time. When stratified by quartile, those in POx Q4 were at increased risk of ESKD compared to POx Q1 across CKD stages 2–3b. As expected, based upon previous prevalence data, patients that progressed to later CKD stages tended to be older and more likely to have PH1. The current study also confirms our previous observation that baseline UOx and UOx over follow-up predict ESKD, with those in the highest quartile at the greatest additional risk [2]. Furthermore, the HRs for the subsequent ESKD of the highest UOx quartile at baseline (2.5) and during follow-up (3.7) were similar to our previous work [2].

Much as the serum creatinine concentration is a net result of creatinine generation from muscle and elimination by the kidneys, POx is the net result of oxalate generated in the liver and absorbed from the GI tract and its elimination by the kidneys. Thus, higher POx can reflect higher hepatic oxalate generation, greater gastrointestinal absorption, lower GFR, or some combination of these. Indeed, our previous publications demonstrated that UOx excretion could be used to predict POx and eGFR [6]. Recent studies also suggest that higher UOx excretion predicts a higher renal tubular fluid oxalate concentration at the S3 segment of the proximal tubule, the anatomic site of nephrocalcinosis in PH [9]. Thus, the results from our current study demonstrating the predictive value of POx across the CKD stage 2–3b spectrum may reflect the fact that POx provides integration of oxalate generation and elimination, and thus becomes a sensitive marker of oxalate burden at the level of the proximal tubule.

One issue with the widespread use of POx is the challenging nature of the available laboratory assays [10]. Under normal circumstances, POx is present in micro-molar concentrations in blood. Thus, sample handling, including prevention of ascorbate conversion to oxalate, is quite important. In addition, methods for measuring oxalate, including sample type, preparation, and analysis, are not interchangeable [10–12]. Our study benefitted from use of a single clinical laboratory over many decades with data to support that POx results could be compared over that time period. However, because of the barriers for analysis in routine laboratories, the POx measurement is not widely available. Additionally, when GFR is normal or near-normal, POx concentrations typically are near or below the limit of quantification in the general population [10]. However, due to a markedly increased oxalate generation, POx is typically above the limit of quantification in most PH patients, even with preserved eGFR [6], suggesting that with a consistent and sensitive assay, POx could be a useful biomarker. Moreover, as GFR declines, POx values rise well within the quantification range with good reproducibility in all PH patients.

The current study has several limitations. Due to the retrospective nature of this analysis based on registry data, laboratory measures and follow-up were limited by availability, and variability in the diagnosis and ability to recruit patients with this rare disease may have introduced bias. There was also no controlled intervention to change POx values. Nevertheless, we were able to analyze a relatively large cohort of over 200 PH patients with available POx values. Furthermore, comorbidities such as obesity, dyslipidemia, hypertension, and albuminuria, which are important CKD risk factors, were not available for multivariate analysis. However, many PH patients progress to ESKD at a very young age, and thus these comorbidities likely play a relatively minimal role in CKD progression, in comparison to common causes of CKD such as diabetic nephropathy in which vascular/microvascular injury and dysfunction play a major role.

In conclusion, there is a need for improved knowledge regarding the utility of biomarkers to predict ESKD risk in PH patients at various stages of CKD. The current study suggests that POx, perhaps in combination with other risk factors, is a useful marker for this purpose.

4. Materials and Methods

Natural history and laboratory data from PH patients enrolled in the RKSC PH Registry were used for analysis [13]. PH1, PH2, and PH3 patients were confirmed by mutations in the AGXT, GRHPR, or HOGA1 genes, respectively. POx was measured in the Mayo Clinic Renal Testing Laboratory (Rochester, MN, USA) by an oxalate oxidase (1991–6/2016) or ion chromatography (6/2016–2019) based-assay per the standard Mayo Renal Testing Laboratory Protocol [10]. Detailed validation data was available to determine that assay results could be compared over the course of this time period. UOx was measured by oxalate oxidase also in the Mayo Renal Testing Laboratory or another accredited clinical laboratory [10,14]. Data for subjects <2 years old were excluded from this analysis due to potential confounding effects of renal maturation in very young children on GFR (and thus POx).

This project was approved by the Mayo Clinic Institutional Review Board (IRB 11-001702; initial approval 16 August 2011). A total of 545 PH patients were identified in the Registry as of March 31, 2019 (Figure 1). After excluding patients who met clinical criteria but had no detectable mutations of AGXT, GRHPR, or HOGA1, ($n = 46$), those with ESKD at diagnosis ($n = 144$), patients less than two years old at ESKD or last follow-up ($n = 22$), and those patients without eGFR data after diagnosis and older than two years before ESKD or death ($n = 106$), a total of 227 patients remained in the final cohort for analysis. Since our previous study suggested an association between POx and CKD stage [6], patients were then divided into four groups based on CKD stage (1, 2, 3a, 3b) in a landmark-style analysis, such that a patient started in a given CKD stage subgroup on their first eGFR observed in that range, while also remaining in any prior groups through all available follow-ups. For instance, a patient whose eGFR measurements were 64, 72, 43, 47, 38, 29, and 21 mL/min/1.73 m^2 would never be included in the CKD stage 1 group, would enter the eGFR 60–89 group with the date of the eGFR = 64 mL/min/1.73 m^2 measurement and be followed until kidney progression or censoring, would enter the eGFR 30–44 group with the date of the eGFR = 43 mL/min/1.73 m^2 measurement and be followed until kidney progression or censoring, and would enter the eGFR 45–59 group with the date of the eGFR = 47 mL/min/1.73 m^2 measurement and be followed until kidney progression or censoring.

Laboratory results were extracted from the registry data, and were from baseline (defined as within one year prior to or within six months of entry into the CKD stage group and prior to kidney progression) or follow-up (defined from six months after the entry into the CKD stage group and prior to kidney progression). None of this patient cohort experienced acute kidney injury events during follow-up. GFR was estimated via the CKD-EPI creatinine equation for adults greater than 18 years old [15] and the Schwartz equation for those less than 18 years old [16]. POx values were manually examined, and outlying transient results not fitting the clinical picture were removed from the analysis.

4.1. Statistical Methods

Plasma Oxalate

Progression to ESKD (eGFR < 15 mL/min/1.73 m^2 or the start of dialysis or renal transplantation) was selected as the primary endpoint. Sensitivity analyses were also performed using a combined endpoint of ESKD or sustained 40% reduction in eGFR from baseline. The results were expressed in terms of the median (25th, 75th percentiles) for continuous variables and as percentages for categorical variables. To maximize available data, the diagnosis/baseline labs were defined as the closest reading between one year before entry and up to six months after entry into a CKD stage group.

The percentage of patients who were free of renal progression (ESKD and > 40% decline in eGFR) after entry into each CKD stage was estimated using the Kaplan–Meier method. The effects of baseline clinical characteristics, as well as Pox on renal progression, were estimated by univariate analyses using the Cox proportional hazard model with log-rank tests. The primary outcome of interest was time to ESKD and was censored on death or loss to follow-up. Hazard ratios (HRs) and 95% confidence intervals (95% CIs) are presented. A time-dependent Cox model was used to explore the effect of POx concentration on renal outcome during follow-up. Times to ESKD by POx quartile during follow-up were estimated for each CKD stage group by dividing individual-patient follow-up time into intervals based on the time between POx measures or last follow-up. Person-time and ESKD events were summed within the POx quartile with the rate = $100 \times$ (Events/Person-time). The proportional hazards assumption was checked for all models using martingale residuals. Generalized estimating equations (GEE) adjusting for time were used to evaluate the association between POx and eGFR throughout follow-up. The effect of follow-up UOx concentration on the risk of renal outcomes were also assessed using a time-dependent Cox model.

Author Contributions: Conceptualization, L.E.V., F.T.E., D.S.M. and J.C.L.; Methodology, L.E.V., F.T.E., D.S.M. and J.C.L. Formal Analysis, L.E.V. and F.T.E.; Investigation, R.J.S., L.E.V., F.T.E., D.S.M. and J.C.L.; Resources, F.T.E., D.S.M., and J.C.L.; Data Curation, R.J.S. and L.E.V.; Writing—Original Draft Preparation, R.J.S.; Writing—Review & Editing, L.E.V., F.T.E., D.S.M., and J.C.L.; Visualization, L.E.V.; Supervision, J.C.L.; Project Administration, J.C.L.; Funding Acquisition, F.T.E., D.S.M., and J.C.L. All authors have read and agreed to the published version of the manuscript.

Acknowledgments: We thank the patients and their families for their gracious participation. We are grateful to the investigators of the RKSC coordinating sites and many additional individual contributors to the PH Registry for generously providing clinical data.

References

1. Cochat, P.; Rumsby, G. Primary hyperoxaluria. *N. Engl. J. Med.* **2013**, *369*, 649–658. [CrossRef] [PubMed]
2. Zhao, F.; Bergstralh, E.J.; Mehta, R.A.; Vaughan, L.E.; Olson, J.B.; Seide, B.M.; Meek, A.M.; Cogal, A.G.; Lieske, J.C.; Milliner, D.S. Predictors of incident ESRD among patients with primary hyperoxaluria presenting prior to kidney failure. *Clin. J. Am. Soc. Nephrol.* **2016**, *11*, 119–126. [CrossRef] [PubMed]
3. Hoppe, B.; Beck, B.B.; Milliner, D.S. The primary hyperoxalurias. *Kidney Int.* **2009**, *75*, 1264–1271. [CrossRef] [PubMed]
4. Dutta, C.; Avitahl-Curtis, N.; Pursell, N.; Larsson Cohen, M.; Holmes, B.; Diwanji, R.; Zhou, W.; Apponi, L.; Koser, M.; Ying, B.; et al. Inhibition of Glycolate Oxidase with Dicer-substrate siRNA Reduces Calcium Oxalate Deposition in a Mouse Model of Primary Hyperoxaluria Type 1. *Mol. Ther.* **2016**, *24*, 770–778. [CrossRef] [PubMed]
5. Edvardsson, V.O.; Goldfarb, D.S.; Lieske, J.C.; Beara-Lasic, L.; Anglani, F.; Milliner, D.S.; Palsson, R. Hereditary causes of kidney stones and chronic kidney disease. *Pediatr. Nephrol.* **2013**. [CrossRef] [PubMed]
6. Perinpam, M.; Enders, F.T.; Mara, K.C.; Vaughan, L.E.; Mehta, R.A.; Voskoboev, N.; Milliner, D.S.; Lieske, J.C. Plasma oxalate in relation to eGFR in patients with primary hyperoxaluria, enteric hyperoxaluria and urinary stone disease. *Clin. Biochem.* **2017**, *50*, 1014–1019. [CrossRef] [PubMed]
7. Elgstoen, K.B.; Johnsen, L.F.; Woldseth, B.; Morkrid, L.; Hartmann, A. Plasma oxalate following kidney transplantation in patients without primary hyperoxaluria. *Nephrol. Dial. Transplant.* **2010**, *25*, 2341–2345. [CrossRef] [PubMed]
8. Bhasin, B.; Ürekli, H.M.; Atta, M.G. Primary and secondary hyperoxaluria: Understanding the enigma. *World J. Nephrol.* **2015**, *4*, 235. [CrossRef] [PubMed]
9. Worcester, E.M.; Evan, A.P.; Coe, F.L.; Lingeman, J.E.; Krambeck, A.; Sommers, A.; Philips, C.L.; Milliner, D. A test of the hypothesis that oxalate secretion produces proximal tubule crystallization in primary hyperoxaluria type I. *Am. J. Physiol.-Ren. Physiol.* **2013**, *305*, F1574–F1584. [CrossRef] [PubMed]
10. Ladwig, P.M.; Liedtke, R.R.; Larson, T.S.; Lieske, J.C. Sensitive spectrophotometric assay for plasma oxalate. *Clin. Chem.* **2005**, *51*, 2377–2380. [CrossRef] [PubMed]
11. Hoppe, B.; Kemper, M.J.; Hvizd, M.G.; Sailer, D.E.; Langman, C.B. Simultaneous determination of oxalate, citrate and sulfate in children's plasma with ion chromatography. *Kidney Int.* **1998**, *53*, 1348–1352. [CrossRef] [PubMed]
12. Elgstoen, K.B. Liquid chromatography-tandem mass spectrometry method for routine measurement of oxalic acid in human plasma. *J. Chromatogr. B Analyt. Technol. Biomed. Life Sci.* **2008**, *873*, 31–36. [CrossRef] [PubMed]
13. Lieske, J.C.; Monico, C.G.; Holmes, W.S.; Bergstralh, E.J.; Slezak, J.M.; Rohlinger, A.L.; Olson, J.B.; Milliner, D.S. International registry for primary hyperoxaluria. *Am. J. Nephrol.* **2005**, *25*, 290–296. [CrossRef] [PubMed]
14. Wilson, D.M.; Liedtke, R.R. Modified enzyme-based colorimetric assay of urinary and plasma oxalate with improved sensitivity and no ascorbate interference: Reference values and specimen handling procedures. *Clin. Chem.* **1991**, *37*, 1229–1235. [CrossRef] [PubMed]
15. Inker, L.A.; Schmid, C.H.; Tighiouart, H.; Eckfeldt, J.H.; Feldman, H.I.; Greene, T.; Kusek, J.W.; Manzi, J.; Van Lente, F.; Zhang, Y.L. Estimating glomerular filtration rate from serum creatinine and cystatin C. *N. Engl. J. Med.* **2012**, *367*, 20–29. [CrossRef] [PubMed]
16. Schwartz, G.J.; Munoz, A.; Schneider, M.F.; Mak, R.H.; Kaskel, F.; Warady, B.A.; Furth, S.L. New equations to estimate GFR in children with CKD. *J. Am. Soc. Nephrol.* **2009**, *20*, 629–637. [CrossRef] [PubMed]

10

One-Year Progression and Risk Factors for the Development of Chronic Kidney Disease in Septic Shock Patients with Acute Kidney Injury

June-sung Kim, Youn-Jung Kim, Seung Mok Ryoo, Chang Hwan Sohn, Dong Woo Seo, Shin Ahn, Kyoung Soo Lim and Won Young Kim *

Department of Emergency Medicine, Asan Medical Center, University of Ulsan College of Medicine, Seoul 05505, Korea; jsmeet09@gmail.com (J.-s.K.); yjkim.em@gmail.com (Y.-J.K.); chrisryoo@naver.com (S.M.R.); schwan97@gmail.com (C.H.S.); leiseo@gmail.com (D.W.S.); ans1023@gmail.com (S.A.); kslim@amc.seoul.kr (K.S.L.)
* Correspondence: wonpia73@naver.com

Abstract: (1) Background: Sepsis-associated acute kidney injury (AKI) can lead to permanent kidney damage, although the long-term prognosis in patients with septic shock remains unclear. This study aimed to identify risk factors for the development of chronic kidney disease (CKD) in septic shock patients with AKI. (2) Methods: A single-site, retrospective cohort study was conducted using a registry of adult septic shock patients. Data from patients who had developed AKI between January 2011 and April 2017 were extracted, and 1-year follow-up data were analysed to identify patients who developed CKD. (3) Results: Among 2208 patients with septic shock, 839 (38%) had AKI on admission (stage 1: 163 (19%), stage 2: 339 (40%), stage 3: 337 (40%)). After one year, kidney function had recovered in 27% of patients, and 6% had progressed to CKD. In patients with stage 1 AKI, 10% developed CKD, and mortality was 13% at one year; in patients with stage 2 and 3 AKI, the CKD rate was 6%, and the mortality rate was 42% and 47%, respectively. Old age, female, diabetes, low haemoglobin levels and a high creatinine level at discharge were seen to be risk factors for the development of CKD. (4) Conclusions: AKI severity correlated with mortality, but it did not correlate with the development of CKD, and patients progressed to CKD, even when initial AKI stage was not severe. Physicians should focus on the recovery of renal function, and ensure the careful follow-up of patients with risk factors for the development of CKD.

Keywords: septic shock; acute kidney injury; acute kidney disease; chronic kidney disease; follow-up

1. Introduction

Sepsis is one of the most common causes of mortality in critically ill patients worldwide [1–3]. Septic shock, the most severe form of sepsis, can lead to multi-system organ failure and is a major risk factor for the development of acute kidney injury (AKI), accounting for more than 50% of cases [4,5]. Although septic AKI has been considered a temporary syndrome [5,6], a growing body of evidence suggests that AKI is likely to lead to continuous or permanent kidney damage, and it can progress to end-stage kidney disease [7,8]. In patients with sepsis and septic shock, the presence of AKI has been shown to be a poor prognostic factor that is associated with higher rates of mortality and short-term adverse consequences, including the prolonged duration of mechanical ventilation, increased intensive care unit stay and death [9,10]. However, few studies have included long-term follow-up periods [11,12], and data describing the relationship between initial severity and the development of chronic kidney disease (CKD) in patients with sepsis-induced AKI are limited [13].

To address this issue, we evaluated data from the Asan Medical Center Emergency Department Septic Shock Registry, to determine the development of CKD in septic shock patients with AKI, and to identify risk factors associated with the development of this condition.

2. Materials and Methods

2.1. Setting and Study Population

This single-center, retrospective, observational, registry-based study was conducted at the Asan Medical Center Emergency Department in South Korea, using data obtained from patients diagnosed between January 2011 and April 2017. The Asan Medical Center is an academic tertiary referral center with 2700 beds; approximately 100,000 patients visit the emergency department annually. The study protocol was approved by the institutional research ethics committee (Study No. 2016-0548), and the requirement for informed consent was waived, due to the retrospective nature of the study.

Adult patients ($\geq$18 years of age) with septic shock were enrolled from the Asan Medical Center Septic Shock Registry. Septic shock was defined as the presence of refractory hypotension (mean arterial pressure $\leq$70 mmHg) requiring treatment with vasopressors, or a blood lactate concentration $\geq$4 mmol/L despite sufficient fluid loading [14]. We excluded individuals who were younger than 18 years and pregnant individuals. Moreover, in addition to evaluate the effect of newly developed AKI to CKD, we also excluded patients who had previously been diagnosed with CKD and end-stage renal disease (ESRD) requiring renal replacement therapy (RRT).

2.2. Data Collection and Definition

Data regarding patient age, sex, previous medical history, laboratory results and infection sites based on clinical and radiological examination were obtained from the registry. Previous CKD or ESRD patients who had outpatient or inpatient diagnosis of pre-existing CKD and ESRD, had code related with hemodialysis and who had a prior diagnosis of AKI or a baseline-estimated glomerular filtration rate (eGFR) lower than 60 mL/min/1.73 m^2 were identified via electronic medical records. AKI on initial admission was defined in accordance with the Kidney Disease: Improving Global Outcomes (KDIGO) guidelines [15], i.e., an increase in serum creatinine (Cr) of 0.3 mg/dL within 48 h, or an increase in creatinine to 1.5 times the lowest known creatinine level during the preceding one week to one year. If baseline Cr levels were not available, an estimated baseline was calculated using the simplified modification of diet in renal disease (MDRD) formula, assuming that a given patient without known renal disease had a normal glomerular filtration rate (GFR) of approximately 75–100 mL/min/1.73 m^2. Serum Cr levels were assessed in all patients at least once each day during the hospital stay, and baseline, initial, peaks within 48 h and discharge values, were recorded. Maximum KDIGO refers to the worst KDIGO stage observed over the 48 h period following admission. Baseline Cr levels were measured preceding one week to one year before admission, and the initial level was measured at admission.

To evaluate the CKD status after one year, serum Cr and eGFR levels were obtained after discharge from the electronic medical records of all patients, 12 $\pm$ 3 months from initial admission. Moreover, in order to reduce missing diagnoses, we collected data of inpatient or outpatient diagnoses of CKD or ESRD and codes related to hemodialysis, via medical records. All eGFRs were calculated by MDRD (GFR = 175 $\times$ serum Cr$^{-1.154}$ $\times$ age$^{-0.203}$ $\times$ 1.212 (if patient is black) $\times$ 0.742 (if female)). When multiple records were present, the highest serum Cr and the lowest GFR values were recorded. CKD risk (based on GFR values, mL/min/1.73 m^2) was then classified according to the KDIGO guidelines: G1 $\geq$90, G2 = 60–89, G3a = 45–59, G3b = 30–44, G4 = 15–29 and G5 <15 [16]. Patients classified as G3a, G3b, G4 and G5 were included in the analysis; those with G1 and G2 disease were excluded, as they were considered to be at a low risk of developing ESRD. The date of the patient's death was extracted from the National Health Insurance Service in South Korea. The primary study outcome was the development of CKD according to the initial and the maximum KDIGO AKI stage. Secondary outcomes included all-cause mortality and RRT dependence within the 1-year follow-up period.

2.3. Statistical Analyses

Statistical analyses were performed using SPSS Statistics for Windows, version 23 (SPSS Inc., Chicago, IL, USA). Continuous variables were reported as the median and interquartile range. Categorical variables were analysed using the chi-square test or Fisher's exact test. The normality of distribution was examined using the Kolmogorov–Smirnov test. The Mann–Whitney U test was used for the comparison of CKD and non-CKD groups after one year of follow-up. Variables with an entry-level significance of $p < 0.2$ in the univariate analysis were included in a stepwise multivariate analysis, because an entry-level of less than 0.2 was more informative than that of 0.1. Possible interactions and collinearities were also tested. To adjust for confounding variables, and to assess possible effect modification, separate multiple logistic regression analyses were performed. The results were reported as odds ratios (OR) and 95% confidence intervals (CI). A p-value <0.05 was considered to be statistically significant.

3. Results

3.1. Patient Characteristics

Between 1 January 2011 and 31 April 2017, 2208 adult patients were enrolled in the Asan Medical Center Emergency Medicine Septic Shock Registry (Figure 1). Of these, 255 who had a pre-existing diagnosis of CKD or ESRD, and 1114 patients with septic shock without AKI, were excluded. The remaining 839 patients (38%) with AKI were categorised according to their KDIGO classification on the day of admission. Among these 839 patients, 163 (19%) had stage 1, 339 (40%) stage 2 and 337 (40%) stage 3. According to the maximum KDIGO criteria, 117 (14%) had stage 1, 337 (40%) stage 2 and 385 (46%) stage 3. Within the first 48 h, maximum serum creatinine was recorded and 35 patients were reassigned from stage 1 to stage 2; 48 patients were additionally included in the stage 3 group. Among them, 151 patients applied continuous RRT during admission, and six patients needed intermittent hemodialysis after stopping continuous RRT.

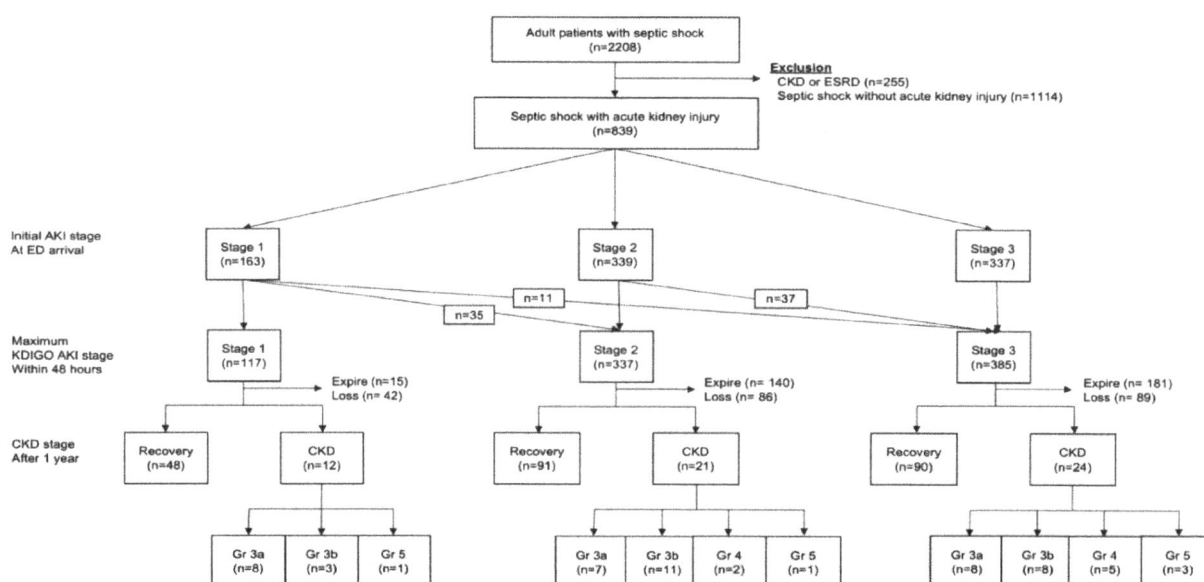

Figure 1. Flowchart of the study population.

The demographic, clinical and laboratory characteristics of patients who developed/did not develop CKD after one year (CKD and non-CKD groups) are summarised in Table 1. Overall, patients were predominantly male (63.3%), with a median age of 64 years. Hypertension and diabetes were more common in the CKD group than the non-CKD group (47.4% vs. 32.8%, $p = 0.045$; 52.6% vs. 23.6%, $p < 0.001$, respectively). No significant differences were seen in other underlying diseases between the two groups. Pulmonary (21.6%) and hepatobiliary (30.9%) infections were most common in both groups, and no statistically significant differences were seen in the locations of the infection sites. Regarding laboratory values, baseline, initial, peak and discharge creatinine, blood urea nitrogen and hemoglobin levels tended to be higher in the CKD group than in the non-CKD group.

Table 1. Characteristics of patients.

Characteristics	Total $n = 286$	Non-CKD after 1 Year $n = 229$	CKD after 1 Year $n = 57$	p-Value
Age	63.7 (56.0–72.0)	64.0 (55.0–70.0)	71.0 (61.3–77.8)	0.001
Male	181 (63.3)	152 (66.4)	29 (50.9)	0.033
Underlying disease				
HTN	102 (35.7)	75 (32.8)	27 (47.4)	0.045
Stroke	24 (8.4)	18 (7.9)	6 (10.5)	0.592
DM	84 (29.4)	54 (23.6)	30 (52.6)	<0.001
Coronary artery disease	22 (7.7)	14 (6.1)	8 (14.0)	0.054
Chronic pulmonary disease	29 (10.1)	22 (9.6)	7 (12.3)	0.623
Liver cirrhosis	43 (15.0)	37 (16.2)	6 (10.5)	0.312
Malignancy	79 (27.6)	56 (25.8)	20 (35.1)	0.186
Infection site				
Unknown	4 (4.1)	2 (8.8)	2 (2.7)	0.788
Pulmonary	21 (21.6)	15 (20.5)	6 (25.0)	0.776
Urinary	23 (23.7)	18 (24.7)	5 (20.8)	0.788
Gastrointestine	15 (15.5)	13 (17.8)	2 (8.3)	0.345
Hepatobiliary	30 (30.9)	21 (28.8)	9 (37.5)	0.452
Others	11 (11.3)	9 (12.3)	2 (8.3)	0.572
Laboratory				
WBC ($\times 10^3$/uL)	10.5 (5.1–17.5)	10.5 (5.7–18.0)	10.6 (4.0–14.9)	0.491
Hb (g/dL)	11.5 (9.3–13.2)	11.9 (9.9–13.6)	14.93 (10.6–22.6)	<0.001
PLT ($\times 10^3$/uL)	137.0 (72.5–207.0)	138.0 (75.5–207.0)	130.0 (66.25–210.5)	0.921
BUN (mg/dL)	32.0 (24.8–45.0)	31.0 (23.0–40.5)	36.0 (29.0–53.0)	0.017
Baseline Cr (mg/dL)	0.72 (0.63–0.86)	0.70 (0.61–0.82)	0.80 (0.72–0.98)	<0.001
Initial Cr (mg/dL)	1.8 (1.4–2.5)	1.8 (1.4–2.4)	2.1 (1.5–3.0)	0.037
Peak Cr (mg/dL)	2.0 (1.5–2.7)	1.9 (1.5–2.6)	2.4 (1.6–3.5)	0.002
Discharge Cr (mg/dL)	0.9 (0.7–1.1)	0.8 (0.6–1.0)	1.1 (0.9–1.8)	<0.001
Lactate (mmol/L)	3.3 (2.0–5.5)	3.3 (2.0–5.6)	3.0 (1.8–4.5)	0.389
CRP (mg/dL)	15.3 (5.9–22.2)	16.1 (6.7–22.3)	11.9 (5.13–22.0)	0.278

Data are presented as n (%) or median with interquartile ranges. HTN = hypertension; DM = diabetes mellitus; CKD = chronic kidney disease; WBC = white blood cells; Hb = hemoglobin; PLT = platelet; BUN = blood urea nitrogen; Cr = creatinine; CRP = c-reactive protein.

3.2. KDIGO Stages and Outcomes

Clinical outcomes in the CKD and non-CKD groups are shown in Figure 1. Among the 117 stage 1 patients, 15 (13%) died, 42 (36%) were lost to follow-up, 48 (41%) recovered full kidney function and 12 (20%) developed CKD (KDIGO CKD stage G3a, $n = 8$ patients; G3b, $n = 3$; G5, $n = 1$). Of the 337 stage 2 patients, 140 (42%) died, 86 (26%) were lost to follow-up within one year, 91 (27%) recovered full kidney function and 21 (6%) developed CKD (stage G3a, $n = 7$; G3b, $n = 11$; G4, $n = 2$; G5, $n = 1$). Of the 385 stage 3 patients, 181 (47%) died, 89 (23%) were lost to follow-up, 90 (23%) recovered full kidney function and 24 (6%) developed CKD (stage G3a, $n = 8$; G3b, $n = 8$; G4, $n = 5$; G5, $n = 3$).

The adjusted ORs of the initial and maximum KDIGO AKI stage for CKD development and all-cause mortality within 1 year are shown in Table 2. Notably, there were no significant differences in the occurrence of CKD by KDIGO classification between the initial and maximum criteria. The OR for CKD development according to the AKI stages increased proportionally, but it was not statistically significant. Meanwhile, all-cause mortality proportionally increased according to KDIGO classification by the initial and maximum Cr levels.

Table 2. Adjusted odds ratios of the AKI stage for CKD development in patients with sepsis-induced AKI.

Variables	Multivariate Analysis		
	OR	95% CI	p-Value
CKD Development			
Initial Cr			
KDIGO stage 1	Reference		
KDIGO stage 2	0.783	0.375–1.635	0.515
KDIGO stage 3	0.924	0.444–1.923	0.832
Maximum Cr			
KDIGO stage 1	Reference		
KDIGO stage 2	0.879	0.396–1.950	0.751
KDIGO stage 3	1.111	0.513–2.405	0.789
All-Cause Mortality			
Initial Cr			
KDIGO stage 1	Reference		
KDIGO stage 2	2.637	1.719–4.046	<0.001
KDIGO stage 3	2.933	1.913–4.499	<0.001
Maximum Cr			
KDIGO stage 1	Reference		
KDIGO stage 2	4.832	2.696–8.668	<0.001
KDIGO stage 3	5.909	3.316–10.530	<0.001

AKI = acute kidney injury; CKD = chronic kidney disease; OR = odds ratio; CI = confidence interval; Cr = creatinine; KDIGO = Kidney Disease Improving Global Outcomes.

3.3. Risk Factors for the Development of CKD

A multivariate logistic regression of factors associated with the occurrence of CKD development within one year is shown in Table 3. Older age (adjusted OR: 1.070, 95% CI: 1.033–1.108, $p < 0.001$), diabetes (adjusted OR: 2.620, 95% CI: 1.352–5.078, $p = 0.004$), low hemoglobin levels (adjusted OR: 0.840, 95% CI: 0.744–0.949, $p = 0.005$) and higher discharge creatinine levels (adjusted OR: 2.686, 95% CI: 1.499–4.812, $p < 0.001$) were associated with the development of CKD.

Table 3. Multivariate logistic regression of factors associated with the occurrence of CKD after one year.

Variables	Univariate Analysis			Multivariate Analysis		
	OR	95% CI	p-Value	OR	95% CI	p-Value
Age	1.066	1.027–1.107	<0.001	1.070	1.033–1.108	<0.001
HTN	0.996	0.487–2.039	0.991			
DM	2.656	1.341–5.257	0.005	2.620	1.352–5.078	0.004
CAD	1.914	0.638–5.745	0.247			
LC	0.992	0.360–2.730	0.987			
Malignancy	1.250	0.601–2.600	0.551			
Hb	0.833	0.734–0.946	0.005	0.840	0.744–0.949	0.005
Discharge Cr	2.503	1.371–4.569	0.003	2.686	1.499–4.812	<0.001

Abbreviations: OR = odds ratio; CI = confidence interval; HTN = hypertension; DM = diabetes mellitus; CAD = coronary artery disease; LC = liver cirrhosis; Hb = hemoglobin; Cr = creatinine.

4. Discussion

In this study, we evaluated the development of CKD in patients with septic shock-associated AKI. In patients who survived and for whom 1-year follow-up data were available, 80% (229/286) recovered full renal function within 1 year and 20% (57/286) had progressed to CKD; 2% (5/286) were dependent on RRT. Long-term all-cause mortality was 40% (336/839), and while the severity of the KDIGO AKI stage was correlated with mortality, it did not correlate with the development of CKD.

In the current study, the incidence of AKI in patients with septic shock was 38% on admission, which is consistent with previous studies reporting an incidence of approximately 35% [17]. AKI can accelerate the progression of CKD [7,18,19], but little is known about the association between AKI severity and the development of CKD. Ishani et al. showed that CKD developed in 6.6%–10.5% of elderly patients with AKI [8]. In addition, they found that elderly individuals, particularly those with previously diagnosed CKD, were at significantly greater risk for end-stage renal disease, suggesting that episodes of AKI may accelerate the progression of renal disease [8].

Few studies have assessed the relationship between AKI severity and CKD progression, and this association therefore remains the subject of some debate [20–22]. Chawla et al. hypothesised that the severity of AKI, according to the Risk, Injury, Failure, Loss and End-stage kidney disease (RIFLE) criteria, correlates with the progression of CKD [23]. In addition, a recent meta-analysis reported that the risk of CKD increased proportionally with mild, moderate and severe AKI (adjusted hazard ratio: 2.0, 3.3 and 28.2, respectively) [18]. However, in the current study, all three stages of AKI were associated with similar rates of recovery and CKD development, suggesting that physicians should focus on the recovery of renal function, even when the initial AKI is not severe. The differing results seen in the present study, in comparison with previous reports, may reflect confounding variables, such as the severity of infection, immune function, duration of exposure to nephrotoxic drugs and timing of RRT initiation, which were not assessed in the current study.

Risk factors for CKD after AKI were seen to include older age, diabetes and higher creatinine level at discharge. Higher creatine levels at discharge indicate delayed or lack of renal function recovery, despite the resolution of the initial infection. Manish et al. suggested that early reversible AKI within the first day of admission was associated with a better survival rate than was no, new or persistent AKI [12]. By contrast, Jones et al. demonstrated that even reversible AKI is strongly associated with an increased risk of progression to CKD [24]. Identifying a direct causative mechanism between AKI and CKD may be impossible, but recent studies demonstrated that persistent kidney injury induced by septic AKI is coupled with systemic inflammation. Renal repair can lead to malfunctions in inflammation and fibrosis and vascular rarefaction that leads to continuous cell and tissue disruption [25,26]. Considering this, protein biomarkers such as neutrophil gelatinase-associated lipocalin and interleukin 6 are likely to have an important role in assessing kidney injury, and aiding the discovery of new treatment targets [26–28].

The current study has several limitations. First, the results are limited by the retrospective study design, and as the data were obtained from a single center, it may not be possible to generalise the findings to other populations. Secondly, because of the long-term study period, patients may not have received consistent prehospital and hospital treatment, which may have affected the outcomes. Thirdly, the diagnosis and classification of AKI based only on serum creatinine values may not have captured all relevant cases of AKI, as extremes in muscle mass or dietary protein consumption may affect serum creatinine, and may not reflect true kidney functioning [29]. A recent study demonstrated that the use of serum creatinine only, urine output only or both factors of the KDIGO criteria showed differing outcomes; for example, hospital mortality within the three groups was 9.2% (serum creatinine only), 7.5% (urine output only) and 26.7% (both serum creatinine and urine output) [30]. Moreover, previous CKD or ESRD, or patients with high risk factors (pre-existing proteinuria, albuminuria, decreased urine output, or long-term usage of medication, which could induce renal dysfunction) could be included in study population. Also, not all patients had baseline serum creatinine or eGFR, so we could not confirm to what extent septic shock was responsible for kidney dysfunction. Because our data did not have urine analysis and renal ultrasonography, which contain other important clues to diagnosis CKD development, there was a potential risk of not having an accurate total number of CKD patients upon follow up. In addition, there is a risk of CKD misclassification, as only single timepoint data were used during the follow-up. Finally, a considerable number of patients (217 of 839, 25%) were lost to follow-up, which may have impacted on the results obtained. To make up for this problem, we compared the baseline characteristics between the study group and the follow-up loss group, and there were no significant differences between the two groups. Moreover, we conducted a sensitivity analysis (Supplementary 1), and found that the trend of ORs for discharge creatinine did not change significantly. These results indirectly imply that follow-up loss patients did not make up a significant bias to our result. However, our results still had the possibility to change if follow-up loss data were included.

5. Conclusions

In conclusion, AKI severity was correlated with mortality, but it did not correlate with the development of CKD, and patients progressed to CKD, even when the initial AKI stage was not severe. Physicians should focus on the recovery of renal function, and ensure the careful follow-up of patients with risk factors for the development of CKD.

Author Contributions: W.Y.K. is the guarantor of the paper. J.-s.K., Y.-J.K., and S.M.R. contributed to the literature search, figures, study design, data collection, data analysis, interpretation and writing, and revisions. S.A., D.W.S., C.H.S., K.S.L. contributed to design, revisions and validation.

References

1. Knoop, S.T.; Skrede, S.; Langeland, N.; Flaatten, H.K. Epidemiology and impact on all-cause mortality of sepsis in Norwegian hospitals: A national retrospective study. *PLoS ONE* **2017**, *12*, e0187990. [CrossRef [PubMed]

2. Kaukonen, K.-M.; Bailey, M.; Suzuki, S.; Pilcher, D.; Bellomo, R. Mortality related to severe sepsis and septic shock among critically ill patients in Australia and New Zealand, 2000–2012. *JAMA* **2014**, *311*, 1308–1309. [CrossRef] [PubMed]

3. Meyer, N.; Harhay, M.O.; Small, D.S.; Prescott, H.C.; Bowles, K.H.; Gaieski, D.F.; Mikkelsen, M.E. Temporal trends in incidence, sepsis-related mortality, and hospital-based acute care after sepsis. *Crit. Care Med.* **2018**, *46*, 354–360. [CrossRef] [PubMed]

4. Fujishima, S. Organ dysfunction as a new standard for defining sepsis. *Inflamm. Regen.* **2016**. [CrossRef] [PubMed]

5. Alobaidi, R.; Basu, R.K.; Goldstein, S.L.; Bagshaw, S.M. Sepsis-associated acute kidney injury. *Semin. Nephrol.* **2015**, *35*, 2–11. [CrossRef] [PubMed]

6. Zarjou, A.; Agarwal, A. Sepsis and acute kidney injury. *J. Am. Soc. Nephrol.* **2011**, *22*, 999–1006. [CrossRef] [PubMed]

7. Kellum, J.A.; Sileanu, F.E.; Bihorac, A.; Hoste, E.A.J.; Chawla, L.S. Recovery after acute kidney injury. *Am. J. Respir. Crit. Care Med.* **2017**, *195*, 784–791. [CrossRef]

8. Ishani, A.; Xue, J.L.; Himmelfarb, J.; Eggers, P.W.; Kimmel, P.L.; Molitoris, B.A.; Collins, A.J. Acute kidney injury increases risk of ESRD among elderly. *J. Am. Soc. Nephrol.* **2009**, *20*, 223–228. [CrossRef]

9. Rhodes, A.; Evans, L.E.; Alhazzani, W.; Levy, M.M.; Antonelli, M.; Ferrer, R.; Kumar, A.; Sevransky, J.E.; Sprung, C.L.; Nunnally, M.E.; et al. Surviving sepsis campaign: International guidelines for management of sepsis and septic shock: 2016. *Intensive Care Med.* **2017**, *43*, 304–377. [CrossRef]

10. Yearly, D.M.; Kellum, J.A.; Huang, D.T.; Barnato, A.E.; Weissfeld, L.A.; Pike, F.; Terndrup, T.; Wang, H.E.; Hou, P.C.; LoVecchio, F.; et al. A randomized trial of protocol-based care for early septic shock. *N. Engl. J. Med.* **2014**, *370*, 1683–1693.

11. Kim, W.Y.; Huh, J.W.; Lim, C.M.; Koh, Y.S.; Hong, S.B. Analysis of progression in risk, injury, failure, loss, and end-stage renal disease classification on outcome in patients with severe sepsis and septic shock. *J. Crit. Care* **2012**, *27*, 104.e1–104.e7. [CrossRef] [PubMed]

12. Sood, M.M.; Shafer, L.A.; Ho, J.; Reslerova, M.; Martinka, G.; Keenan, S.; Dial, S.; Wood, G.; Rigatto, C.; Kumar, A. Early reversible acute kidney injury is associated with improved survival in septic shock. *J. Crit. Care* **2014**, *29*, 711–717. [CrossRef] [PubMed]

13. Xu, J.-R.; Zhu, J.-M.; Jiang, J.; Ding, X.-Q.; Fang, Y.; Shen, B.; Liu, Z.-H.; Zou, J.-Z.; Liu, L.; Wang, C.-S.; et al. Risk factors for long-term mortality and progressive chronic kidney disease associated with acute kidney injury after cardiac surgery. *Medicine* **2015**, *94*, e2025. [CrossRef] [PubMed]

14. Levy, M.M.; Fink, M.P.; Marshall, J.C.; Abraham, E.; Angus, D.; Cook, D.; Cohen, J.; Opal, S.M.; Vincent, J.-L.; Ramsay, G. 2001 SCCM/ESICM/ACCP/ATS/SIS international sepsis definitions conference. *Crit. Care Med.* **2003**, *31*, 1250–1256. [CrossRef] [PubMed]

15. KDIGO. KDIGO Clinical Practice Guideline for Acute Kidney Injury. Available online: https://kdigo.org/guidelines/ (accessed on 15 December 2018).

16. KDIGO. KDIGO 2017 Clinical Practice Guideline Update for the Diagnosis, Evaluation, Prevention, and Treatment of Chronic Kidney Disease–Mineral and Bone Disorder (CKD-MBD). Available online: https://kdigo.org/guidelines/ (accessed on 15 December 2018).

17. Singbartl, K.; Kellum, J.A. AKI in the ICU: Definition, epidemiology, risk stratification, and outcomes. *Kidney Int.* **2012**, *81*, 819–825. [CrossRef] [PubMed]

18. Coca, S.G.; Singanamala, S.; Parikh, C.R. Chronic kidney disease after acute kidney injury: A systematic review and meta-analysis. *Kidney Int.* **2012**, *81*, 442–448. [CrossRef] [PubMed]

19. Pereira, B.J.; Barreto, S.; Gentil, T.; Assis, L.S.; Soeiro, E.M.; de Castro, I.; Laranja, S.M. Risk factors for the progression of chronic kidney disease after acute kidney injury. *J. Bras. Nefrol.* **2017**, *39*, 1–7. [CrossRef]

20. Fujii, T.; Uchino, S.; Doi, K.; Sato, T.; Kawamura, T. Diagnosis, management, and prognosis of patients with acute kidney injury in Japanese intensive care units: The JAKID study. *J. Crit. Care* **2018**, *47*, 1–7. [CrossRef]

21. Chawla, L.S.; Amdur, R.L.; Amodeo, S.; Kimmel, P.L.; Palant, C.E. The severity of acute kidney injury predicts progression to chronic kidney disease. *Kidney Int.* **2011**, *79*, 1361–1369. [CrossRef]

22. Heung, M.; Chawla, L.S. Acute kidney injury: Gateway to chronic kidney disease. *Nephron Clin. Pract.* **2014**, *127*, 30–34. [CrossRef]

23. Chawla, L.S.; Amdur, R.L.; Shaw, A.D.; Faselis, C.; Palant, C.E.; Kimmel, P.L. Association between acute kidney injury and long-term renal and cardiovascular outcomes in United States Veterans. *Clin. J. Am. Soc. Nephrol.* **2014**, *9*, 448–456. [CrossRef] [PubMed]

24. Jones, J.; Holmen, J.; De Graauw, J.; Jovanovich, A.; Thornton, S.; Chonchol, M. Association of complete recovery from acute kidney injury with incident CKD Stage 3 and all-cause mortality. *Am. J. Kidney Dis.* **2012**, *60*, 402–408. [CrossRef] [PubMed]

25. Murugan, R.; Wen, X.; Shah, N.; Lee, M.; Kong, L.; Pike, F.; Keener, C.; Unruh, M.; Finkel, K.; Vijayan, A.; et al. Plasma inflammatory and apoptosis markers are associated with dialysis dependence and death among critically ill patients receiving renal replacement therapy. *Nephrol. Dial. Transplant.* **2014**, *29*, 1854–1864. [CrossRef] [PubMed]

26. Mårtensson, J.; Vaara, S.T.; Pettilä, V.; Ala-Kokko, T.; Karlsson, S.; Inkinen, O.; Uusaro, A.; Larsson, A.; Bell, M. Assessment of plasma endostatin to predict acute kidney injury in critically ill patients. *Acta Anaesthesiol. Scand.* **2017**, *61*, 1286–1295. [CrossRef] [PubMed]

27. Kellum, J.A.; Prowle, J.R. Paradigms of acute kidney injury in the intensive care setting. *Nat. Rev. Nephrol.* **2018**, *14*, 217–230. [CrossRef] [PubMed]

28. Forni, L.G.; Darmon, M.; Ostermann, M.; Straaten, H.M.O.-V.; Pettilä, V.; Prowle, J.R.; Schetz, M.; Joannidis, M. Renal recovery after acute kidney injury. *Intensive Care Med.* **2017**, *43*, 855–866. [CrossRef] [PubMed]

29. Carlier, M.; Dumoulin, A.; Janssen, A.; Picavet, S.; Vanthuyne, S.; Van Eynde, R.; Vanholder, R.; Delanghe, J.; De Schoenmakere, G.; De Waele, J.J.; et al. Comparison of different equations to assess glomerular filtration in critically ill patients. *Intensive Care Med.* **2015**, *41*, 427–435. [CrossRef] [PubMed]

30. Kaddourah, A.; Basu, R.K.; Bagshaw, S.M.; Goldstein, S.L. Epidemiology of acute kidney injury in critically ill children and young adults. *N. Engl. J. Med.* **2017**, *376*, 11–20. [CrossRef] [PubMed]

11

Derivation and Validation of Machine Learning Approaches to Predict Acute Kidney Injury after Cardiac Surgery

Hyung-Chul Lee, Hyun-Kyu Yoon, Karam Nam, Youn Joung Cho, Tae Kyong Kim, Won Ho Kim * **and Jae-Hyon Bahk**

Department of Anesthesiology and Pain Medicine, Seoul National University Hospital, Seoul National University College of Medicine, Seoul 03080, Korea; azong@hanmail.net (H.-C.L.); hyunkyu18@gmail.com (H.-K.Y.); karamnam@gmail.com (K.N.); mingming7@gmail.com (Y.J.C.); ktkktk@gmail.com (T.K.K.); bahkjh@snu.ac.kr (J.-H.B.)
* Correspondence: wonhokim@snu.ac.kr

Abstract: Machine learning approaches were introduced for better or comparable predictive ability than statistical analysis to predict postoperative outcomes. We sought to compare the performance of machine learning approaches with that of logistic regression analysis to predict acute kidney injury after cardiac surgery. We retrospectively reviewed 2010 patients who underwent open heart surgery and thoracic aortic surgery. Baseline medical condition, intraoperative anesthesia, and surgery-related data were obtained. The primary outcome was postoperative acute kidney injury (AKI) defined according to the Kidney Disease Improving Global Outcomes criteria. The following machine learning techniques were used: decision tree, random forest, extreme gradient boosting, support vector machine, neural network classifier, and deep learning. The performance of these techniques was compared with that of logistic regression analysis regarding the area under the receiver-operating characteristic curve (AUC). During the first postoperative week, AKI occurred in 770 patients (38.3%). The best performance regarding AUC was achieved by the gradient boosting machine to predict the AKI of all stages (0.78, 95% confidence interval (CI) 0.75–0.80) or stage 2 or 3 AKI. The AUC of logistic regression analysis was 0.69 (95% CI 0.66–0.72). Decision tree, random forest, and support vector machine showed similar performance to logistic regression. In our comprehensive comparison of machine learning approaches with logistic regression analysis, gradient boosting technique showed the best performance with the highest AUC and lower error rate. We developed an Internet–based risk estimator which could be used for real-time processing of patient data to estimate the risk of AKI at the end of surgery.

Keywords: acute kidney injury; cardiovascular surgery; machine learning

1. Introduction

Generalized linear models, such as logistic regression analysis, have been used to predict postoperative morbidity. However, the logistic regression model requires the statistical assumption of a linear relationship between the covariates and the risk of morbidity. Furthermore, the limitation of overfitting and multicollinearity of regression analysis preclude the analysis of many explanatory variables. These limitations have restricted the analysis model to select a small set of variables that are known to be clinically relevant.

Recently, the machine learning technique has been applied in areas of medicine, including detecting a specific clinical finding on medical imaging and has shown excellent performance with high sensitivity and specificity [1,2]. Additionally, there were reports about the use of machine learning techniques to predict postoperative clinical outcomes including specific morbidity or in-hospital mortality [3–5]. Machine learning techniques showed better performance and low error rates to predict clinical outcomes compared to the logistic regression or Cox regression analysis. However, there was also a study reporting that the machine learning technique did not show a better performance that a previous risk prediction model for in-hospital mortality [5].

Postoperative acute kidney injury (AKI) after cardiovascular surgery is known to be a relevant complication because it is associated with increased long-term mortality and development of chronic kidney disease [6–8]. To find a risk factor and develop a risk prediction model, previous studies reported the results of multivariable logistic regression analysis [9–17]. Although many risk factors and risk scores were reported by multivariable logistic regression analysis, their performance in terms of the area under the receiver operating characteristic curves (AUC) was about 0.70 to 0.83 with room for further improvement [9,10,13,14,18]. Furthermore, previous prediction models may have included an insufficient number of perioperative variables owing to overfitting and multi-collinearity of the logistic regression analysis. Additionally, the potential non-linear relationship between the covariates and the risk of outcome cannot be considered. However, machine learning techniques are relatively free of these limitations of statistical analysis and may demonstrate better performance than that of logistic regression analysis.

Therefore, we attempted to directly compare the performance and error rate of prediction with machine learning techniques with that of prediction with multivariable logistic regression analysis. We hypothesized that prediction with machine learning techniques involving many perioperative variables may demonstrate better performance and low error rate than that of logistic regression analysis. We evaluated as many machine learning techniques as possible that are currently available in the statistical software package R (version 3.4.4., R Development Core Team, Vienna, Austria) because the R software package is easily and freely accessible to investigators and many packages for machine learning approaches are currently available.

2. Materials and Methods

2.1. Study Design

This retrospective observational study was approved by the institutional review board of Seoul National University Hospital (1805-170-948). We retrospectively reviewed the electronic medical records of 2010 consecutive patients who underwent coronary artery surgery, valve replacement, or thoracic aortic surgery at our institution between 2008 and 2015. The need for informed consent was waived because of the retrospective design of the study.

2.2. Anesthesia, Surgical Technique

General anesthesia was maintained using a target-controlled infusion of propofol and remifentanil, or inhalational anesthetics during the study period. Standard monitoring devices were applied, including pulmonary artery catheters (Swan-Ganz CCOmbo CCO/SvO2™; Edward Lifesciences LLC, Irvine, CA, USA), in all patients.

2.3. Data Collection

On the basis of previous studies, data related to demographic or perioperative variables known to be related to postoperative renal dysfunction were collected (Table 1) [6,9–17,19–23]. The following perioperative clinical variables were collected: patient demographics, medical history, medication history, baseline laboratory finding, surgery type, operation time, type of anesthesia, intraoperative fluid and colloid administration, intraoperative transfusion amount, and intraoperative hemodynamic variables.

Table 1. Patient characteristics and postoperative renal function in the dataset.

Variables	All	Training Set	Test Set	p-Value
Patient population, n	2010	1005	1005	
Demographic data				
Age (years)	64 (56–71)	64 (56–71)	64 (55–71)	0.884
Female (n)	553 (27.5)	279 (27.8)	274 (27.3)	0.803
Body-mass index (kg/m^2)	23.8 (21.6–25.9)	23.9 (21.7–25.9)	23.7 (21.5–25.9)	0.563
Surgery type				
Coronary artery bypass (n)	911 (45.3)	473 (47.1)	438 (43.6)	0.117
Valvular heart surgery (n)	1052 (52.3)	503 (50.0)	549 (54.6)	0.060
Thoracic aortic surgery (n)	47 (2.3)	29 (2.9)	18 (1.8)	0.104
Emergency (n)	51 (2.5)	26 (2.6)	25 (2.5)	0.887
Previous cardiac surgery (n)	149 (7.4)	75 (7.5)	74 (7.4)	0.932
Medical history				
Hypertension (n)	1057 (52.6)	538 (53.5)	519 (51.6)	0.396
Diabetes mellitus (n)	588 (29.3)	302 (30.0)	286 (28.5)	0.433
Three vessel disease (n)	602 (30.0)	306 (30.4)	296 (29.5)	0.626
Previous coronary stent insertion (n)	235 (11.7)	118 (11.7)	117 (11.6)	0.945
Cerebrovascular accident (n)	228 (11.3)	101 (10.0)	127 (12.6)	0.078
COPD (n)	100 (5.0)	49 (4.9)	51 (5.1)	0.837
Pulmonary hypertension (n)	129 (6.4)	60 (6.0)	69 (6.9)	0.413
Chronic kidney disease (n)	121 (6.0)	57 (5.7)	64 (6.4)	0.512
Preoperative Medication				
ACEi (n)	114 (5.7)	58 (5.8)	56 (5.6)	0.847
ARB (n)	249 (12.4)	122 (12.1)	127 (12.6)	0.735
β-blocker (n)	289 (19.4)	199 (19.8)	190 (18.9)	0.611
Diuretics (n)	297 (14.8)	133 (13.2)	164 (16.3)	0.059
Calcium channel blocker (n)	287 (14.3)	151 (15.0)	136 (13.5)	0.339
Statins (n)	506 (25.2)	255 (25.4)	251 (25.0)	0.837
Aspirin (n)	957 (47.6)	498 (49.6)	459 (45.7)	0.090
Baseline laboratory findings				
Preoperative LVEF (%)	58 (52–63)	58 (53–63)	57 (52–63)	0.427
Hematocrit (%)	38 (34–42)	38 (34–42)	38 (34–42)	0.844
Serum creatinine (mg/dL)	0.94 (0.80–1.12)	0.93 (0.80–1.10)	0.94 (0.80–1.13)	0.613
Serum Albumin (g/dL)	4.1 (3.8–4.3)	4.1 (3.9–4.3)	4.1 (3.8–4.3)	0.183
Serum uric acid (mg/dL)	4.6 (3.7–5.6)	4.6 (3.7–5.7)	4.5 (3.6–5.5)	0.190
Blood glucose (mg/dL)	115 (96–146)	116 (96–146)	113 (96–147)	0.500
Surgery and anaesthesia details				
Operation time (h)	6.25 (5.33–7.25)	6.25 (5.41–7.27)	6.25 (5.33–7.24)	0.654
Anesthesia time (h)	7.50 (6.25–8.50)	7.50 (6.50–8.50)	7.50 (6.50–8.42)	0.608
Total intravenous anesthesia (n)	1858 (92.4)	937 (93.2)	921 (91.6)	0.206
Inhalational anesthesia (n)	152 (7.6)	68 (6.8)	84 (8.4)	0.206
Intraoperative crystalloid infusion (L)	2150 (1150–3000)	2200 (1100–3100)	2150 (1200–2950)	0.656
Intraoperative colloid use (mL)	900 (350–1500)	1000 (350–1550)	800 (350–1500)	0.067
pRBC transfusion during surgery (units)	2 (0–3)	2 (0–3)	2 (0–3)	0.725
FFP transfusion during surgery (units)	0 (0–3)	0 (0–3)	0 (0–3)	0.589
Intraoperative mean arterial pressure (mmHg)	72 (67–78)	72 (67–78)	72 (67–78)	0.974
Intraoperative mean cardiac index (L/min)	2.3 (2.1–2.7)	2.3 (2.1–2.7)	2.3 (2.1–2.7)	0.257
Intraoperative mean SvO$_2$ (%)	73 (69–76)	73 (69–76)	73 (68–76)	0.207
Intraoperative diuretics use (n)	204 (10.1)	91 (9.1)	113 (11.2)	0.107
Postoperative renal function				
AKI according to KDIGO criteria (n)				0.596
Stage 1	591 (29.4)	282 (28.1)	309 (30.7)	
Stage 2	114 (5.7)	60 (6.0)	54 (5.4)	
Stage 3	65 (3.2)	33 (3.3)	32 (3.2)	
Hemodialysis dependent (n)	125 (6.2)	60 (6.0)	65 (6.5)	0.644
GFR at postoperative day one (ml/min/1.73m^2)	79 (58–94)	79 (57–95)	78 (58–94)	0.864

Data are presented as median (interquartile range) or number (%). COPD = chronic obstructive pulmonary disease, ACEi = angiotensin-converting-enzyme inhibitor, AKI = acute kidney injury, ARB = angiotensin II receptor blocker, LVEF = left ventricular ejection fraction, pRBC = packed red blood cell transfusion, FFP = fresh-frozen plasma, SvO$_2$ = mixed venous oxygen saturation, KDIGO = kidney disease improving global outcomes, GFR = glomerular filtration rate.

The primary outcome variable was postoperative AKI defined according to the Kidney Disease Improving Global Outcomes (KDIGO) criteria, which was determined according to the maximal change in serum creatinine level during the first seven postoperative days [6,24]. The most recent serum creatinine level measured before surgery was used as the baseline value. The detailed diagnostic criteria are shown in Table S1. We did not use the urine output criteria because previous studies suggested that different cutoffs of oliguria may be required for AKI after surgery [25,26]. We also analyzed the stage 2 or 3 AKI as secondary outcomes because stage 1 AKI may only be transient and functional and stage 2 or 3 AKI is more strongly associated with patient mortality [27]. The prediction of severe stages of AKI would be practically more important.

2.4. Statistical Analysis

R software version 3.4.4. (R Development Core Team, Vienna, Austria) was used for our analysis. The following R packages for machine learning approaches were used: Tree, rpart, ROSE (Random Over-Sampling Examples), randomForest, DMwR (Data Mining with R), XGBoost (eXtreme Gradient Boosting), e1071, UBL (utility-based learning), Kernlab, nnet, neuralnet, and h2o. Tree, rpart, and ROSE packages with CART (Classification And Regression Tree) analysis were used for decision tree analysis; randomForest and DMwR were used for random forest; XGboost was used for extreme gradient boosting; e1071, UBL, and kernlab were used for support vector machine; nnet and neuralnet were used for neural network regression; and h2o was used for deep belief networks (Text S1). Seventy-two explanatory variables including variables in Table 1 were used to machine learning. Our sample was randomly divided into a training and test set with a ratio of 1:1. The coefficients of machine learning techniques were trained with the training set and tested with the test set. Our primary analysis attempted to compare the predictive accuracy of machine learning approaches with traditional analytic techniques for classification, and previous risk scores for AKI after cardiac surgery [9–16]. To evaluate and compare the predictive accuracy of prediction by machine learning techniques and logistic regression models, we calculated the areas under the receiver operating characteristics curve (AUCs) [28,29] and compared AUCs of all classifiers and models using De Long's method [30]. We also compared the error rate, which was defined as the sum of the number of cases with false positive and false negative divided by the size of the test set. The error rates of the logistic regression model and other previous risk scores were calculated by using a cutoff where the sum of sensitivity and specificity was maximal.

For decision tree analysis, the number of terminal nodes was determined considering the scree plot showing the relationship between the tree size and coefficient of variance. We considered several decision trees with some terminal nodes that were associated with a small coefficient of variance. The final decision tree model that is clinically acceptable was chosen. The decision tree was pruned based on cross-validated error results using the complexity parameter associated with the minimal error. The ROSE package generates a synthetic balanced dataset with both over- and under-sampling and allows strengthening of the subsequent estimation of any binary outcomes [31].

The randomForest package provided a variable importance plot which shows the relative importance of the explanatory variables according to the mean decrease in accuracy or Gini. DMwR package is a technique to improve predictive ability by increasing the number of positive cases, which is called SMOTE (Synthetic Minority Over-sampling Technique). The XGBoost provides extreme and efficient gradient boosting [32–34]. The e1071 package was used for the support vector machine. The UBL package provides an over-sampling technique of SMOTE, which was also used to handle the class imbalance in the training set for the support vector machine [35]. The parameters of the support vector machine for classification was tuned based on balance data after SMOTE. The best parameters were determined to be a gamma of 0.1 at a cost of 10. The kernlab package provided the least square support vector machine. The neuralnet package provided the neural network classification and the number of hidden layers was defined as 6 with minimal error. The h2o deep learning package was used for deep learning.

Multivariable logistic regression analysis, including the variables in Table 1, was performed to identify independent predictors used for the development of a multivariable prediction model. To avoid multicollinearity, variables that were closely correlated with each other were excluded before being entered into the multivariable analysis. Backward stepwise variable selection was conducted using cutoff of $p < 0.10$. Previous risk scores of Palomba, Wijeysundera, Mehta, Thakar, Brown, Aronson, Fortescue, and Rhamanian et al. [9–16] were also applied to our study data and their performance was also compared with logistic models of ours, as well as other machine learning techniques. As a sensitivity analysis, logistic regression analysis without stepwise variable selection was performed to evaluate the performance.

Missing data were noted in <8% of records. We imputed the missing values according to the incidence of the missing values for each predictor. If the incidence of the missing was <2%, the missing values were substituted by the mean of continuous variables and by the mode for the incidence variable. The missing values of variables with a missing ratio of >2% and <8% were replaced using multiple imputations. Multiple imputations were performed separately in the training and test dataset. Multiple imputed training and test datasets were combined for a single run of the machine learning classifiers or logistic regression analysis.

We developed a risk estimator based on our gradient boosting model [36]. This estimator calculates the risk of developing AKI after cardiac surgery and classifies the risk into three classes of low, moderate, and high risk of AKI.

3. Results

A total of 2010 cases including 911 (45.3%) coronary artery bypass and 1052 (52.3%) valve replacement surgery cases were included in our analysis. During the first seven postoperative days, AKI, as determined according to the KDIGO criteria, was observed in 770 patients (38.3%) and stage 2 or 3 AKI developed in 179 patients (8.9%). The incidence of AKI was 37.3% (375/1005) for the training set and 39.3% (395/1005) for the test set. The incidences of stage 2 or 3 AKI were 9.3% (93/1005) and 8.6% (86/1005) for training and test set, respectively. Patient demographics and surgery-related variables in both training and test set are compared in Table 1.

The error rate and AUCs of all machine techniques, logistic regression model, and risk scores to predict AKI of all stages in the test data set were compared in Table 2 and Figure 1. Extreme gradient boosting classification showed the lowest test error rate (26.0%) and the largest AUC (0.78, 95% confidence interval (CI) 0.75–0.80), which was significantly greater than AUCs of other machine learning techniques or risk scores compared ($p < 0.001$). The deep belief network classifier showed the highest test error rate (47.2%) and smallest test AUC (0.55) among all machine learning techniques compared. The error rate and AUCs to predict AKI of stage 2 or 3 in the test set were compared in Table S2. Gradient boosting classification showed lowest test error rate (8.5%) and the largest AUC (0.74). The results of multivariable logistic regression analysis with and without stepwise variable selection was shown in Table 3 and Table S3. The AUC of the multivariable logistic prediction model with stepwise variable selection was 0.69 (95% CI 0.66 to 0.72) and the model without variable selection showed similar AUC (Table 2).

Table 2. Comparison of area under receiver-operating characteristic curve among the different models.

Model	Software or R Packages	Error Rate of Test Data Set	AUC in the Test Set
Machine learning techniques			
Decision tree, CART	tree, rpart	28.9%	0.71 (0.67–0.74)
ROSE decision tree	ROSE	30.6%	0.66 (0.65–0.72)
Random forest model	randomForest	30.4%	0.68 (0.64–0.71)
Random forest SMOTE model	DMwR	33.5%	0.68 (0.65–0.71)
Gradient boosting classification	XGBoost	26.0%	0.78 (0.75–0.80) *
Support vector machine, classifier	e1071	31.4%	0.67 (0.63–0.70)
Support vector machine, SMOTE model	UBL	33.3%	0.68 (0.65–0.71)
Support vector machine, least square	Kernlab	30.2%	0.69 (0.66–0.72)
Neural network classifier	nnet	38.4%	0.64 (0.61–0.68)
Neural network classifier	neuralnet	43.9%	0.57 (0.53–0.61)
Deep belief network	h2o	47.2%	0.55 (0.51–0.59)
Risk scores from logistic regression analysis			
Logistic regression model, stepwise variable selection	R	33.6%	0.69 (0.66–0.72)
Logistic regression model, without variable selection	R	32.8%	0.70 (0.68–0.73)
AKICS score	R	43.4%	0.57 (0.53–0.60)
Wijeysundera and colleagues	R	45.2%	0.55 (0.51–0.59)
Metha and colleagues	R	45.8%	0.55 (0.52–0.59)
Thakar and colleagues	R	45.3%	0.56 (0.53–0.60)
Brown and colleagues	R	43.1%	0.58 (0.54–0.61)
Aronson and colleagues	R	43.3%	0.58 (0.51–0.62)
Fortescue and colleagues	R	44.2%	0.56 (0.52–0.60)
Rhamanian and colleagues	R	47.0%	0.55 (0.52–0.58)

Error rate was defined as sum of the number of cases with false positive and false negative divided by all test set. * Significantly greater than AUC of all the other techniques, AUC = area under the receiver operating characteristic curve, CART = Classification And Regression Tree, ROSE = Random Over-Sampling Examples, SMOTE = Synthetic Minority Over-sampling Technique, DMwR = Data Mining with R, XGBoost = eXtreme Gradient Boosting, UBL = utility-based learning, AKICS = acute kidney injury following cardiac surgery.

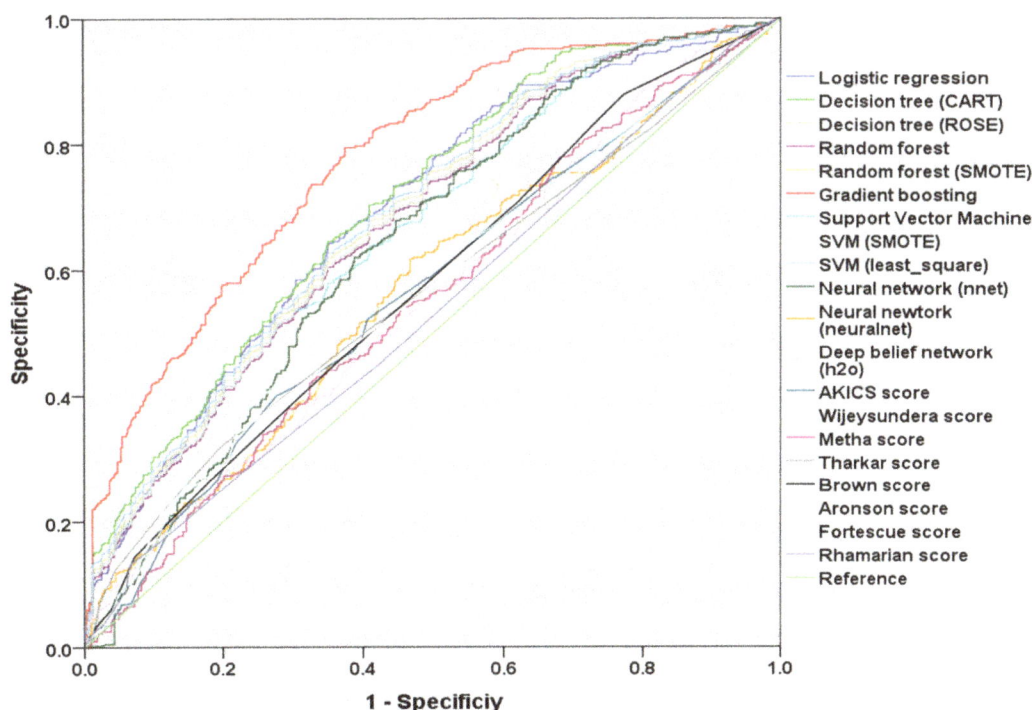

Figure 1. Comparison of AUC among the different machine learning models and logistic regression model. AKICS = acute kidney injury after cardiac surgery.

Table 3. Development of multivariable logistic regression model to predict acute kidney injury using stepwise variable selection.

Variable	Beta-Coefficient	Odds Ratio	95% CI	*p*-Value
Age per 10 year	0.128	1.14	1.04–1.61	0.004
History of hypertension	0.320	1.38	1.12–1.69	0.002
Baseline chronic kidney disease	0.907	2.48	1.62–3.78	<0.001
Preoperative E/e′ > 15	0.454	1.58	1.27–1.96	<0.001
Preoperative hematocrit, %	−0.062	0.94	0.92–0.96	<0.001
Surgery time, per 1 h	0.073	1.08	1.01–1.15	0.036
Intraoperative red blood cell transfusion, unit	0.056	1.06	1.01–1.11	0.022
Intraoperative fresh frozen plasma transfusion, unit	0.085	1.09	1.03–1.15	0.001
Intraoperative diuretics use	0.630	1.88	1.36–2.60	<0.001

Multivariable logistic regression analysis was performed using all the variables in Table 1. Stepwise backward variable selection process was used for this analysis using cutoff of *p*-value of less than 0.10. Nagelkerke's R^2 was 0.32 and Hosmer-Lemeshow goodness-of-fit test showed good calibration (chi-square = 12.1, $p = 0.231$). CI = confidence interval, E/e′ = ratio of early transmitral flow velocity to early diastolic velocity of the mitral annulus.

Simple decision tree model showing the classification of patients with and without AKI is shown in Figure 2. The importance matrix plot of gradient boosting is shown in Figure 3 and the amount of Intraoperative red blood cells transfusion and preoperative hematocrit level were ranked the first and second. The variables of importance plot of random forest model was shown in Figure S1. The same variables were ranked first and second in terms of both mean decreases in accuracy and Gini. The matrix of classification of extreme gradient boosting was visualized in Figure S2. Figure S3 shows an example of the support vector machine classification plot.

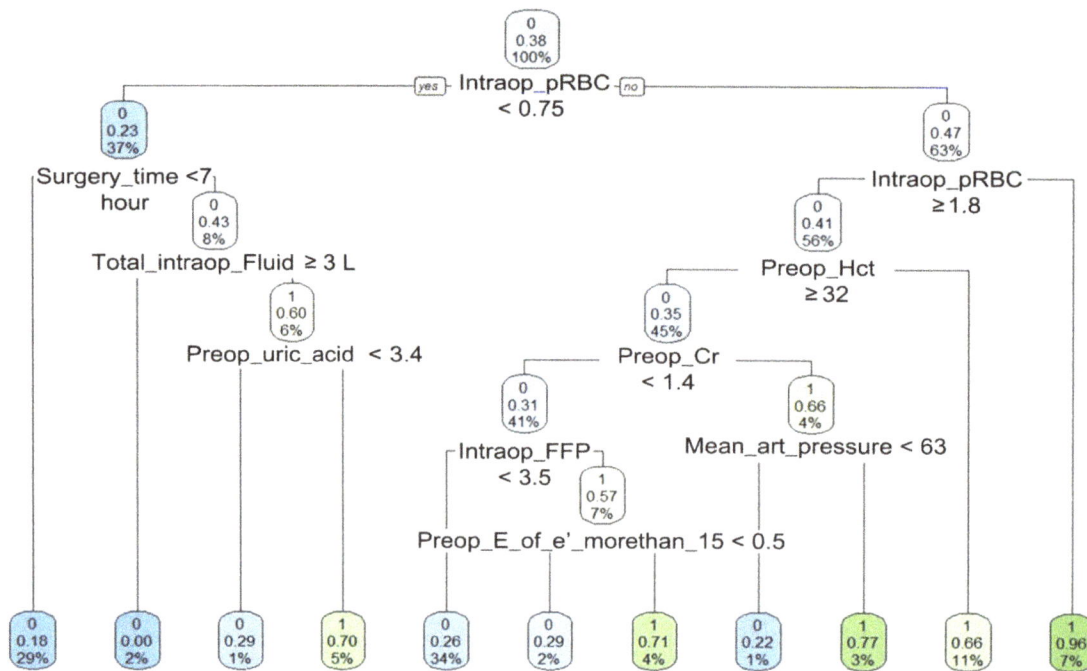

Figure 2. Simple decision tree model showing the classification of patients with (1) and without (0) acute kidney injury (AKI). The numbers with two decimals in each cell means the probability of developing AKI in each classification tree. The blue or green color becomes dense when it is more likely to develop acute kidney injury or not. The % number in the boxes denotes the percentage of patients with each discriminating variable from CART (Classification And Regression Tree) analysis. Intraop = intraoperative, preop = preoperative, pRBC = packed red blood cells, Hct = hematocrit, Cr = creatinine, FFP = fresh frozen plasma, E_or_e_prime = preoperative ratio of early transmitral flow velocity to early diastolic velocity of the mitral annulus.

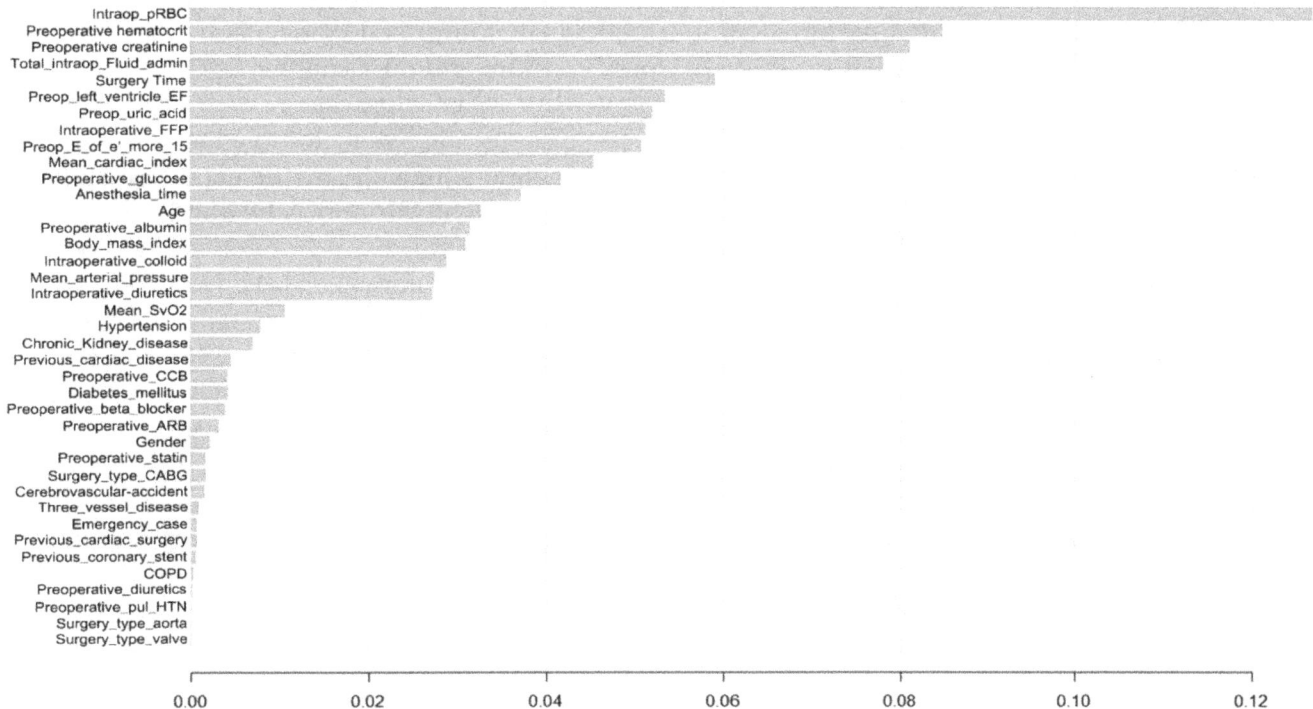

Figure 3. Importance matrix plot of the gradient boosting machine. This figure shows the importance of each covariates in the final model. ARB = angiotensin receptor blocker, BMI = body-mass index, CABG = coronary artery bypass graft, CCB = calcium channel blocker, CKD = chronic kidney disease, Cr = creatinine, CVA = history of cerebrovascular accident, EF = ejection fraction, E_or_e_prime = preoperative ratio of early transmitral flow velocity to early diastolic velocity of the mitral annulus, FFP = fresh frozen plasma, hct = hematocrit, HTN = hypertension, intraop = intraoperative, mean SvO2 = intraoperative mean mixed venous oxygen saturation, three_VD = three vessel coronary disease, preop = preoperative, pRBC = packed red blood cells.

4. Discussion

We compared the predictive accuracy of the prediction for AKI after cardiovascular surgery among the machine learning techniques, traditional statistical approach, and previous risk scoring models. We included currently available machine learning techniques, including decision tree, random forest, support vector machines, neural networks, and deep belief networks. Logistic regression analysis was used as the traditional approach. The results showed that extreme gradient boosting machine showed the lowest error rate and largest AUC among all techniques and risk scores, which was consistent for the prediction of stage 2 or 3 AKI. Extreme gradient boosting machine based prediction may result in significant improvement in the prediction of AKI after cardiac surgery. A risk estimator based on our gradient boosting model was developed for clinical use to determine the risk of AKI at the end of surgery.

Extreme gradient boosting showed the best predictive ability in our analysis [32,33,37]. While the random forest builds an ensemble of independent recursive partitioning tress of unlimited depth, extreme gradient boosting builds a sequential series of shallow trees, where each tree corrects for the residuals in the predictions made by all the previous tress (Figure S2). Gradient boosting uses techniques to reduce overfitting such as shrinkage and column resampling. After each step of boosting, the algorithm scales the newly added weights, which reduces the influence of each tree and allowing the model to learn better. Column resampling considers only a random subset of descriptors in building a given tree, which also fastens the training process by reducing the number of descriptors to consider [32]. It may be determined in further multicenter larger studies whether the better performance of boosting could be applied to data of other institutions or other surgical populations.

Decision tree analysis showed a similar performance to that of logistic regression model in our study. Decision trees are a hierarchical model that are comprised of decision rules based on the optimal feature cutoff values. It recursively classifies independent variables into different small groups based on the Gini impurity measure or entropy, while logistic regression analysis analyzes the interaction of included variables [38–40]. The odds ratio of a specific risk factor in a logistic regression model is applied to all study population rather than a single subgroup, while each branch of the decision tree may have different covariates from another branch. Variable selection in the process of decision tree is not based on probabilistic methods, which may result in overestimation of the importance of explanatory variables or may miss other potential confounders [41]. Decision trees can improve the predictive ability achieved by logistic regression models under certain circumstances. With sufficiently many terminal nodes with a low coefficient of variance, the decision tree model enables the detection of some individual cases that would have been unnoticed applying conventional logistic regression models. However, the clinical interpretation of variable selection and their cutoffs is often difficult, because the decision tree classification does not consider the clinical relevance. Decision trees are susceptible to fluctuations in the training set and are, thus, prone to overfitting and poor generalizability [4]. Additionally, decision tree models may not be practically useful if it includes too many variables. However, for the low error rate and high AUC, more classifying variables are needed.

The performance of random forest was also similar to that of logistic regression analysis in our dataset. Random forest is considered to have advantages, especially in handling electronic medical records. It is an extension to traditional decision tree classifiers [42], and attempts to mitigate the limitations of decision tree through an ensemble-based technique using multiple decision trees. Each tree is constructed from a random subset of the original training data and a random subset of a total number of variables is analyzed at each node for splitting. Random forests can minimize the problem of overfitting by taking the mode of decisions of a large number of these randomly generated trees [43]. Other advantages of random forests to analyze electronic medical records include running efficiently on large samples with thousands of input variables, the ability to accommodate different data scales, and robustness to the inclusion of irrelevant variables. There was no significant performance gain of the random forest over that of the simple decision tree in our study, which may be because the number of input variables was insufficient to demonstrate any difference in performance.

The deep neural network model showed a good performance to predict in-hospital mortality in a previous study, although it was not superior to previous risk score [5]. Contrary to our expectations, the performance of neural network in our study was inferior to the performances of all other machine learning techniques. This may be explained because our data for learning the relationship between the covariates and risk of AKI may not be sufficient. Although the multilayer perceptron is mathematically proven to be able to approximate any nonlinear function, it requires a large amount of learning data. Therefore, the dataset of our study may not be large enough and the number of covariates was not sufficient to train the multilayer perceptron [44].

The performance of previous eight risk scoring models was poor in our test dataset [9–16]. The AUCs of these risk scores were similar possibly because similar predictors were used to construct the risk score [6], and the poor performance may be due to the small number of predictors and lack of intraoperative variables, such as transfusion amounts or hemodynamic variables. A previous study showed that the performance of the logistic regression model could be improved when we consider many perioperative variables as possible [19].

Several previous studies reported that the AUCs of machine learning techniques were not superior to previous risk scores or logistic regression models to predict postoperative mortality [5,45]. However, our study demonstrated that the AUCs of machine learning techniques could be significantly greater than the AUC of logistic regression model to predict AKI. Previous studies compared the predictive ability for in-hospital mortality in a population with a very low incidence (<1%) [5,45]. The difference in AUC or error rate may be small for an outcome with low incidence, and this small difference in performance would be difficult to be demonstrated. It seems that any difference in error rate and AUC would be more pronounced in our study sample with a postoperative AKI of higher incidence (38.3%). This could also be the reason why the SMOTE model of random forests or support vector machines did not significantly increase the AUC in our test dataset. SMOTE model increases the incidence of outcome cases and balancing the case with and without outcome variables. However, our test set already had a nearly balanced dataset for AKI.

The importance matrix plot of the gradient boosting machine shows the similar predictors that were known to be associated with the development of AKI after cardiac surgery [6,9–14,16,19–21,46]. However, the plot additionally gives the relative importance of each predictor, which was similar to the variance importance plot of random forest model. This analysis may help to find a new risk factor for postoperative morbidity or mortality.

Our study has several limitations. First, our analysis used only single-center data and included a relatively small number of cases and covariates. The performance of machine learning techniques might be different when they are applied to a much larger sample with a different distribution of the covariates. The external validity of our results may be limited. Furthermore, important predictors may be different according to different institutions. However, the relative performance of logistic regression and machine learning techniques would be similar to our results. Each institution may need to develop their own prediction model with the machine learning approach, by using historical data from their electronic medical records and updating the model periodically. Real-time processing of patient data would produce risk prediction for each patient after surgery. Second, machine learning techniques are often difficult to interpret the results. Inferences about the explanatory variables are more difficult than logistic regression analysis [4]. However, the gradient boosting machine and random forest provided for some interpretability through the importance matrix plot and variable importance plot. Third, it is not certain that our results could translate into improved clinical outcomes for the patients. Most of our important variables reported are not clinically modifiable and accurate risk prediction may not be followed by improved patient outcomes. However, further prospective trials may evaluate whether adjustment of potentially modifiable predictors, such as hemodynamic variables could decrease the risk of AKI [46–48].

5. Conclusions

In conclusion, our study demonstrated that the machine learning technique of extreme gradient boosting showed significantly better performance than the traditional logistic regression analysis or previous risk scores in predicting both AKI of all stages and stage 2 or 3 AKI after cardiac surgery. Gradient boosting machine may be used for real-time processing of patient data to estimate the risk of AKI after cardiac surgery at the end of surgery. Our Internet-based risk estimator may help to evaluate the risk of AKI at the end of surgery. However, prospective multicenter trials are required to validate the better prediction by gradient boosting. Further studies may apply extreme gradient boosting machine to the other important clinical outcomes after cardiac surgeries and may prospectively validate our results.

Supplementary Materials:
Figure S1, Variable importance plot using the random forest model. The abbreviations were the same as the legends of Figure 3; Figure S2, Gradient boosting tree plot showing the matrix of classification. Extreme gradient boosting builds a sequential series of shallow trees; Figure S3, Support vector machine classification plot. This figure shows a simple two-dimensional visual illustration of support vector machine classification. Each triangle and circle means a binomial classification of acute kidney injury or not. The open circle or triangle means a correct classification and closed circle or triangle means an incorrect classification. This figure was drawn by Kernlab package of R; Table S1, KDIGO (Kidney Disease Improving Global Outcomes) serum creatinine diagnostic criteria of acute kidney injury; Table S2, Comparison of area under receiver-operating characteristic curve among the different models for predicting stage 2 or 3 acute kidney injury; Table S3, Results of multivariable logistic regression analysis for acute kidney injury without stepwise variable selection; Text S1, R source code to perform machine learning techniques.

Author Contributions: Formal analysis: W.H.K. and H.-C.L.; data curation: W.H.K., and H.-C.L.; methodology: W.H.K.; supervision: J.-H.B.; writing—original draft: W.H.K.; writing—review and editing: H.-C.L., H.-K.Y., K.N., Y.J.C., and T.K.K.

References

1.   Bejnordi, B.E.; Veta, M.; van Diest, P.J.; van Ginneken, B.; Karssemeijer, N.; Litjens, G.; van der Laak, J.A.W.M. Diagnostic Assessment of Deep Learning Algorithms for Detection of Lymph Node Metastases in Women With Breast Cancer. *Jama* **2017**, *318*, 2199–2210. [CrossRef] [PubMed]
2.   Ting, D.S.W.; Cheung, C.Y.L.; Lim, G.; Tan, G.S.W.; Quang, N.D.; Gan, A.; Hamzah, H.; Garcia-Franco, R.; San Yeo, I.Y.; Lee, S.Y.; et al. Development and Validation of a Deep Learning System for Diabetic Retinopathy and Related Eye Diseases Using Retinal Images From Multiethnic Populations With Diabetes. *Jama* **2017**, *318*, 2211–2223. [CrossRef] [PubMed]
3.   Fei, Y.; Hu, J.; Li, W.Q.; Wang, W.; Zong, G.Q. Artificial neural networks predict the incidence of portosplenomesenteric venous thrombosis in patients with acute pancreatitis. *J. Thromb. Haemost.* **2017**, *15*, 439–445. [CrossRef] [PubMed]
4.   Taylor, R.A.; Pare, J.R.; Venkatesh, A.K.; Mowafi, H.; Melnick, E.R.; Fleischman, W.; Hall, M.K. Prediction of In-hospital Mortality in Emergency Department Patients with Sepsis: A Local Big Data-Driven, Machine Learning Approach. *Acad. Emerg. Med.* **2016**, *23*, 269–278. [CrossRef] [PubMed]
5.   Lee, C.K.; Hofer, I.; Gabel, E.; Baldi, P.; Cannesson, M. Development and Validation of a Deep Neural Network Model for Prediction of Postoperative In-hospital Mortality. *Anesthesiology* **2018**, in press. [CrossRef] [PubMed]
6.   Shin, S.R.; Kim, W.H.; Kim, D.J.; Shin, I.W.; Sohn, J.T. Prediction and Prevention of Acute Kidney Injury after Cardiac Surgery. *Biomed Res. Int.* **2016**, *2016*, 2985148. [CrossRef] [PubMed]
7.   Hobson, C.E.; Yavas, S.; Segal, M.S.; Schold, J.D.; Tribble, C.G.; Layon, A.J.; Bihorac, A. Acute kidney injury is associated with increased long-term mortality after cardiothoracic surgery. *Circulation* **2009**, *119*, 2444–2453. [CrossRef] [PubMed]
8.   Chawla, L.S.; Eggers, P.W.; Star, R.A.; Kimmel, P.L. Acute kidney injury and chronic kidney disease as interconnected syndromes. *N. Engl. J. Med.* **2014**, *371*, 58–66. [CrossRef] [PubMed]
9.   Thakar, C.V.; Arrigain, S.; Worley, S.; Yared, J.P.; Paganini, E.P. A clinical score to predict acute renal failure after cardiac surgery. *J. Am. Soc. Nephrol.* **2005**, *16*, 162–168. [CrossRef] [PubMed]
10. Mehta, R.H.; Grab, J.D.; O'Brien, S.M.; Bridges, C.R.; Gammie, J.S.; Haan, C.K.; Ferguson, T.B.; Peterson, E.D. Bedside tool for predicting the risk of postoperative dialysis in patients undergoing cardiac surgery. *Circulation* **2006**, *114*, 2208–2216. [CrossRef] [PubMed]
11. Palomba, H.; de Castro, I.; Neto, A.L.; Lage, S.; Yu, L. Acute kidney injury prediction following elective cardiac surgery: AKICS Score. *Kidney Int.* **2007**, *72*, 624–631. [CrossRef] [PubMed]
12. Wijeysundera, D.N.; Karkouti, K.; Dupuis, J.Y.; Rao, V.; Chan, C.T.; Granton, J.T.; Beattie, W.S. Derivation and validation of a simplified predictive index for renal replacement therapy after cardiac surgery. *Jama* **2007**, *297*, 1801–1809. [CrossRef] [PubMed]
13. Aronson, S.; Fontes, M.L.; Miao, Y.; Mangano, D.T. Risk index for perioperative renal dysfunction/failure: Critical dependence on pulse pressure hypertension. *Circulation* **2007**, *115*, 733–742. [CrossRef] [PubMed]
14. Brown, J.R.; Cochran, R.P.; Leavitt, B.J.; Dacey, L.J.; Ross, C.S.; MacKenzie, T.A.; Kunzelman, K.S.; Kramer, R.S.; Hernandez, F.; Helm, R.E.; et al. Multivariable prediction of renal insufficiency developing after cardiac surgery. *Circulation* **2007**, *116*, I139–I143. [CrossRef] [PubMed]
15. Fortescue, E.B.; Bates, D.W.; Chertow, G.M. Predicting acute renal failure after coronary bypass surgery: Cross-validation of two risk-stratification algorithms. *Kidney Int.* **2000**, *57*, 2594–2602. [CrossRef] [PubMed]
16. Rahmanian, P.B.; Kwiecien, G.; Langebartels, G.; Madershahian, N.; Wittwer, T.; Wahlers, T. Logistic risk model predicting postoperative renal failure requiring dialysis in cardiac surgery patients. *Eur. J. Cardiothorac. Surg.* **2011**, *40*, 701–707. [PubMed]
17. Vives, M.; Callejas, R.; Duque, P.; Echarri, G.; Wijeysundera, D.N.; Hernandez, A.; Sabate, A.; Bes-Rastrollo, M.; Monedero, P. Modern hydroxyethyl starch and acute kidney injury after cardiac surgery: A prospective multicentre cohort. *Br. J. Anaesth.* **2016**, *117*, 458–463. [CrossRef] [PubMed]
18. Kim, W.H.; Lee, J.H.; Kim, E.; Kim, G.; Kim, H.J.; Lim, H.W. Can We Really Predict Postoperative Acute Kidney Injury after Aortic Surgery? Diagnostic Accuracy of Risk Scores Using Gray Zone Approach.

Thorac. Cardiovasc. Surg. **2016**, *64*, 281–289. [CrossRef] [PubMed]

19. Parolari, A.; Pesce, L.L.; Pacini, D.; Mazzanti, V.; Salis, S.; Sciacovelli, C.; Rossi, F.; Alamanni, F. Risk factors for perioperative acute kidney injury after adult cardiac surgery: Role of perioperative management. *Ann. Thorac. Surg.* **2012**, *93*, 584–591. [CrossRef] [PubMed]

20. Kim, W.H.; Lee, S.M.; Choi, J.W.; Kim, E.H.; Lee, J.H.; Jung, J.W.; Ahn, J.H.; Sung, K.I.; Kim, C.S.; Cho, H.S. Simplified clinical risk score to predict acute kidney injury after aortic surgery. *J. Cardiothorac. Vasc. Anesth.* **2013**, *27*, 1158–1166. [CrossRef] [PubMed]

21. Kim, W.H.; Park, M.H.; Kim, H.J.; Lim, H.Y.; Shim, H.S.; Sohn, J.T.; Kim, C.S.; Lee, S.M. Potentially modifiable risk factors for acute kidney injury after surgery on the thoracic aorta: A propensity score matched case-control study. *Medicine* **2015**, *94*, e273. [CrossRef] [PubMed]

22. Hur, M.; Koo, C.H.; Lee, H.C.; Park, S.K.; Kim, M.; Kim, W.H.; Kim, C.S.; Lee, S.M. Preoperative aspirin use and acute kidney injury after cardiac surgery: A propensity-score matched observational study. *PLoS ONE* **2017**, *12*, E0177201. [CrossRef] [PubMed]

23. Hur, M.; Nam, K.; Jo, W.Y.; Kim, G.; Kim, W.H.; Bahk, J.H. Association Between Elevated Echocardiographic Index of Left Ventricular Filling Pressure and Acute Kidney Injury After Off-Pump Coronary Artery Surgery. *Circ. J.* **2018**, *82*, 857–865. [CrossRef] [PubMed]

24. Thomas, M.E.; Blaine, C.; Dawnay, A.; Devonald, M.A.; Ftouh, S.; Laing, C.; Latchem, S.; Lewington, A.; Milford, D.V.; Ostermann, M. The definition of acute kidney injury and its use in practice. *Kidney Int.* **2015**, *87*, 62–73. [CrossRef] [PubMed]

25. Hori, D.; Katz, N.M.; Fine, D.M.; Ono, M.; Barodka, V.M.; Lester, L.C.; Yenokyan, G.; Hogue, C.W. Defining oliguria during cardiopulmonary bypass and its relationship with cardiac surgery-associated acute kidney injury. *Br. J. Anaesth.* **2016**, *117*, 733–740. [CrossRef] [PubMed]

26. Mizota, T.; Yamamoto, Y.; Hamada, M.; Matsukawa, S.; Shimizu, S.; Kai, S. Intraoperative oliguria predicts acute kidney injury after major abdominal surgery. *Br. J. Anaesth.* **2017**, *119*, 1127–1134. [CrossRef] [PubMed]

27. Kellum, J.A.; Zarbock, A.; Nadim, M.K. What endpoints should be used for clinical studies in acute kidney injury? *Intensive Care Med.* **2017**, *43*, 901–903. [CrossRef] [PubMed]

28. Hanley, J.A.; McNeil, B.J. The meaning and use of the area under a receiver operating characteristic (ROC) curve. *Radiology* **1982**, *143*, 29–36. [CrossRef] [PubMed]

29. Zou, K.H.; O'Malley, A.J.; Mauri, L. Receiver-operating characteristic analysis for evaluating diagnostic tests and predictive models. *Circulation* **2007**, *115*, 654–657. [CrossRef] [PubMed]

30. DeLong, E.R.; DeLong, D.M.; Clarke-Pearson, D.L. Comparing the areas under two or more correlated receiver operating characteristic curves: A nonparametric approach. *Biometrics* **1988**, *44*, 837–845. [CrossRef] [PubMed]

31. Zavrsnik, J.; Kokol, P.; Maleiae, I.; Kancler, K.; Mernik, M.; Bigec, M. ROSE: Decision trees, automatic learning and their applications in cardiac medicine. *Medinfo* **1995**, *8*, 1688. [PubMed]

32. Sheridan, R.P.; Wang, W.M.; Liaw, A.; Ma, J.; Gifford, E.M. Extreme Gradient Boosting as a Method for Quantitative Structure-Activity Relationships. *J. Chem. Inf. Model.* **2016**, *56*, 2353–2360. [CrossRef] [PubMed]

33. Gao, C.; Sun, H.; Wang, T.; Tang, M.; Bohnen, N.I.; Muller, M.L.; Herman, T.; Giladi, N.; Kalinin, A.; Spino, C.; et al. Model-based and Model-free Machine Learning Techniques for Diagnostic Prediction and Classification of Clinical Outcomes in Parkinson's Disease. *Sci. Rep.* **2018**, *8*, 7129. [CrossRef] [PubMed]

34. Available online: https://github.com/dmlc/xgboost (accessed on 3 October 2018).

35. Chawla, N.V.; Bowyer, K.W.; Hall, L.O.; Kegelmeyer, W.P. SMOTE: Synthetic minority over-sampling technique. *J. Artif. Intell. Res.* **2002**, *16*, 321–357. [CrossRef]

36. Available online: https://vitaldb.net/aki (accessed on 3 Octber 2018).

37. Lei, T.; Sun, H.; Kang, Y.; Zhu, F.; Liu, H.; Zhou, W.; Wang, Z.; Li, D.; Li, Y.; Hou, T. ADMET Evaluation in Drug Discovery. 18. Reliable Prediction of Chemical-Induced Urinary Tract Toxicity by Boosting Machine Learning Approaches. *Mol. Pharm.* **2017**, *14*, 3935–3953. [CrossRef] [PubMed]

38. Aviles-Jurado, F.X.; Leon, X. Prognostic factors in head and neck squamous cell carcinoma: Comparison of CHAID decision trees technology and Cox analysis. *Head Neck* **2013**, *35*, 877–883. [CrossRef] [PubMed]

39. Kasbekar, P.U.; Goel, P.; Jadhav, S.P. A Decision Tree Analysis of Diabetic Foot Amputation Risk in Indian Patients. *Front. Endocrinol.* **2017**, *8*, 25. [CrossRef] [PubMed]

40. Zintzaras, E.; Bai, M.; Douligeris, C.; Kowald, A.; Kanavaros, P. A tree-based decision rule for identifying profile groups of cases without predefined classes: Application in diffuse large B.-cell lymphomas. *Comput. Biol. Med.* **2007**, *37*, 637–641. [CrossRef] [PubMed]

41. Lemon, S.C.; Roy, J.; Clark, M.A.; Friedmann, P.D.; Rakowski, W. Classification and regression tree analysis in public health: Methodological review and comparison with logistic regression. *Ann. Behav. Med.* **2003**, *26*, 172–181. [CrossRef] [PubMed]

42. Li, K.; Yu, N.; Li, P.; Song, S.; Wu, Y.; Li, Y.; Liu, M. Multi-label spacecraft electrical signal classification method based on DBN and random forest. *PLoS ONE* **2017**, *12*, E0176614. [CrossRef] [PubMed]

43. Hsu, P.L.; Robbins, H. Complete Convergence and the Law of Large Numbers. *Proc. Natl. Acad. Sci. USA* **1947**, *33*, 25–31. [CrossRef] [PubMed]

44. Hornik, K. Approximation capabilities of multilayer feedforward networks. *Neural. Networks.* **1991**, *4*, 251–257. [CrossRef]

45. Kuo, P.J.; Wu, S.C.; Chien, P.C.; Rau, C.S.; Chen, Y.C.; Hsieh, H.Y.; Hsieh, C.H. Derivation and validation of different machine-learning models in mortality prediction of trauma in motorcycle riders: A cross-sectional retrospective study in southern Taiwan. *BMJ Open* **2018**, *8*, e018252. [CrossRef] [PubMed]

46. Karkouti, K.; Wijeysundera, D.N.; Yau, T.M.; Callum, J.L.; Cheng, D.C.; Crowther, M.; Dupuis, J.Y.; Fremes, S.E.; Kent, B.; Laflamme, C.; et al. Acute kidney injury after cardiac surgery: Focus on modifiable risk factors. *Circulation* **2009**, *119*, 495–502. [CrossRef] [PubMed]

47. Lee, E.H.; Kim, W.J.; Kim, J.Y.; Chin, J.H.; Choi, D.K.; Sim, J.Y.; Choo, S.J.; Chung, C.H.; Lee, J.W.; Choi, I.C. Effect of Exogenous Albumin on the Incidence of Postoperative Acute Kidney Injury in Patients Undergoing Off-pump Coronary Artery Bypass Surgery with a Preoperative Albumin Level of Less Than 4.0 g/dl. *Anesthesiology* **2016**, *124*, 1001–1011. [CrossRef] [PubMed]

48. Yoo, Y.C.; Shim, J.K.; Kim, J.C.; Jo, Y.Y.; Lee, J.H.; Kwak, Y.L. Effect of single recombinant human erythropoietin injection on transfusion requirements in preoperatively anemic patients undergoing valvular heart surgery. *Anesthesiology* **2011**, *115*, 929–937. [CrossRef] [PubMed]

12

Preadmission Statin Therapy is Associated with a Lower Incidence of Acute Kidney Injury in Critically Ill Patients: A Retrospective Observational Study

Tak Kyu Oh [1],*, In-Ae Song [1], Young-Jae Cho [2], Cheong Lim [3], Young-Tae Jeon [1], Hee-Joon Bae [4] and You Hwan Jo [5]

[1] Department of Anesthesiology and Pain Medicine, Seoul National University Bundang Hospital, Gumi-ro 173 Beon-gil, Bundang-gu, Seongnam 13620, Korea; songoficu@outlook.kr (I.-A.S.); ytjeon@snubh.org (Y.-T.J.)
[2] Division of Pulmonary and Critical Care Medicine, Department of Internal Medicine, Seoul National University Bundang Hospital, Gumi-ro 173 Beon-gil, Bundang-gu, Seongnam 13620, Korea; lungdrcho@snubh.org
[3] Department of Thoracic and Cardiovascular Surgery, Seoul National University Bundang Hospital, Gumi-ro 173 Beon-gil, Bundang-gu, Seongnam 13620, Korea; mluemoon@snubh.org
[4] Department of Neurology, Stroke Center, Seoul National University Bundang Hospital, Gumi-ro 173 Beon-gil, Bundang-gu, Seongnam 13620, Korea; braindoc@snubh.org
[5] Department of Emergency Medicine, Seoul National University Bundang Hospital, Gumi-ro 173 Beon-gil, Bundang-gu, Seongnam 13620, Korea; drakejo@snubh.org
* Correspondence: airohtak@hotmail.com

Abstract: This study aimed to investigate the association between preadmission statin use and acute kidney injury (AKI) incidence among critically ill patients who needed admission to the intensive care unit (ICU) for medical care. Medical records of patients admitted to the ICU were reviewed. Patients who continuously took statin for >1 month prior to ICU admission were defined as statin users. We investigated whether preadmission statin use was associated with AKI incidence within 72 h after ICU admission and whether the association differs according to preadmission estimated glomerular filtration rate (eGFR; in mL min^{-1} 1.73 m^{-2}). Among 21,236 patients examined, 5756 (27.1%) were preadmission statin users and 15,480 (72.9%) were non-statin users. Total AKI incidence within 72 h after ICU admission was 31% lower in preadmission statin users than in non-statin users [odds ratio (OR), 0.69; 95% confidence interval (CI), 0.61–0.79; $p < 0.001$]. This association was insignificant among individuals with eGFR <30 mL min^{-1} 1.73 m^{-2} ($p > 0.05$). Our results suggested that preadmission statin therapy is associated with a lower incidence of AKI among critically ill patients; however, this effect might not be applicable for patients with eGFR <30 mL min^{-1} 1.73 m^{-2}.

Keywords: acute kidney injury; statins; chronic kidney disease

1. Introduction

Acute kidney injury (AKI) is defined as a rapid worsening of renal functions [1] and affects 2–18% of inpatients and 57% of critical care patients [2–4]. AKI in critically ill patients in the intensive care unit (ICU) is an important issue because it delays recovery and increases hospital mortality [5]. Thus, appropriately preventing AKI in the ICU is currently an important task in ICU patient management [6].

Statin, known as a 3-hydroxy-3-methylglutaryl-coenzyme A inhibitor, is one of the most commonly prescribed drugs worldwide [7] that lowers the risk of cardiovascular death by reducing the serum cholesterol level [8]. Furthermore, statin has anti-inflammatory, antithrombotic, and immunomodulating effects [9,10], also known as "pleiotropic effects" [11]. These pleiotropic effects are reported to lower the incidence of surgery-related [12,13], contrast-induced [14], and sepsis-related AKI [15]. However, some study findings show that statin failed to improve the outcomes of kidney disease, and the debate regarding the relationship between statin use and AKI is ongoing [16]. Thus, further studies are needed to substantiate the inhibitory effects of statin on AKI. Additionally, considering that statin therapy may be discontinued for many patients based on their states after ICU admission, it is important to clarify the association between preadmission statin use and AKI incidence after ICU admission.

This study aimed to investigate the association between preadmission statin use and AKI incidence after ICU admission in the general adult population. Additionally, we examined whether this association differs with respect to pre-ICU kidney function.

2. Materials and Method

This retrospective observational study was approved by the Institutional Review Board (IRB) of Seoul National University Bundang Hospital (IRB approval number: B-1806/474-105). Because of the retrospective nature of the study, the IRB waived the need to obtain informed consent from the patients. All data for the study were collected by a medical records technician who was blinded to the purpose of this study.

2.1. Patients

The medical records of adult patients aged ≥18 years who were admitted to the ICU between January 2012 and December 2017 were analyzed. When a patient was admitted to the ICU more than once during the study period, only data from the last ICU admission case, which might be the most severe, were included in the analysis. The exclusion criteria were as follows: (1) patients with an estimated glomerular filtration rate (eGFR; in mL min^{-1} 1.73 m^{-2}) of <15 or those with end-stage renal disease (ESRD) who were undergoing renal replacement therapy (RRT) prior to admission because they usually received RRT after ICU admission regardless of AKI development; (2) patients lacking information on baseline creatinine or creatinine level within 72 h after ICU admission; and (3) patients diagnosed with AKI prior to ICU admission.

2.2. Preadmission Statin Use (Main Independent Variables)

Preadmission statin users were defined as patients who confirmed taking statins as maintenance treatment as prescribed by their physicians at least one month before ICU admission. The other cases were classified as non-statin users. Statin was classified as atorvastatin, rosuvastatin, simvastatin, pitavastatin, and other statins (pravastatin, fluvastatin, and lovastatin).

2.3. Measurements (Covariates)

Demographic information (sex, age, and body mass index) of the patients and comorbidities at ICU admission, including Acute Physiology and Chronic Health Evaluation II score and eGFR, total serum cholesterol at ICU admission (mg dL^{-1}), and data regarding admission to the emergency department and other departments (internal medicine, neurologic center, cardiothoracic surgical department, and other surgical departments) were collected. Pre-ICU admission eGFR was computed using the Modification of Diet in Renal Disease formula [17]: eGFR (mL min^{-1} 1.73 m^{-2}) = 186 × (creatinine level)$^{-1.154}$ × (age)$^{-0.203}$ × (0.742 if female). Using the cut-off points of total cholesterol as 160 and 200 mg/dL, which are known to be clinically meaningful, the subjects were divided into three groups (<160, 160–199, and ≥200) [18,19].

2.4. Diagnosis of AKI (Dependent Variable)

AKI was diagnosed based on the Kidney Disease: Improving Global Outcomes criteria and grading (Appendix A) [20]. Considering the varying lengths of urinary catheters used across patients, only serum creatinine (mg dL^{-1}) was used for diagnosing AKI. Serum creatinine level measured at least within a month prior to ICU admission was defined as baseline creatinine, and AKI was diagnosed using serum creatinine levels measured within 72 h after ICU admission.

2.5. Outcomes

This study investigated how preadmission statin use is associated with the incidence of total AKI and stage ≥ 2 AKI after ICU admission. Additionally, we examined how this association differs according to preadmission eGFR.

2.6. Statistical Analysis

The baseline characteristics of the patients were presented as means with standard deviation or numbers with percentage. To compare preadmission statin users and non-statin users, continuous variables were tested using the two-sample t-test, while categorical variables were tested using the chi-square test. First, the individual association between each covariate and total AKI was examined with univariable logistic regression analysis. The covariates with $p < 0.1$ in the univariable logistic regression model were selected for adjustment in the final multivariable logistic regression analysis. Considering that baseline kidney function is a risk factor of AKI [21], we investigated the interaction between eGFR before ICU admission and preadmission statin use, and when there was an interaction, we performed a subgroup analysis by dividing the participants according to eGFR (≥ 90, 60–90, 30–60, and <30 mL min^{-1} 1.73 m^{-2}). In the subgroup analysis, the Bonferroni correction was used to prevent type I errors that resulted from multiple comparisons [22]. The same method was used for analyzing stage ≥ 2 AKI as the dependent variable. All analyses were performed using IBM SPSS version 24.0 (IBM Corp., Armonk, NY, USA), and $p < 0.05$ was considered statistically significant.

3. Results

A total of 30,398 patients were admitted to the ICU 40,533 times between January 2012 and December 2017. These 30,398 patients were selected after excluding 10,135 cases involving the same patient being admitted to the ICU more than once. Next, we excluded 5440 patients aged <18 years, 47 ESRD patients who were undergoing RRT prior to ICU admission, 970 patients without baseline creatinine data, 2170 patients whose creatinine level was not measured within 72 h after ICU admission, and 535 patients who were diagnosed with AKI prior to ICU admission. As a result, 21,236 patients were included in the analysis, of whom 5756 (27.1%) were preadmission statin users and 15,480 (72.9%) were non-statin users (Figure 1). Their baseline characteristics are presented in Table 1. A total of 5469 (25.8%) patients developed AKI within 72 h after ICU admission, and 2216 (10.4%) of them had stage ≥ 2 AKI. Another 488 (2.3%) patients began postoperative RRT within 72 h after ICU admission.

3.1. Preadmission Statin Use and AKI Incidence

Table 2 shows the differences in characteristics between statin and non-statin users. The incidence of total AKI and stage ≥ 2 AKI among statin users was 1301/5756 (22.6%) and 439/5756 (7.6%), respectively, which was significantly lower than that in non-statin users [4168/15,480 (26.9%) and 1777/15,480 (11.5%), respectively] ($p < 0.001$). Table 3 shows the results of the multivariable logistic analysis after adjusting for the covariates selected in the univariate logistic regression analysis for total AKI incidence (Appendix B). AKI incidence within 72 h after ICU admission was 31% lower in preadmission statin users than in non-statin users [odds ratio (OR), 0.69; 95% confidence interval (CI), 0.61–0.79; $p < 0.001$]. Additionally, AKI incidence was 1.63-fold higher in patients with total cholesterol <160 mg dL^{-1} (OR: 1.63, 95% CI, 1.45–1.83; $p < 0.001$) than in those with total cholesterol of 160–200 mg dL^{-1} at ICU admission. There was no significant difference in patients with total cholesterol >200 mg dL^{-1} ($p = 0.111$).

Table 1. Baseline characteristics of adults patients who were admitted to ICU in 2012–2017.

Variable		Total (21,236)	Mean	SD
Sex: male		12,434 (58.6%)		
Age, year			64.0	15.8
Body mass index, kg m^{-2}			23.7	3.9
APACHE II			20.0	10.0
Comorbidities at ICU admission				
	eGFR ^{a} $\geq$ 90	12,993 (61.2%)		
	60 $\leq$ eGFR ^{a} < 90	4527 (21.3%)		
	30 $\leq$ eGFR ^{a} < 60	2364 (11.1%)		
	eGFR ^{a} < 30	1352 (6.4%)		
	Hypertension	9346 (44.0%)		
	Diabetes mellitus	1969 (9.3%)		
	Ischemic heart disease	538 (2.5%)		
	Cerebrovascular disease	945 (4.4%)		
	Chronic obstructive lung disease	921 (4.3%)		
	Liver disease (LC, hepatitis, fatty liver)	683 (3.2%)		
	Anemia (Hb < 10 g dL^{-1})	7569 (35.6%)		
	Cancer	4308 (20.3%)		
Characteristics of ICU admission				
	Admission through emergency department	12,042 (56.7%)		
	Admission department			
	Internal medicine	4671 (22.0%)		
	Neurologic center	4975 (23.4%)		
	Cardiothoracic surgical department	6875 (32.4%)		
	Other surgical department	4715 (22.2%)		
	Length of ICU stay, day		3.1	10.0
	Length of hospital stay, day		12.9	20.1
Preadmission statin use		5756 (27.1%)		
Total serum cholesterol at ICU adm, mg dL^{-1}			138.2	47.9
	<160, mg dL^{-1}	8584 (40.4%)		
	160–200 mg dL^{-1}	10,751 (50.6%)		
	>200 mg dL^{-1}	1901 (9.0%)		
Type of statin				
	Atorvastatin	3456 (16.3%)		
	Rosuvastatin	1391 (6.6%)		
	Simvastatin	396 (1.9%)		
	Pitavastatin	346 (1.6%)		
	Other statin ^{b}	167 (0.8%)		
Total acute kidney injury		5469 (25.8%)		
Acute kidney injury stage $\geq$2		2216 (10.4%)		
RRT after ICU adm within 72 h		488 (2.3%)		

Presented as Number (percentage) or Mean value (standard deviation): ^{a}: eGFR (mL min $^{-1}$ 1.73 m^{-2}): 186 × (Creatinine)$^{-1.154}$ × (Age)$^{-0.203}$ × (0.742 if female); ^{b}: Other statin: Pravastatin, Fluvastatin, and Lovastatin; ICU, intensive care unit; APACHE, acute physiology and chronic health evaluation; eGFR, estimated glomerular filtration rate; LC, liver cirrhosis; Hb, hemoglobin; RRT, renal replacement therapy.

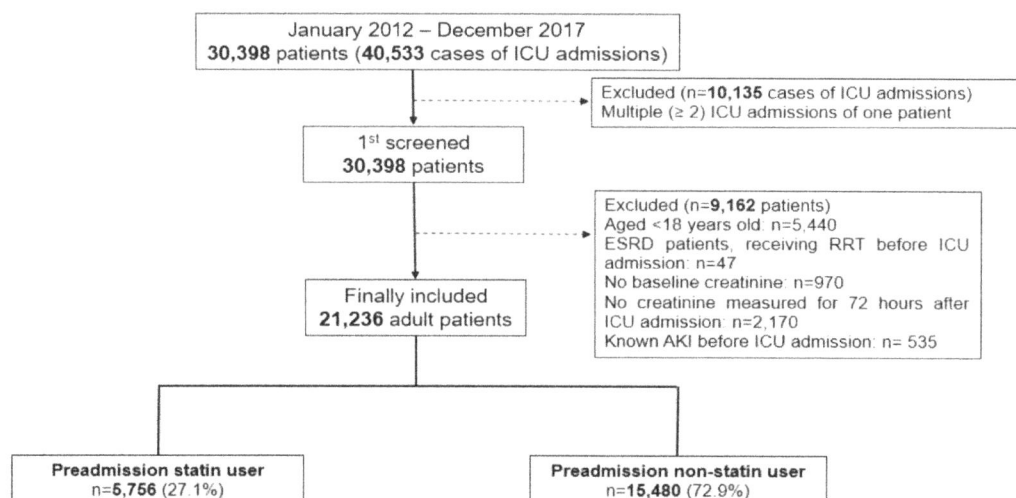

Figure 1. Flowchart of patient selection. ICU, Intensive Care Units; ESRD, End Stage Renal Disease; AKI, Acute Kidney Injury.

Table 2. Comparison of characteristics between preadmission statin user and non-statin user.

Variables	Statin Group $n = 5756$	Non-Statin Group $n = 15,480$	p-Value
Sex: male	3398 (59.0%)	9036 (58.4%)	0.384
Age, year	68.6 (12.0)	62.2 (16.6)	<0.001
Body Mass Index, kg m^{-2}	24.6 (3.8)	23.3 (3.8)	<0.001
Comorbidities at ICU admission			
APACHE II	19.8 (9.8)	20.2 (10.1)	0.012
eGFR ^{a}			<0.001
≥90	3073 (53.4%)	9920 (64.1%)	
60–90	1488 (25.9%)	3039 (19.6%)	
30–60	764 (13.3%)	1.600 (10.3%)	
<30	431 (7.5%)	921 (5.9%)	
Hypertension	3672 (63.8%)	5674 (36.7%)	<0.001
Diabetes mellitus	830 (14.4%)	1139 (7.4%)	<0.001
Ischemic heart disease	314 (5.5%)	224 (1.4%)	<0.001
Cerebrovascular disease	505 (8.8%)	440 (2.8%)	<0.001
Chronic obstructive lung disease	229 (4.0%)	692 (4.5%)	0118
Liver disease (LC, hepatitis, fatty liver)	87 (1.5%)	596 (3.9%)	<0.001
Anemia (Hb < 10 g dL^{-1})	1774 (30.8%)	5795 (37.4%)	<0.001
Cancer	875 (15.22%)	3433 (22.2%)	<0.001
Admission through ED	2640 (45.9%)	9402 (60.7%)	<0.001
Admission department			<0.001
Internal medicine	1317 (22.9%)	3354 (21.7%)	
Neurologic center	1252 (21.8%)	3723 (24.1%)	
Cardiothoracic surgical department	2166 (37.6%)	4709 (30.4%)	
Other surgical department	1021 (17.7%)	3694 (23.9%)	
Total serum cholesterol at ICU adm, mg dL^{-1}	125.2 (37.6)	143.1 (50.4)	<0.001
Length of hospital stay, day	11.3 (22.5)	13.5 (19.0)	<0.001
Length of ICU stay, day	2.5 (15.3)	3.3 (7.2)	<0.001
Total acute kidney injury	1301 (22.6%)	4168 (26.9%)	<0.001
Acute kidney injury stage ≥2	439 (7.6%)	1777 (11.5%)	<0.001
RRT after ICU adm within 72 h	140 (2.4%)	348 (2.2%)	0.426

Presented as number (percentage) or mean value (standard deviation). Two sample t-test for continuous variables and chi-square test for categorical variables were used: ^{a}: eGFR (mL min $^{-1}$ 1.73 m^{-2}): 186 × (Creatinine)$^{-1.154}$ × (Age)$^{-0.203}$ × (0.742 if female); ICU, intensive care unit; APACHE, acute physiology and chronic health evaluation; eGFR, estimated glomerular filtration rate; LC, liver cirrhosis; Hb, hemoglobin; ED, emergency department; RRT, renal replacement therapy.

Table 3. Multivariable logistic regression analysis for occurrence of acute kidney injury during 72 h after ICU admission.

Variable	Multivariable Model	
	Odds Ratio (95% CI)	p-Value
Dependent Variable: Total AKI		
Model 1: Preadmission statin use	0.69 (0.61, 0.79)	<0.001
Total serum cholesterol at ICU adm		
160–200 mg dL^{-1}	1	<0.001
<160, mg dL^{-1}	1.63 (1.45, 1.83)	<0.001
>200 mg dL^{-1}	0.86 (0.72, 1.04)	0.111
Interaction: eGFR ^{a} ≥ 90 × Non-statin use	1	0.001
60 ≤ eGFR ^{a} < 90 × Statin use	1.19 (0.95, 1.49)	0.132
30 ≤ eGFR ^{a} < 60 × Statin use	0.97 (0.74, 1.26)	0.801
eGFR ^{a} < 30 × Statin use	1.89 (1.35, 2.65)	<0.001
Dependent Variable: Stage ≥2 AKI		
Model 3: Preadmission statin use	0.69 (0.57, 0.84)	<0.001
Total serum cholesterol at ICU adm		
160–200 mg dL^{-1}	1	<0.001
<160 mg dL^{-1}	1.66 (1.38, 1.99)	<0.001
>200 mg dL^{-1}	0.85 (0.63, 1.15)	0.295
Interaction: eGFR ^{a} ≥ 90 × Non-statin use	1	
60 ≤ eGFR ^{a} < 90 × Statin use	0.95 (0.64, 1.40)	0.788
30 ≤ eGFR ^{a} < 90 × Statin use	1.04 (0.67, 1.61)	0.856
eGFR ^{a} < 30 × Statin use	1.27 (0.85, 1.91)	0.242

All covariates of $p < 0.1$ in univariable logistic regression analysis were included in multivariable logistic regression analysis. ^{a}: eGFR (mL min $^{-1}$ 1.73 m^{-2}): 186 × (Creatinine)$^{-1.154}$ × (Age)$^{-0.203}$ × (0.742 if female) ICU, intensive care unit; AKI, acute kidney injury; eGFR, estimated glomerular filtration rate.

An interaction occurred between eGFR before ICU admission and total AKI after ICU admission with respect to preadmission statin use (overall $p = 0.001$, in Table 3; model 1); thus, additional subgroup analysis was performed (Table 4). When the patients were divided according to eGFR at ICU admission, total AKI incidence within 72 h after ICU admission was 28% lower among statin users with eGFR $\geq$90 mL min $^{-1}$ 1.73 m^{-2} (OR, 0.72; 95% CI, 0.63–0.82; $p < 0.001$), 26% lower among statin users with $60 \leq$ eGFR $<$90 mL min $^{-1}$ 1.73 m^{-2} (OR, 0.74; 95% CI, 0.61–0.91; $p = 0.004$), and 35% lower among statin users with $30 \leq$ eGFR $<$60 mL min $^{-1}$ 1.73 m^{-2} (OR, 0.65; 95% CI, 0.51–0.83; $p = 0.001$) than among non-statin users. Meanwhile, there were no significant differences in total AKI incidence between groups with eGFR $<$30 mL min $^{-1}$ 1.73 m^{-2} ($p = 0.095$).

Table 4. Multivariable logistic regression analysis for occurrence of acute kidney injury during 72 h after ICU admission according to eGFR at ICU admission.

Variable	Multivariable Model	
	Odds Ratio (95% CI)	***p*-Value ***
eGFR [a] $\geq$ 90 ($n = 12{,}993$)		
Preadmission statin use	0.72 (0.63, 0.82)	<0.001
$60 \leq$ eGFR [a] < 90 ($n = 4527$)		
Preadmission statin use	0.74 (0.61, 0.91)	0.004
$30 \leq$ eGFR [a] < 60 ($n = 2364$)		
Preadmission statin use	0.65 (0.51, 0.83)	0.001
eGFR [a] < 30 ($n = 1340$)		
Preadmission statin use	1.33 (0.95, 1.86)	0.095

p * < 0.013 was considered as statistical significance after Bonferroni correction. [a]: eGFR (mL min $^{-1}$ 1.73 m^{-2}): $186 \times (\text{Creatinine})^{-1.154} \times (\text{Age})^{-0.203} \times (0.742 \text{ if female})$. ICU, intensive care unit; eGFR, estimated glomerular filtration rate.

3.2. Preadmission Statin Use and Stage $\geq$2 AKI Incidence

Table 3 also shows the results of the multivariable logistic regression analysis for stage $\geq$2 AKI incidence, including the covariates selected in the univariable logistic regression analysis (Appendix C). Stage $\geq$2 AKI incidence within 72 h after ICU admission was 31% lower among preadmission statin users than among non-statin users (OR, 0.69; 95% CI, 0.57–0.84; $p < 0.001$; model 3). Additionally, stage $\geq$2 AKI incidence was 1.66-fold higher in patients with total cholesterol $<$160 mg dL^{-1} (OR: 1.66, 95% CI, 1.38–1.99; $p < 0.001$) than in those with total cholesterol of 160–200 mg dL^{-1} at ICU admission. There was no significant difference in patients with total cholesterol $>$200 mg dL^{-1} ($p = 0.295$). Moreover, no interaction occurred between eGFR at ICU admission and stage $\geq$2 AKI with resto preadmission statin use (overall $p = 0.788$).

4. Discussion

This study showed that preadmission statin use is associated with a lower incidence of AKI after ICU admission. This association was also evident with stage $\geq$2 AKI. However, the association was not significant among patients with severe kidney dysfunction (eGFR $<$30 mL min^{-1} 1.73 m^{-2}) prior to ICU admission. Although the study results were derived from a retrospective observational study, it is striking because the statin group was comprised of significantly older and sicker patients and had a higher proportion of patients with renal dysfunction, more diabetes mellitus, ischemic heart disease, and cerebrovascular disease. Therefore, the study results suggested that clinicians who did not favor statin would consider prescribing statins to patients with respect to preventive effects for the development of AKI in critically ill patients.

The most interesting finding of this study was that an interaction occurred between eGFR at ICU admission and total AKI incidence with respect to preadmission statin use. In subsequent analyses, the potential benefit of preadmission statin use on AKI was not significant among patients with stage $\geq$4 chronic kidney disease (CKD). A meta-analysis, published in 2015, reported that statin therapy does not improve the overall kidney function of CKD patients with eGFR <60 mL min^{-1} 1.73 m^{-2} and that high-dose statin therapy leads to limited improvement in kidney function [23]. Another meta-analysis, published in 2017, concluded that statin therapy was not beneficial in reducing major cardiovascular events, cardiovascular death, and all-cause mortality of patients with CKD 4 or 5 (eGFR <30 mL min^{-1} 1.73 m^{-2}) [24]. Although the primary endpoints were different from those used in our study, the previous meta-analysis suggested that statin therapy did not improve outcomes of patients with severe kidney dysfunction (CKD stage ≥4), which is consistent with our study finding. Patients with stage ≥4 CKD have worse baseline renovascular function than patients with normal kidney function and thus are more susceptible to ischemic oxidative damage, which is a major mechanism of AKI [25]. Furthermore, it was possible that treating patients with CKD stage ≥4 would be ineffective and the course of AKI could no longer be affected. However, it is difficult to completely explain the renal outcomes according to CKD stage solely based on this cohort study; hence, additional studies are needed.

This study suggested that preadmission statin therapy causes immunomodulatory effects, which were explained based on the pleiotropic effect of statin therapy [26]. We defined preadmission statin users as patients who confirmed taking statins as maintenance treatment as prescribed by their physicians at least one month before ICU admission. Most preadmission statin users received statin therapy for a long time, and there was some evidence that showed a clinical benefit of long-term statin therapy in patients with septic shock [27], pneumonia [28], or acute respiratory distress syndrome [29]. Although the immunomodulatory effect of statin therapy on critically ill patients remains controversial [30,31], it might affect the study results.

There is another important finding that should be carefully interpreted. The total incidence of AKI was higher in patients with <160 mg dL^{-1} of total serum cholesterol than in those with 160–200 mg dL^{-1} of total serum cholesterol, while patients with >200 mg dL^{-1} of total serum cholesterol had no association with the incidence of total AKI. In general, hyperlipidemia is an associated factor for renal damage [32]; however, hyperlipidemia was not associated with a lower incidence of AKI in this study. This can be explained based on the characteristics of ICU patients in this study. Lower cholesterol is a known factor that negatively affects the outcomes of critically ill patients [33,34], which is also coincident with our current study. Therefore, the effect of total serum cholesterol level on the incidence of AKI might be influenced by the characteristics of critically ill patients.

This study has a few limitations. First, a selection bias may have occurred due to the retrospective observational nature of the study. Second, the findings have limited generalizability because the study was conducted in a single center. For example, as previously mentioned, ethnical differences may have been involved in the effects of rosuvastatin. Lastly, because the duration of preadmission statin use differed among patients, we could not consider it in the analysis.

5. Conclusions

This study showed that preadmission statin use is associated with a lower incidence of total AKI and stage ≥ 2 AKI among critically ill patients after ICU admission. This association was most significantly evident among rosuvastatin users, but was absent among CKD patients with eGFR <30 mL min^{-1} 1.73 m^{-2}.

Author Contributions: T.K.O. contributed to the study design, analyzed the data, and drafted the first manuscript; I.-A.S., Y.-J.C., C.L., Y.-T.J., H.-J.B., and Y.H.J. contributed to the acquisition of data and provided critical revision of the manuscript; All authors have given final approval for the final version of the manuscript.

Appendix A. Staging of Postoperative Acute Kidney Injury (KDIGO)

Stage	Serum Creatinine
1	1.5–1.9 times baseline or $\geq$0.3 mg dL^{-1} increase within 72 h after ICU admission
2	2.0–2.9 times baseline within 72 h after ICU admission
3	3.0 times baseline or increase in serum creatinine to $\geq$4.0 mg dL^{-1} or initiation of RRT within 72 h after ICU admission

KDIGO, Kidney Disease: Improving Global Outcomes; RRT, Renal Replacement Therapy.

Appendix B. Univariable Logistic Regression Analysis of Covariates for Occurrence of Total Acute Kidney Injury during 72 h after ICU Admission

Variables	Odds Ratio (95% CI)	p-Value
Sex: male	1.06 (1.00–1.13)	0.066
Age, year	1.02 (1.02–1.02)	<0.001
Body mass index, kg m^{-2}	0.96 (0.95–0.97)	<0.001
APACHE II	1.04 (1.04–1.04)	<0.001
Comorbidities at ICU admission		
Hypertension	1.26 (1.18–1.34)	<0.001
Diabetes mellitus	1.46 (1.32–1.61)	<0.001
Ischemic heart disease	1.17 (0.97–1.42)	0.101
Cerebrovascular disease	1.31 (1.14–1.51)	<0.001
Chronic obstructive lung disease	1.13 (0.97–1.31)	0.109
Liver disease (LC, hepatitis, fatty liver)	2.48 (2.13–2.89)	<0.001
Anemia (Hb < 10 g dL^{-1})	3.82 (3.58–4.07)	<0.001
Cancer	1.90 (1.77–2.05)	<0.001
eGFR mL min^{-1} 1.73 m^{-2}		
$\geq$90	1	<0.001
60–90	0.99 (0.91–1.07)	0.731
30–60	2.08 (1.89–2.28)	<0.001
<30	5.18 (4.61–5.82)	<0.001
Admission through emergency department	1.52 (1.43–1.62)	<0.001
Total serum cholesterol at ICU adm		
160–200 mg dL^{-1}	1	<0.001
<160, mg dL^{-1}	2.21 (2.01, 2.43)	<0.001
>200 mg dL^{-1}	0.81 (0.69, 0.94)	<0.001
Admission department		
Internal medicine	1	<0.001
Neurologic center	0.25 (0.23–0.28)	<0.001
Cardiothoracic surgical department	0.78 (0.72–0.84)	<0.001
Other surgical department	0.83 (0.76–0.90)	<0.001
Year at ICU admission		
2012	1	<0.001
2013	1.31 (1.16–1.48)	<0.001
2014	1.26 (1.12–1.42)	<0.001
2015	1.09 (0.97–1.23)	0.150
2016	1.02 (0.91–1.15)	0.690
2017	0.96 (0.86–1.08)	0.535

All covariates of $p < 0.1$ in univariable logistic regression analysis were included in multivariable logistic regression analysis; ICU, intensive care unit; AKI, acute kidney injury; APACHE, acute physiology and chronic health evaluation; LC, liver cirrhosis; Hb, hemoglobin.

Appendix C. Univariable Logistic Regression Analysis of Covariates for Occurrence of Stage ≥ 2 AKI Acute Kidney Injury during 72 h after ICU Admission

Variables	Odds Ratio (95% CI)	p-Value
Sex: male	1.04 (0.95–1.13)	0.452
Age, year	1.01 (1.01–1.02)	<0.001
Body mass index, kg m^{-2}	0.94 (0.92–0.95)	<0.001
APACHE II	1.04 (1.04–1.04)	<0.001
Comorbidities at ICU admission		
Hypertension	1.08 (0.99–1.18)	0.106
Diabetes mellitus	1.25 (1.09–1.44)	0.002
Ischemic heart disease	0.94 (0.70–1.25)	0.654
Cerebrovascular disease	1.03 (0.83–1.27)	0.795
Chronic obstructive lung disease	0.97 (0.78–1.21)	0.816
Liver disease (LC, hepatitis, fatty liver)	3.26 (2.73–3.88)	<0.001
Anemia (Hb < 10 g dL^{-1})	4.86 (4.42–5.35)	<0.001
Cancer	2.23 (2.03–2.46)	<0.001
eGFR mL min^{-1} 1.73 m^{-2}		
≥90	1	<0.001
60–90	0.73 (0.64–0.82)	<0.001
30–60	1.10 (0.96–1.27)	0.171
<30	2.84 (2.47–3.26)	<0.001
Admission through emergency department	2.00 (1.82–2.21)	<0.001
Total serum cholesterol at ICU adm		
160–200 mg dL^{-1}	1	
<160, mg dL^{-1}	2.34 (2.02, 2.70)	<0.001
>200 mg dL^{-1}	0.81 (0.64, 1.04)	0.095
Admission department		
Internal medicine	1	<0.001
Neurologic center	0.20 (0.17–0.24)	<0.001
Cardiothoracic surgical department	0.52 (0.46–0.58)	<0.001
Other surgical department	0.67 (0.60–0.75)	<0.001
Year at ICU admission		
2012	1	<0.001
2013	1.52 (1.27–1.80)	<0.001
2014	1.38 (1.16–1.63)	<0.001
2015	1.19 (1.00–1.41)	0.053
2016	1.05 (0.88–1.24)	0.605
2017	1.00 (0.84–1.19)	0.999

All covariates of $p < 0.1$ in univariable logistic regression analysis were included in multivariable logistic regression analysis. ICU, intensive care unit; APACHE, acute physiology and chronic health evaluation; eGFR, estimated glomerular filtration rate; LC, liver cirrhosis; Hb, hemoglobin; RRT, renal replacement therapy.

References

1. Waikar, S.S.; Bonventre, J.V. Creatinine kinetics and the definition of acute kidney injury. *J. Am. Soc. Nephrol.* **2009**, *20*, 672–679. [CrossRef] [PubMed]
2. Bellomo, R.; Kellum, J.A.; Ronco, C. Acute kidney injury. *Lancet* **2012**, *380*, 756–766. [CrossRef]
3. Lewington, A.J.; Cerda, J.; Mehta, R.L. Raising awareness of acute kidney injury: A global perspective of a silent killer. *Kidney Int.* **2013**, *84*, 457–467. [CrossRef] [PubMed]
4. Nash, K.; Hafeez, A.; Hou, S. Hospital-acquired renal insufficiency. *Am. J. Kidney Dis.* **2002**, *39*, 930–936. [CrossRef] [PubMed]
5. Thakar, C.V.; Christianson, A.; Freyberg, R.; Almenoff, P.; Render, M.L. Incidence and outcomes of acute kidney injury in intensive care units: A veterans administration study. *Crit. Care Med.* **2009**, *37*, 2552–2558. [CrossRef]
6. Macedo, E.; Mehta, R.L. Preventing acute kidney injury. *Crit. Care Clin.* **2015**, *31*, 773–784. [CrossRef] [PubMed]
7. Santodomingo-Garzon, T.; Cunha, T.M.; Verri, W.A., Jr.; Valerio, D.A.; Parada, C.A.; Poole, S.; Ferreira, S.H.; Cunha, F.Q. Atorvastatin inhibits inflammatory hypernociception. *Br. J. Pharmacol.* **2006**, *149*, 14–22. [CrossRef] [PubMed]

8. Rosenson, R.S. Low high-density lipoprotein cholesterol and cardiovascular disease: Risk reduction with statin therapy. *Am. Heart J.* **2006**, *151*, 556–563. [CrossRef]

9. Novack, V.; Terblanche, M.; Almog, Y. Do statins have a role in preventing or treating sepsis? *Crit. Care* **2006**, *10*, 113. [CrossRef]

10. Terblanche, M.; Almog, Y.; Rosenson, R.S.; Smith, T.S.; Hackam, D.G. Statins and sepsis: Multiple modifications at multiple levels. *Lancet Infect Dis.* **2007**, *7*, 358–368. [CrossRef]

11. Wang, C.Y.; Liu, P.Y.; Liao, J.K. Pleiotropic effects of statin therapy: Molecular mechanisms and clinical results. *Trends Mol. Med.* **2008**, *14*, 37–44. [CrossRef] [PubMed]

12. Molnar, A.O.; Coca, S.G.; Devereaux, P.J.; Jain, A.K.; Kitchlu, A.; Luo, J.; Parikh, C.R.; Paterson, J.M.; Siddiqui, N.; Wald, R.; et al. Statin use associates with a lower incidence of acute kidney injury after major elective surgery. *J. Am. Soc. Nephrol.* **2011**, *22*, 939–946. [CrossRef] [PubMed]

13. Campbell, J. Hmg coa reductase inhibitors (statins) for preventing acute kidney injury after surgical procedures requiring cardiac bypass. *J. Perioper. Pract.* **2018**, *28*, 142–143. [CrossRef] [PubMed]

14. Han, Y.; Zhu, G.; Han, L.; Hou, F.; Huang, W.; Liu, H.; Gan, J.; Jiang, T.; Li, X.; Wang, W.; et al. Short-term rosuvastatin therapy for prevention of contrast-induced acute kidney injury in patients with diabetes and chronic kidney disease. *J. Am. Coll. Cardiol.* **2014**, *63*, 62–70. [CrossRef] [PubMed]

15. Yasuda, H.; Yuen, P.S.; Hu, X.; Zhou, H.; Star, R.A. Simvastatin improves sepsis-induced mortality and acute kidney injury via renal vascular effects. *Kidney Int.* **2006**, *69*, 1535–1542. [CrossRef] [PubMed]

16. Su, X.; Zhang, L.; Lv, J.; Wang, J.; Hou, W.; Xie, X.; Zhang, H. Effect of statins on kidney disease outcomes: A systematic review and meta-analysis. *Am. J. Kidney Dis.* **2016**, *67*, 881–892. [CrossRef] [PubMed]

17. Hallan, S.; Asberg, A.; Lindberg, M.; Johnsen, H. Validation of the modification of diet in renal disease formula for estimating gfr with special emphasis on calibration of the serum creatinine assay. *Am. J. Kidney Dis.* **2004**, *44*, 84–93. [CrossRef] [PubMed]

18. Neaton, J.D.; Blackburn, H.; Jacobs, D.; Kuller, L.; Lee, D.J.; Sherwin, R.; Shih, J.; Stamler, J.; Wentworth, D. Serum cholesterol level and mortality findings for men screened in the multiple risk factor intervention trial. Multiple risk factor intervention trial research group. *Arch. Intern. Med.* **1992**, *152*, 1490–1500. [CrossRef] [PubMed]

19. Sempos, C.T.; Cleeman, J.I.; Carroll, M.D.; Johnson, C.L.; Bachorik, P.S.; Gordon, D.J.; Burt, V.L.; Briefel, R.R.; Brown, C.D.; Lippel, K.; et al. Prevalence of high blood cholesterol among us adults. An update based on guidelines from the second report of the national cholesterol education program adult treatment panel. *JAMA* **1993**, *269*, 3009–3014. [CrossRef] [PubMed]

20. Kellum, J.A.; Lameire, N.; Group, K.A.G.W. Diagnosis, evaluation, and management of acute kidney injury: A kdigo summary (part 1). *Crit. Care* **2013**, *17*, 204. [CrossRef] [PubMed]

21. Chawla, L.S.; Eggers, P.W.; Star, R.A.; Kimmel, P.L. Acute kidney injury and chronic kidney disease as interconnected syndromes. *N. Engl. J. Med.* **2014**, *371*, 58–66. [CrossRef]

22. Armstrong, R.A. When to use the bonferroni correction. *Ophthalmic Physiol. Opt.* **2014**, *34*, 502–508. [CrossRef]

23. Sanguankeo, A.; Upala, S.; Cheungpasitporn, W.; Ungprasert, P.; Knight, E.L. Effects of statins on renal outcome in chronic kidney disease patients: A systematic review and meta-analysis. *PLoS ONE* **2015**, *10*, e0132970. [CrossRef]

24. Messow, C.M.; Isles, C. Meta-analysis of statins in chronic kidney disease: Who benefits? *QJM* **2017**, *110*, 493–500. [CrossRef] [PubMed]

25. Basile, D.P.; Anderson, M.D.; Sutton, T.A. Pathophysiology of acute kidney injury. *Compr. Physiol.* **2012**, *2*, 1303–1353. [PubMed]

26. Liao, J.K.; Laufs, U. Pleiotropic effects of statins. *Annu. Rev. Pharmacol. Toxicol.* **2005**, *45*, 89–118. [CrossRef] [PubMed]

27. Fuller, B.M.; Gajera, M.; Schorr, C.; Gerber, D.; Dellinger, R.P.; Zanotti, S. The association of prior statin use in septic shock treated with early goal directed therapy. *Eur. J. Emerg. Med.* **2012**, *19*, 226–230. [CrossRef] [PubMed]

28. Thomsen, R.W.; Riis, A.; Kornum, J.B.; Christensen, S.; Johnsen, S.P.; Sorensen, H.T. Preadmission use of statins and outcomes after hospitalization with pneumonia: Population-based cohort study of 29,900 patients. *Arch. Intern. Med.* **2008**, *168*, 2081–2087. [CrossRef]

29. Craig, T.; O'Kane, C.; McAuley, D. Potential mechanisms by which statins modulate the development of acute lung injury. In *Intensive Care Medicine*; Springer: Berlin, Germany, 2007; pp. 276–288.

30. Nagendran, M.; McAuley, D.F.; Kruger, P.S.; Papazian, L.; Truwit, J.D.; Laffey, J.G.; Thompson, B.T.; Clarke, M.; Gordon, A.C. Statin therapy for acute respiratory distress syndrome: An individual patient data meta-analysis of randomised clinical trials. *Intensive Care Med.* **2017**, *43*, 663–671. [CrossRef]

31. Thomas, G.; Hraiech, S.; Loundou, A.; Truwit, J.; Kruger, P.; McAuley, D.F.; Papazian, L.; Roch, A. Statin therapy in critically-ill patients with severe sepsis: A review and meta-analysis of randomized clinical trials. *Minerva Anestesiol.* **2015**, *81*, 921–930.

32. Sastre, C.; Rubio-Navarro, A.; Buendia, I.; Gomez-Guerrero, C.; Blanco, J.; Mas, S.; Egido, J.; Blanco-Colio, L.M.; Ortiz, A.; Moreno, J.A. Hyperlipidemia-associated renal damage decreases klotho expression in kidneys from apoe knockout mice. *PLoS ONE* **2013**, *8*, e83713. [CrossRef] [PubMed]

33. Wilson, R.F.; Barletta, J.F.; Tyburski, J.G. Hypocholesterolemia in sepsis and critically ill or injured patients. *Crit. Care* **2003**, *7*, 413–414. [CrossRef] [PubMed]

34. Gui, D.; Spada, P.L.; De Gaetano, A.; Pacelli, F. Hypocholesterolemia and risk of death in the critically ill surgical patient. *Intensive Care Med.* **1996**, *22*, 790–794. [CrossRef] [PubMed]

13

Nephrocalcinosis: A Review of Monogenic Causes and Insights they Provide into this Heterogeneous Condition

Fay J. Dickson [1] and John A. Sayer [2,3,4,*]

[1] Hull University Teaching Hospitals, Anlaby Road, Hull HU3 2JZ, UK; fayhill@gmail.com
[2] Translational and Clinical Research Institute, Faculty of Medical Sciences, Newcastle University, Central Parkway, Newcastle upon Tyne NE1 3BZ, UK
[3] The Newcastle upon Tyne NHS Hospitals Foundation Trust, Newcastle upon Tyne NE7 7DN, UK
[4] NIHR Newcastle Biomedical Research Centre, Newcastle upon Tyne NE4 5PL, UK
[*] Correspondence: john.sayer@ncl.ac.uk

Abstract: The abnormal deposition of calcium within renal parenchyma, termed nephrocalcinosis, frequently occurs as a result of impaired renal calcium handling. It is closely associated with renal stone formation (nephrolithiasis) as elevated urinary calcium levels (hypercalciuria) are a key common pathological feature underlying these clinical presentations. Although monogenic causes of nephrocalcinosis and nephrolithiasis are rare, they account for a significant disease burden with many patients developing chronic or end-stage renal disease. Identifying underlying genetic mutations in hereditary cases of nephrocalcinosis has provided valuable insights into renal tubulopathies that include hypercalciuria within their varied phenotypes. Genotypes affecting other enzyme pathways, including vitamin D metabolism and hepatic glyoxylate metabolism, are also associated with nephrocalcinosis. As the availability of genetic testing becomes widespread, we cannot be imprecise in our approach to nephrocalcinosis. Monogenic causes of nephrocalcinosis account for a broad range of phenotypes. In cases such as Dent disease, supportive therapies are limited, and early renal replacement therapies are necessitated. In cases such as renal tubular acidosis, a good renal prognosis can be expected providing effective treatment is implemented. It is imperative we adopt a precision-medicine approach to ensure patients and their families receive prompt diagnosis, effective, tailored treatment and accurate prognostic information.

Keywords: nephrocalcinosis; nephrolithiasis; hypercalciuria; monogenic; precision medicine

1. Introduction

Nephrocalcinosis can broadly be defined as the deposition of calcium, either as calcium phosphate or calcium oxalate, within the interstitium of the kidney [1]. Whilst Oliver Wrong's original classification sub-divided nephrocalcinosis into being either molecular, microscopic or macroscopic, in clinical practice the term commonly refers to macroscopic nephrocalcinosis that can be detected radiologically [2]. Rarely, asymmetric presentation of nephrocalcinosis localised to the renal cortex may represent calcium release from tissue breakdown, for example in renal transplant rejection or renal infarction [3]. However, in the majority of cases, nephrocalcinosis affects the renal medulla and can be detected as bilateral, symmetrical increased echogenicity within the renal pyramids on ultrasound imaging [4]. This non-invasive imaging modality is utilised either as a screening tool, or as a method of assessing disease progression/response to treatment, as medullary nephrocalcinosis can be reliably graded (Grade I–III) according to the extent of increased echogenicity affecting the medullary pyramids [5].

Whilst the exact pathogenesis of nephrocalcinosis remains under investigation, it is acknowledged medullary nephrocalcinosis is a consequence of hypercalciuria. Increased urinary calcium load arises either through increased calcium absorption (extra-renal causes) or impaired calcium reabsorption within the renal tubule [2]. The majority of calcium reabsorption (~65%) occurs in the proximal tubule, whilst ~25% is reabsorbed in the thick ascending limb of the loop of Henle [6] and ~5% is reabsorbed from the cortical collecting duct [2]. Identification of monogenic causes of nephrocalcinosis affecting these areas has provided valuable insights into the pathogenesis of this heterogeneous condition. Interestingly, although a further ~7–10% of calcium is reabsorbed within the distal convoluted tubule, no monogenic causes of nephrocalcinosis have been identified which affect this section of the renal tubule [2].

Hypercalciuria, in addition to being part of the underlying pathological process for nephrocalcinosis, also predisposes patients to renal stone formation (nephrolithiasis). Nephrocalcinosis and nephrolithiasis will therefore commonly co-exist within the phenotypes of these rare monogenic conditions, and nephrolithiasis onset at a young age may prompt investigations for nephrocalcinosis and uncover an inherited condition [7].

Nephrocalcinosis in itself is a rare disorder, and consequently monogenic forms affect even smaller numbers of the population. For those individuals affected by nephrocalcinosis, however, a tailored, individualised approach to their initial diagnostic work-up is imperative. Presentation at a young age, a family history of an affected individual or carrier, or a history of consanguinity in the family is often suggestive of an inherited tubulopathy. Several factors, including recessive inheritance patterns and varied phenotype presentation, dictate that a family history is often not present, and suspicion of a monogenic cause should not be dismissed simply due to absence of the above factors.

The morbidity associated with nephrolithiasis and nephrocalcinosis is widely accepted [8]. Whilst an overall approach may focus upon slowing progression of associated chronic kidney disease (CKD), specific treatment strategies, such as dietary modifications or use of thiazide diuretics, will vary depending upon the underlying disease process. Widespread adoption of precision medicine within this field is likely to have significant advantages for both current and future patients. Several monogenic causes of nephrocalcinosis are associated with rapid progression of CKD, often requiring initiation of renal replacement therapies before adulthood. Early diagnosis of a monogenic cause is vital for providing accurate prognostic information for the patient and their family, including the opportunity to screen other family members or offer pre-implantation genetic diagnosis (PGD) testing for subsequent pregnancies. Perhaps most significantly, a prompt diagnosis may also avoid the individual being exposed to unnecessary or harmful treatments. For example, a patient with OCRL mutations (Dent disease 2) was reported to receive immunosuppressive therapies including corticosteroids and cyclophosphamide, based on a misdiagnosis of nephrotic syndrome, before their inherited tubulopathy was correctly identified [9]. Commonly used medications may easily inadvertently worsen the condition of patients with other inherited tubulopathies: loop diuretic use can potentiate hypercalciuria and worsen nephrolithiasis/nephrocalcinosis burden, whereas use of potassium-sparing diuretics should be avoided in patients with distal renal tubular acidosis [10]. Furthermore, in cases where a proactive approach to personalised genetic medicine has been taken, next generation sequencing has identified CLCN5 mutations (Dent disease 1) in patients for whom only low-molecular weight proteinuria was present at diagnosis, i.e., before the full phenotype had emerged [11]. Finally, given the current paucity of treatment options for nephrocalcinosis, it is potentially from the study of these rare monogenic causes that key future therapeutic targets may emerge which could revolutionise our management of the condition (Table A1).

2. Monogenic Causes of Nephrocalcinosis

2.1. CLCN5 Mutations

The proximal tubule represents the site of greatest calcium reabsorption within the renal tubule, and it is mutations in the ClC-5 chloride transporter in this region, encoded by *CLCN5*, that give rise to Dent disease type 1 [12]. This condition demonstrates an X-linked recessive pattern of inheritance; affected males usually display a triad of low molecular weight (LMW) proteinuria, hypercalciuria and nephrocalcinosis, although the triad may be incomplete at initial presentation [11]. Female carriers are usually asymptomatic, but may occasionally have LMW proteinuria, hypercalciuria or nephrolithiasis [12].

Dent disease 1 (*CLCN5* mutations) accounts for 60% of Dent disease cases. *OCRL* mutations, which may result in a spectrum of phenotypes ranging from Dent disease 2 to the more severe Lowe oculocerebrorenal syndrome, account for a further 15% of cases, whilst the underlying genetic mutation remains unascertained in 25% of cases [12]. The varied phenotypes of Dent disease may also include a partial Fanconi syndrome as the initial clue indicating proximal tubular dysfunction [13], whilst nephrolithiasis or haematuria can also feature alongside the cardinal LMW proteinuria [11]. Although genetic conditions with a Fanconi syndrome, including Lowe oculocerebrorenal syndrome (*OCRL* mutations) and cystinosis (*CTNS* mutations) may also feature nephrocalcinosis [14,15], it remains more commonly associated with Dent disease 1 (*CLCN5* mutations) [16].

Patients with Dent disease carry a poor prognosis in terms of renal function: 30–80% of males develop end-stage renal disease (ESRD) by middle-age [12]. The development of CKD has been hypothesised to be linked to nephrocalcinosis, although this theory does not explain Dent disease patients without nephrocalcinosis who also develop progressive CKD, and it is probable more than one mechanism exists [16,17].

Treatment options for Dent disease are limited. Early diagnosis is crucial in order to prioritise preservation of renal function for as long as possible and offer accurate prognostic information [11]. Patients should undergo careful CKD monitoring with control of variables such as blood pressure. A strategy to try and reduce nephrocalcinosis development is to reduce urinary calcium excretion; thiazide diuretics may be used but in some patients their role is limited by unacceptable side effects including hypokalaemia, muscle cramps and dehydration [12]. The majority of patients will reach ESRD by the age of 40 [18]; renal transplantation offers the best outcomes as there is no recurrence in the renal allograft due to the donor kidney not carrying the causative mutation [12].

2.2. CYP24A1 Mutations

Nephrocalcinosis occurs as a result of impaired renal calcium handling; disorders of vitamin D metabolism can result in elevated calcium levels and represent a different pathway predisposing to nephrocalcinosis formation. The second stage of vitamin D activation takes place within the kidney, resulting in production of the active metabolite 1,25-dihydroxyvitamin D^3. Mutations in *CYP24A1*, which encodes 1,25-hydroxyvitamin-D_3-24-hydroxylase, result in an inability to catabolise this active vitamin D metabolite [19]. *CYP24A1* mutations were first detected following reports of a small cohort of babies developing adverse effects (including hypercalcemia and nephrocalcinosis) as a result of the public health intervention to routinely supplement formula milk with vitamin D [20]. Following further analysis, two distinct phenotypes resulting from *CYP24A1* mutations have been recognised, both of which frequently include nephrocalcinosis [19].

The first phenotype, idiopathic infantile hypercalcaemia (IIH) presents in childhood, and is classified as hypercalcaemia, infantile 1 (HCINF1). Affected infants often present with symptomatic hypercalcaemia, severe dehydration, vomiting and failure to thrive [21]. Nephrocalcinosis is often detectable on ultrasound imaging at diagnosis [21]. Management of these patients focusses upon removing exogenous sources of vitamin D (e.g., supplements), fluid resuscitation and future conservative measures (high fluid intake, dietary adjustments, avoidance of tanning beds) to prevent further nephrolithiasis/nephrocalcinosis formation.

A second, later-onset, phenotype has also been demonstrated in adults who present with nephrolithiasis, hypercalciuria or incidentally detected nephrocalcinosis [22]. This phenotype is usually less severe, and a history of vitamin D supplementation is not universally present. Treatment strategies focus upon low calcium and oxalate diet, avoidance of vitamin D supplementation and excessive sunlight exposure [19]. Use of azole antifungal agents (fluconazole, ketoconazole) have shown benefit as non-specific P450 enzyme inhibitors which inhibit 1α-hydroxylase (encoded by $CYP27B1$), thereby reducing production of the active form of vitamin D [19,23]. However, lifelong treatment with these agents may be undesirable owing to their side effect profile, including hepatotoxicity. Recently, rifampicin was demonstrated to reduce hypercalcaemia and effectively control 1,25-dihydroxyvitamin D^3 levels in patients with $CYP24A1$ mutations [24]. Rifampicin acts upon an alternative vitamin D catabolism pathway as a potent inducer of $CYP3A4$ [24]. This provides an alternative therapy that may be better tolerated as a lifelong treatment.

2.3. SLC34A1 Mutations

Autosomal recessive inheritance of mutations in the sodium-phosphate co-transporter NaPi2a, encoded by $SLC34A1$, cause idiopathic infantile hypercalcaemia (IIH), classified as hypercalcaemia, infantile 2 (HCINF2), in a subgroup of patients without $CYP24A1$ mutations [25]. In addition to the classic biochemical features associated with IIH of hypercalcaemia, hypercalciuria and high levels of 1,25-dihydroxyvitamin D$_3$, patients with $SLC34A1$ loss-of-function mutations exhibit hypophosphatemia [26]. This hypophosphatemia arises as a result of renal phosphate wasting within the proximal tubule, driving excessive production of 1,25-dihydroxyvitamin D$_3$ and subsequent hypercalcaemia and hypercalciuria.

Nephrocalcinosis is a common phenotypical feature in patients with $SLC34A1$ mutations [27]. In the acute presentation, where patients may have classical features of IIH such as failure to thrive, dehydration and vomiting, they should be fluid resuscitated and may receive loop diuretics (furosemide) to induce calciuresis [27]. Similar to patients with $CYP24A1$ mutations, an azole antifungal agent (ketoconazole or fluconazole) may be used to inhibit 1α-hydroxylase, thereby reducing the high calcium levels predisposing to nephrocalcinosis through reduction in levels of 1,25-dihydroxyvitamin D$_3$ [26]. The long-term management of these patients, however, should focus upon a low calcium diet and avoidance of vitamin D supplementation or heightened vitamin D exposure, in order to minimise the risk of nephrocalcinosis.

2.4. CLDN16 and CLDN19 Mutations

The thick ascending limb (TAL) of loop of Henle, where ~25% of calcium reabsorption [6] and ~60% of magnesium reabsorption usually takes place [28], is the site of two rare autosomal recessive channelopathies affecting calcium and magnesium absorption. Mutations in $CLDN16$ and $CLDN19$, which encode the tight junction proteins claudin-16 and claudin-19 respectively, give rise to the condition familial hypomagnesaemia with hypercalciuria and nephrocalcinosis (FHHNC) [29].

Patients are symptomatic from a young age, although initial presenting features may be non-specific such as polyuria/polydipsia, failure to thrive and vomiting. The biochemical profile of FHHNC phenotypes includes excessive loss of calcium and magnesium in the urine, with normal serum calcium levels and low serum magnesium levels [28]. Importantly, serum hypomagnesaemia is not universally present, and a fractional excretion value of magnesium (FeMg%) should be calculated using serum magnesium, serum creatinine and urinary magnesium levels to ensure diagnostic accuracy [30]. Nephrocalcinosis is a universal feature which develops early in the disease course of FHHNC, and hypercalciuria is one predisposing factor for this [30]. A further predisposing factor for nephrolithiasis and nephrocalcinosis in FHHNC is hypocitraturia, which removes the protective effect of urinary citrate against precipitation of calcium salts in the urine [30]. The renal prognosis for FHHNC is poor;

many patients progress to ESRD during adolescence [28]. Rapid progression of CKD in these patients may not be attributable solely to nephrocalcinosis, as their renal dysfunction is more severe/presents earlier than that observed in other tubulopathies predisposing to nephrocalcinosis such as primary distal renal tubular acidosis or Bartter syndrome [30]. *CLDN19* mutations are associated with severe ocular abnormalities as claudin-19 is also expressed in the retinal epithelium [28].

Treatment strategies for FHHNC patients focus initially on supportive measures aimed at reducing hypercalciuria and replacing magnesium; thiazide diuretics and oral magnesium supplements are used for this respectively, although their impact on total urine calcium and serum magnesium levels is not always significant [28,30]. Overall, these supportive treatments do not negate the progression of renal dysfunction, and renal replacement therapies are commonly necessitated before adulthood. Renal transplantation is the ideal option: the loss-of-function channelopathy is not present in the renal allograft so renal calcium and magnesium handling are normalised and there is no disease recurrence [31].

2.5. Bartter Syndromes

The Bartter syndromes describe five channelopathies affecting thick ascending limb (TAL) transporter proteins involved in sodium chloride (NaCl) re-absorption. Autosomal recessive inheritance of these gene mutations results in salt-losing tubulopathies characterised by excessive urinary sodium losses, with corresponding hypokalaemia, metabolic alkalosis and secondary hyperaldosteronism [32]. Nephrocalcinosis has been described in all Bartter syndromes but is most frequently associated with Bartter I, II and V [2]. The pathogenesis of nephrocalcinosis in Bartter syndromes is not fully understood, although it is most probably a consequence of hypercalciuria seen within the Bartter syndrome phenotypes [33]. Early identification of the Bartter syndrome genotype is clinically advantageous, especially given the fact nephrocalcinosis and other renal manifestations are not uniformly represented across the different Bartter syndrome phenotypes. Several clinical features, including age of onset, presence of transient hyperkalaemia, severity of hypokalaemia, sensorineural deafness and renal impairment may provide vital clues about the likely underlying genotype which can guide genetic testing.

Bartter syndromes I and II, caused by mutations in *SLC12A1* and *KCNJ1* respectively, usually present during the antenatal/postnatal period, and have been traditionally referred to as antenatal Bartter syndromes (aBS). Polyhydramnios, premature birth and low-birth weight are classic features of aBS, and nephrocalcinosis is frequently already detectable at this young age [34]. *KCNJ1* mutations, encoding the ROMK potassium channel, often display transient hyperkalaemia in the neonatal period prior to development of classic hypokalaemia [32]. Early treatment to correct electrolyte disturbance, rehydrate patients and minimise growth retardation is necessitated [35]. Cyclo-oxygenase inhibitors (e.g., indomethacin), which target the elevated prostaglandin levels seen within aBS, are an effective treatment and can lead to effective catch-up growth [33,35].

Our understanding of Bartter syndrome II has recently expanded to include a late-onset phenotype following case reports of two adults found to have *KCNJ1* mutations after incidental nephrocalcinosis detection. Both patients had nephrocalcinosis and mild renal impairment at diagnosis, and were treated with oral potassium supplementation, and either a potassium-sparing diuretic or angiotensin-converting enzyme inhibitor respectively [33,35].

Bartter syndrome III occurs as a result of mutations in *CLCNKB* which encode the chloride channel ClC-Kb. The syndrome often has a milder phenotype with later-onset of symptoms, although presentations within the neonatal period have been reported [32]. Patients with Bartter III often have a more severe hypokalaemic alkalosis which is the most likely clinical clue to their underlying genotype [32]. Hypercalciuria and nephrocalcinosis are less frequently associated with the Bartter III phenotype compared to Bartter I and II [32].

Mutations in *BSND*, which encode Barttin (a chaperone protein for ClC-Ka and ClC-Kb) account for Bartter syndrome IV. Sensorineural deafness is part of the Bartter IV phenotype [36]. An association between Bartter syndrome IV and renal impairment has been reported. Patients frequently develop CKD at a very young age, and may not respond to indomethacin, in contrast to those with other aBS genotypes [36].

Although the term Bartter syndrome V is sometimes used in the literature to describe gain-of-function mutations in *CASR* encoding the calcium-sensing receptor (CaSR), according to OMIM classification Bartter syndrome V instead refers to mutations in the *MAGED2* gene, causing an X-linked recessively inherited transient antenatal BS [37]. To avoid this nomenclature issue, CaSR mutations are described separately in the section below.

2.6. CASR Mutations

The calcium-sensing receptor (CaSR), expressed in the parathyroid gland and kidney, responds to changes in serum calcium levels, acting to inhibit parathyroid hormone (PTH) secretion and renal tubular calcium reabsorption [38]. A total of 112 mutations of the *CASR* gene have been reported, of which 48 are gain-of-function mutations, including those associated with autosomal dominant hypocalcaemia (ADH)/autosomal dominant hypocalcemic hypercalciuria (ADHH) [38].

Patients with ADH exhibit a biochemical phenotype which includes serum hypocalcemia, low-normal levels of PTH, hypercalciuria, and polyuria [39]. It is essential to distinguish these patients from those with hypoparathyroidism: ADH patients given vitamin D supplementation are likely to develop worsening hypercalciuria, nephrocalcinosis and renal impairment as 1,25-dihydroxyvitamin D upregulates transcription of the *CASR* gene [40]. Instead, a low-normal serum PTH (in contrast to a very low or undetectable level) and low urinary calcium levels in a hypocalcemic patient should prompt clinicians to screen for *CASR* mutations [40]. Patients with ADH should receive treatment for their hypocalcemia only if it is symptomatic, and should aim for symptom control rather than normalised serum calcium levels [40]. Gain-of-function *CASR* mutations that inhibit activity of NKCC2 and ROMK channels in the thick ascending limb (TAL) of loop of Henle have been reported to produce a Bartter-like phenotype, which may include hypokalaemia and hyperreninemic hyperaldosteronism, in addition to hypocalcemia [41,42].

2.7. ADCY10 Mutations

Mutations in *ADCY10*, which encodes the soluble adenylyl cyclase gene, have been linked to familial idiopathic hypercalciuria, also known as Absorptive Hypercalciuria, 2 (HCA2) [43]. HCA2 displays autosomal dominant inheritance, with a phenotype including frequent calcium nephrolithiasis [44]. The underlying aetiology of the condition has not been fully delineated, but it is known increased intestinal calcium absorption is responsible for the hypercalciuria seen in these patients. Alongside the common clinical finding of calcium nephrolithiasis, increased renal calcium handling predisposes these patients to nephrocalcinosis formation [44].

2.8. Primary Distal Renal Tubular Acidosis

In distal renal tubular acidosis (dRTA), affected patients have a hyperchloremic normal anion-gap metabolic acidosis and alkaline urine (pH > 5.3) [10]. This characteristic biochemical profile arises as a consequence of type A intercalated cells in the collecting duct failing to acidify the urine [45].

Under normal physiological conditions, H^+ and HCO_3^- are produced within the type A intercalated cells. Mutations in either the vacuolar H^+-ATPase pump, which excretes H^+ into the urine, or the chloride bicarbonate counter transporter anion exchanger (AE1), which reabsorbs HCO_3^- into the circulation, account for 85% of known causes of primary dRTA [10]. Mutations in the B1 and A4 subunit of the vacuolar H^+-ATPase pump, encoded by *ATP6V1B1* and *ATP6V0A4* respectively, demonstrate autosomal recessive transmission and produce a phenotype frequently associated with sensorineural hearing loss as well as the commonly recognised biochemical abnormalities [45]. Mutations in *SLC4A1*, which encodes AE1, can occur with either autosomal dominant or autosomal recessive transmission: autosomal recessive cases are associated with earlier age of symptom onset and a more severe phenotype [10]. Red blood cell abnormalities may also form part of the phenotype for patients with *SLC4A1* mutations [45]. More recently, mutations in Forkhead box protein Il (encoded by *FOXI1)* and WD repeat-containing protein 72 (encoded by *WDR72)* have been recognised as alternative underlying genetic mutations in a small number of families with autosomal recessive inheritance of dRTA [46,47]. At present the underlying genetic defect remains unknown in approximately 15% of cases of primary dRTA [10].

Nephrocalcinosis is an extremely common feature within the phenotype of primary dRTA patients [48]. Calcium phosphate precipitates at higher pH; the alkaline urine of dRTA patients acts as a predisposing factor for nephrolithiasis and nephrocalcinosis formation [45]. In addition, chronic metabolic acidosis leads to excessive bone demineralisation often resulting in hypercalciuria: this also increases the likelihood of nephrocalcinosis developing if patients do not receive early diagnosis and treatment [48].

Treatment strategies for dRTA focus primarily on correcting the underlying metabolic acidosis; patients are maintained on oral potassium citrate which must be taken at regular intervals given its short half-life. This treatment may soon become less cumbersome for patients, as a controlled-release preparation of potassium bicarbonate and potassium citrate designed to be taken twice daily is undergoing phase three trials [10]. Primary distal renal tubular acidosis carries a good prognosis providing prompt diagnosis and treatment initiation are achieved. In patients on treatment with a corrected metabolic acidosis, it has been noted nephrocalcinosis does not progress and their renal function usually remains preserved [10]. However, potassium citrate treatment cannot reverse nephrocalcinosis if already present. Long-term follow-up of dRTA patients should include annual ultrasound screening to monitor for nephrocalcinosis and nephrolithiasis, as well as monitoring of their renal function [45].

2.9. Primary Hyperoxaluria

Primary hyperoxaluria describes a group of inborn errors of metabolism where defective liver enzymes involved in glyoxylate metabolism result in excess production of oxalate [49]. The predominant route of oxalate excretion is via the kidneys, with enteric excretion also playing a role when renal function is impaired [50]. In primary hyperoxaluria, excessive oxalate levels supersaturate renal excretion mechanisms, leading initially to calcium oxalate deposition within the kidney, and subsequently systemic oxalosis (deposition of oxalate within other systems) affecting the skeleton, heart, liver and other organs [49].

Currently there are three known types of primary hyperoxaluria which all display autosomal recessive inheritance. Reports of phenotypically similar cases with no proven monogenic cause increase the likelihood of further pathogenic mutations being discovered over time [49]. Recurrent calcium-oxalate nephrolithiasis and nephrocalcinosis are a central feature of primary hyperoxaluria phenotypes. Treatment options and renal prognosis vary considerably between the three genotypes however, making early genetic diagnosis imperative.

Primary hyperoxaluria type 1 (PH1) is the commonest form of primary hyperoxaluria and displays the most severe phenotype, with 50% of patients developing ESRD before the age of 25 [51]. Mutations in *AGXT*, which encode the hepatic alanine-glyoxylate aminotransferase (AGT) enzyme, result in an inability to break down glyoxylate into glycine. Instead, glyoxylate is converted to oxalate, leading to pathological hyperoxaluria [49]. Pyridoxine (vitamin B6) is a co-factor for AGT, and therefore offers a therapeutic target unique to PH1. An estimated 10–40% of PH1 patients respond to pyridoxine supplementation, which can delay progression to ESRF and allow consideration of isolated renal transplantation rather than simultaneous liver/kidney transplantation providing the patient is fully pyridoxine sensitive [51,52]. Early initiation of conservative measures such as high fluid intake and use of potassium citrate may reduce the incidence of nephrolithiasis and delay progression to ESRD [51]. However, due to the risk of systemic oxalosis, renal replacement therapy (RRT) must be initiated once plasma oxalate levels > 30–45 μmol/L, often resulting in patients commencing dialysis at much higher GFR levels than for other renal conditions [52].

PH1 is far more prevalent in developing countries (likely related to higher consanguinity rates) meaning access to liver transplantation is limited [51]. Even in countries where transplantation is more accessible, it carries significant risks for the patient [52]. The evolution of our treatment of this condition therefore hinges upon identifying therapeutic targets which do not necessitate organ transplantation to replace the defective enzyme. Trials utilising the oxalate-metabolising bacterium *Oxabacter formigenes* to increase gut excretion of oxalate and reduce urinary oxalate excretion reached phase II/III trials but did not significantly reduce urinary oxalate excretion [50]. Animal studies have shown oxalate decarboxylase enzymes can effectively reduce urinary oxalate levels, providing an alternative potential future therapy for reduction of calcium-oxalate nephrocalcinosis in primary hyperoxaluria [53,54].

Primary hyperoxaluria type 2 (PH2) occurs as a result of mutations in *GRHPR* which encodes the glyoxylate reductase/hydroxypyruvate reductase enzyme. PH2 exhibits a less severe phenotype, with lower incidence of nephrolithiasis and nephrocalcinosis. It is rare for PH2 patients to progress to ESRD or develop systemic oxalosis [51].

Primary hyperoxaluria type 3 (PH3) account for only 10% of PH patients [49]. Mutations in *HOGA1*, which encodes the hepatic enzyme 4-hydroxy-2-oxoglutarate aldolase, underlie the condition. PH3 has a milder phenotype, with lower nephrolithiasis burden, and nephrocalcinosis and renal impairment being less common

2.10. GDNF Mutations

Medullary sponge kidney (MSK) is a congenital disorder resulting in ectatic collecting ducts within one or both kidneys. The clinical sequelae of nephrolithiasis, nephrocalcinosis, recurrent urinary tract infections and urinary acidification defects are often not apparent until adulthood [55]. The underlying pathogenesis of MSK is yet to be fully elicited. Whilst once considered a sporadic disorder, evidence of MSK cases showing likely autosomal dominant inheritance have emerged, intensifying the search for underlying genetic causes [56]. Identification of mutations in *GDNF*, which encodes glial cell-derived neurotrophic factor, have now been identified in some MSK patients and may account for the underlying pathophysiological process in a subset of MSK patients [57].

3. Other Genetic Conditions That May Feature Nephrocalcinosis within Their Clinical Phenotype

Hypercalciuria acts as a predisposing factor for medullary nephrocalcinosis formation; any condition associated with excess urinary calcium excretion may lead to cases of nephrocalcinosis. Hypercalciuria and nephrocalcinosis have been described in association with the inherited conditions Wilson's disease, Williams-Beuren syndrome and cystic fibrosis.

Wilson's disease, a rare autosomal recessive condition characterised by *ATP7B* mutations leading to defective copper excretion, can feature a renal Fanconi syndrome [58,59]. In Wilson's disease patients exhibiting hypercalciuria, nephrolithiasis and nephrocalcinosis have been described [59].

Williams-Beuren syndrome is a developmental disorder occurring as a result of a microdeletion on the q arm of chromosome 7. The classical phenotype includes a distinctive facial appearance, intellectual disability and cardiovascular problems. However, patients with this syndrome have been found to be at increased risk of hypercalcaemia; the combination of resulting dehydration and hypercalciuria have led to cases of nephrocalcinosis being described [60].

Cystic fibrosis, caused by mutations in the *CFTR* gene, has been associated with hypercalciuria and microscopic nephrocalcinosis. However, the patients described did not demonstrate any signs of renal dysfunction associated with their microscopic nephrocalcinosis [61].

Amelogenesis Imperfecta describes a group of inherited enamel defects; there have been case reports of nephrocalcinosis detection in some of these patients in association with a distal renal tubular acidosis. However, in contrast to Wilson's disease, Williams-Beuren syndrome and cystic fibrosis, these patients have not demonstrated hypercalciuria, indicating different underlying pathophysiology [62].

4. Conclusions

Monogenic causes of nephrocalcinosis account for a rare set of conditions with a low population frequency. However, the clinical course for affected patients is very different depending on their underlying genotype. Accurate, prompt diagnosis allows early initiation of conservative measures, which in some cases can halt nephrocalcinosis or delay progression of renal impairment. Establishing the underlying genetic mutation also allows accurate prognostic information to be given and can help facilitate screening of other family members. As our understanding of these rare inherited conditions increases, it is hoped further treatment targets that address underlying enzymatic/protein defects will emerge. However, at present for the majority of cases treatment strategies focus upon supportive treatments to correct biochemical parameters, and careful monitoring of disease progression.

Appendix A

Table A1. Monogenic causes of nephrocalcinosis.

Gene	Encoded Protein	Site of Action	Clinical Condition	Inheritance	Phenotype
CLCN5	ClC-5 chloride transporter	Renal proximal tubule	Dent disease 1	X-linked recessive	Low molecular-weight (LMW) proteinuria, hypercalciuria, nephrocalcinosis/nephrolithiasis, progression to ESRD [1] by middle-age
OCRL	Inositol polyphosphate 5-phosphatase OCRL-1	Renal proximal tubule	Dent disease 2; Lowe oculocerebrorenal syndrome	X-linked recessive	Low molecular-weight (LMW) proteinuria, hypercalciuria, nephrocalcinosis/nephrolithiasis (less frequently than in Dent disease 1) Mild intellectual disability, cataracts Lowe oculocerebrorenal syndrome: more severe phenotype including ocular abnormalities, intellectual disability, amino aciduria, renal dysfunction, vitamin-D resistant rickets
CYP24A1	1,25-hydroxyvitamin-D_3-24-hydroxylase	Kidney	Hypercalcemia, Infantile, 1: HCINF1 2	AR [3]	Hypercalcemia, hypercalciuria, high 1,25-dihydroxyvitamin D_3 (a) Early presentation with vomiting, dehydration, failure to thrive, nephrocalcinosis (b) Adult presentation with nephrocalcinosis, nephrolithiasis
SLC34A1	Sodium-phosphate co-transporter NaPi2a	Renal proximal tubule	Hypercalcemia, Infantile 2: HCINF2 [4]	AR	Hypercalcemia, hypercalciuria, high 1,25-dihydroxyvitamin D_3, hypophosphatemia, vomiting, dehydration, failure to thrive, nephrocalcinosis
CLDN16	Tight junction protein claudin-16	Thick ascending limb (TAL)	FHHNC [5]	AR	Hypomagnesaemia, high urinary Mg^{2+}/Ca^{2+}, polyuria/polydipsia, failure to thrive, nephrocalcinosis, progression to ESRD in adolescence
CLDN19	Tight junction protein claudin-19	Thick ascending limb (TAL)	FHHNC with severe ocular involvement	AR	Hypomagnesaemia, high urinary Mg^{2+}/Ca^{2+}, polyuria/polydipsia, failure to thrive, nephrocalcinosis, progression to ESRD in adolescence severe ocular abnormalities
SLC12A1	Sodium-potassium-chloride cotransporter NKCC2	Thick ascending limb (TAL)	Bartter syndrome Type 1, Antenatal (BARTS1)	AR	Antenatal/neonatal presentation with polyhydramnios, premature birth and low-birth weight, nephrocalcinosis, hypokalaemia, metabolic alkalosis, secondary hypoaldosteronism

Table A1. *Cont.*

Gene	Encoded Protein	Site of Action	Clinical Condition	Inheritance	Phenotype
KCNJ1	ROMK potassium channel	Thick ascending limb (TAL)	Bartter syndrome Type 2, Antenatal (BARTS2)	AR	Often antenatal/neonatal presentation with polyhydramnios, premature birth and low-birth weight, nephrocalcinosis, hypokalaemia, metabolic alkalosis, secondary hypoaldosteronismFew reports of later-onset (adult) presentation with nephrocalcinosis and CKD [6]
CLCNKB	Chloride channel ClC-Kb	Thick ascending limb (TAL)	Bartter syndrome, Type 3 (BARTS3)	AR	Severe hypokalaemic metabolic alkalosis, secondary hypoaldosteronism Usually later symptom-onset but few cases of neonatal onset
BSND	Barttin, chaperone protein for ClC-Ka and ClC-Kb	Thick ascending limb (TAL)	Bartter syndrome, Type 4: BSND [7]	AR	Severe hypokalaemic metabolic alkalosis, secondary hypoaldosteronism, sensorineural deafness, development of CKD in childhood
CASR	Gain-of-function mutation in Calcium-sensing receptor (CaSR)	Thick ascending limb (TAL), parathyroid gland	Hypocalcemia, autosomal dominant 1 (HYPOC1)	AD [8]	Serum hypocalcaemia, low serum PTH, hypercalciuria, nephrocalcinosis
ADCY10	Soluble Adenylate cyclase 10	Increased intestinal calcium reabsorption	Familial idiopathic hypercalciuria	AD	Hypercalciuria, calcium nephrolithiasis, nephrocalcinosis
ATP6V1B1	B1 subunit vacuolar H+-ATPase pump	Collecting duct	distal RTA [9] with deafness	AR	Hyperchloremic normal anion-gap metabolic acidosis, alkaline urine sensorineural deafness, nephrocalcinosis Good renal prognosis once on treatment
ATP6V0A4	A4 subunit vacuolar H+-ATPase pump	Collecting duct	distal RTA	AR	Hyperchloremic normal anion-gap metabolic acidosis, alkaline urine, sensorineural deafness, nephrocalcinosis Good renal prognosis once on treatment
SLC4A1	AE1	Collecting duct	distal RTA	AD or AR	Hyperchloremic normal anion-gap metabolic acidosis, alkaline urine nephrocalcinosis, red blood cell abnormalities Good renal prognosis once on treatment
FOXI1	Forkhead box protein I1	Collecting duct	distal RTA	AR	Hyperchloremic normal anion-gap metabolic acidosis, alkaline urine, nephrocalcinosis. Good renal prognosis once on treatment
WDR72	WD repeat-containing protein 72	Collecting duct	distal RTA	AR	Hyperchloremic normal anion-gap metabolic acidosis, alkaline urine nephrocalcinosis. Good renal prognosis once on treatment

Table A1. *Cont.*

Gene	Encoded Protein	Site of Action	Clinical Condition	Inheritance	Phenotype
AGXT	Alanine-glyoxylate aminotransferase	Hepatic peroxisomes	Hyperoxaluria, primary, type 1	AR	Early onset recurrent calcium oxalate nephrolithiasis, nephrocalcinosis Frequent progression to ESRD Systemic oxalosis affecting multiple organs including kidney, bones, heart, liver
GRHPR	Glyoxylate reductase/hydroxypyruvate reductase	Liver, leucocytes, kidney	Hyperoxaluria, primary, type 2	AR	Recurrent nephrolithiasis, nephrocalcinosis Milder phenotype than PH1, only some patients progress to ESRD
HOGA1	4-hydroxy-2-oxoglutarate aldolase	Liver	Hyperoxaluria, primary, type 3	AR	Nephrolithiasis ± rarely nephrocalcinosis, renal impairment rare
GDNF	Glial cell-derived neurotrophic factor	Kidney	Medullary sponge kidney	Sporadic or AD	Nephrolithiasis, nephrocalcinosis, recurrent urinary tract infection, urinary acidification defects

[1] ESRD = End stage renal disease, [2] HCINF1 = Hypercalcemia, idiopathic, of infancy type 1, [3] AR = Autosomal Recessive, [4] HCINF2 = Hypercalcaemia, idiopathic, of infancy type 2, [5] FHHNC = Familial hypomagnesaemia with hypercalciuria and nephrocalcinosis, [6] CKD = Chronic kidney disease, [7] BSND = Bartter Syndrome, Neonatal, with Sensorineural Deafness, [8] AD = Autosomal Dominant, [9] Distal RTA = distal renal tubular acidosis.

References

1. Shavit, L.; Jaeger, P.; Unwin, R.J. What is nephrocalcinosis? *Kidney Int.* **2019**, *88*, 35–43. [CrossRef]

2. Oliveira, B.; Kleta, R.; Bockenhauer, D.; Walsh, S.B. Genetic, pathophysiological, and clinical aspects of nephrocalcinosis. *Am. J. Physiol.* **2016**, *311*, F1243–F1252. [CrossRef] [PubMed]

3. Barratt, J.; Harris, K.; Topham, P. *Oxford Desk Reference Nephrology*; Oxford University Press: New York, NY, USA, 2008; pp. 278–279.

4. Glazer, G.M.; Callen, P.W.; Filly, R.A. Medullary nephrocalcinosis: Sonographic evaluation. *Am. J. Roentgenol.* **1982**, *138*, 55–57. [CrossRef] [PubMed]

5. Dick, P.T.; Shuckett, B.M.; Tang, B.; Daneman, A.; Kooh, S.W. Observer reliability in grading nephrocalcinosis on ultrasound examinations in children. *Pediatr. Radiol.* **1999**, *29*, 68–72. [CrossRef] [PubMed]

6. Moor, M.B.; Bonny, O. Ways of calcium reabsorption in the kidney. *Am. J. Physiol.* **2016**, *310*, F1337–F1350. [CrossRef] [PubMed]

7. Daga, A.; Majmundar, A.J.; Braun, D.A.; Gee, H.Y.; Lawson, J.A.; Shril, S.; Jobst-Schwan, T.; Vivante, A.; Schapiro, D.; Tan, W.; et al. Whole exome sequencing frequently detects a monogenic cause in early onset nephrolithiasis and nephrocalcinosis. *Kidney Int.* **2018**, *93*, 204–213. [CrossRef]

8. Weigert, A.; Hoppe, B. Nephrolithiasis and nephrocalcinosis in childhood- risk factor related current and future treatment options. *Front. Pediatr.* **2018**, *6*, 98. [CrossRef]

9. He, G.; Zhang, H.; Cao, S.; Xiao, H.; Yao, Y. Dent's disease complicated by nephrotic syndrome: A case report. *Intractable Rare Dis. Res.* **2016**, *5*, 297–300. [CrossRef]

10. Alexander, R.; Law, L.; Gil-Pena, H.; Greenbaum, L.; Santos, F. Hereditary distal tubular acidosis. In *GeneReviews, 2019*; Adam, M., Ardinger, H., Pagon, R., Wallace, S., Bean, L., Stephens, K., Amemiya, A., Eds.; University of Washington: Seattle, WA, USA, 2019. Available online: https://www.ncbi.nlm.nih.gov/pubmed/31600044/ (accessed on 24 November 2019).

11. Wen, M.; Shen, T.; Wang, Y.; Li, Y.; Shi, X.; Dang, X. Next-Generation Sequencing in Early Diagnosis of Dent Disease 1: Two Case Reports. *Front. Med.* **2018**, *5*, 347. [CrossRef]

12. Lieske, J.C.; Milliner, D.S.; Beara-Lasic, L.; Harris, P.; Cogal, A.; Abrash, E. Dent Disease. In *GeneReviews, 2017*; Adam, M., Ardinger, H., Pagon, R., Wallace, S., Bean, L., Stephens, K., Amemiya, A., Eds.; University of Washington: Seattle, WA, USA, 2019. Available online: https://www.ncbi.nlm.nih.gov/books/NBK99494/ (accessed on 20 November 2019).

13. Hodgin, J.B.; Corey, H.E.; Kaplan, B.S.; D'Agati, V.D. Dent disease presenting as partial Fanconi syndrome and hypercalciuria. *Kidney Int.* **2008**, *73*, 1320–1323. [CrossRef]

14. Bökenkamp, A.; Ludwig, M. The oculocerebrorenal syndrome of Lowe: An update. *Pediatr. Nephrol.* **2016**, *31*, 2201–2212. [CrossRef]

15. Elmonem, M.A.; Veys, K.R.; Soliman, N.A.; van Dyck, M.; van den Heuvel, L.P.; Levtchenko, E. Cystinosis: A review. *Orphanet J. Rare Dis.* **2016**, *11*, 47. [PubMed]

16. Anglani, F.; D'Angelo, A.; Bertizzolo, L.M.; Tosetto, E.; Ceol, M.; Cremasco, D.; Bonfante, L.; Addis, M.A.; Del Prete, D. Nephrolithiasis, kidney failure and bone disorders in Dent disease patients with and without CLCN5 mutations. *Springerplus* **2015**, *4*, 492. [CrossRef] [PubMed]

17. Anglani, F.; Gianesello, L.; Beara-Lasic, L.; Lieske, J. Dent disease: A window into calcium and phosphate transport. *J. Cell. Mol. Med.* **2019**, *23*, 7132–7142. [CrossRef] [PubMed]

18. Blanchard, A.; Curis, E.; Guyon-Roger, T.; Kahila, D.; Treard, C.; Baudouin, V.; Bérard, E.; Champion, G.; Cochat, P.; Dubourg, J.; et al. Observations of a large Dent disease cohort. *Kidney Int.* **2016**, *90*, 430–439. [CrossRef]

19. Hill, F.; Sayer, J.A. Clinical and biochemical features of patients with CYP24A1 mutations. In *A Critical Evaluation of Vitamin D*, 1st ed.; Gowder, S., Ed.; IntechOpen: London, UK, 2017; pp. 91–101. [CrossRef]

20. British Paediatric Association. Hypercalcemia in infants and vitamin D. *Br. Med. J.* **1956**, *2*, 149. [CrossRef]

21. Schlingmann, K.P.; Kaufmann, M.; Weber, S.; Irwin, A.; Goos, C.; John, U.; Misselwitz, J.; Klaus, G.; Kuwertz-Bröking, E.; Fehrenbach, H.; et al. Mutations in CYP24A1 and Idiopathic Infantile Hypercalcemia. *N. Engl. J. Med.* **2011**, *365*, 410–421. [CrossRef]

22. Dganit, D.; Pazit, B.; Liat, G.; Karen, T.; Zemach, E.; Holtzman, E.J. Loss-of-Function Mutations of CYP24A1, the Vitamin D 24-Hydroxylase Gene, Cause Long-standing Hypercalciuric Nephrolithiasis and Nephrocalcinosis. *J. Urol.* **2013**, *190*, 552–557.

23. Sayers, J.; Hynes, A.M.; Srivastava, S.; Dowen, F.; Quinton, R.; Datta, H.K.; Sayer, J.A. Successful treatment of hypercalcaemia associated with a CYP24A1 mutation with fluconazole. *Clin. Kidney J.* **2018**, *8*, 453–455. [CrossRef]

24. Hawkes, C.P.; Li, D.; Hakonarson, H.; Meyers, K.E.; Thummel, K.E.; Levine, M.A. CYP3A4 Induction by Rifampin: An Alternative Pathway for Vitamin D Inactivation in Patients With CYP24A1 Mutations. *J. Clin. Endocrinol. Metab.* **2017**, *102*, 1440–1446. [CrossRef]

25. Schlingmann, K.P.; Ruminska, J.; Kaufmann, M.; Dursun, I.; Patti, M.; Kranz, B.; Pronicka, E.; Ciara, E.; Akcay, T.; Bulus, D.; et al. Autosomal-Recessive Mutations in SLC34A1 Encoding Sodium-Phosphate Cotransporter 2A Cause Idiopathic Infantile Hypercalcemia. *J. Am. Soc. Nephrol.* **2016**, *27*, 604–614. [CrossRef] [PubMed]

26. De Paolis, E.; Scaglione, G.; De Bonis, M.; Minucci, A.; Capoluongo, E. CYP24A1 and SLC34A1 genetic defects associated with idiopathic infantile hypercalcemia: From genotype to phenotype. *Clin. Chem. Lab. Med.* **2019**, *57*, 1650. [CrossRef]

27. Kang, S.J.; Lee, R.; Kim, H.S. Infantile hypercalcemia with novel compound heterozygous mutation in SLC34A1 encoding renal sodium-phosphate cotransporter 2a: A case report. *Ann. Pediatr. Endocrinol. Metab.* **2019**, *24*, 64–67. [CrossRef]

28. Claverie-Martin, F. Familial hypomagnesaemia with hypercalciuria and nephrocalcinosis: Clinical and molecular characteristics. *Clin. Kidney J.* **2015**, *8*, 656–664. [CrossRef] [PubMed]

29. Viering, D.H.H.M.; de Baaij, J.H.F.; Walsh, S.B.; Kleta, R.; Bockenhauer, D. Genetic causes of hypomagnesemia, a clinical overview. *Pediatr. Nephrol.* **2017**, *32*, 1123–1135. [CrossRef] [PubMed]

30. Sikora, P.; Zaniew, M.; Haisch, L.; Pulcer, B.; Szczepańska, M.; Moczulska, A.; Rogowska-Kalisz, A.; Bieniaś, B.; Tkaczyk, M.; Ostalska-Nowicka, D.; et al. Retrospective cohort study of familial hypomagnesaemia with hypercalciuria and nephrocalcinosis due to CLDN16 mutations. *Nephrol. Dial. Transplant.* **2014**, *30*, 636–644. [CrossRef]

31. Vianna, J.G.P.; Simor, T.G.; Senna, P.; De Bortoli, M.R.; Costalonga, E.F.; Seguro, A.C.; Luchi, W.M. Atypical presentation of familial hypomagnesemia with hypercalciuria and nephrocalcinosis in a patient with a new claudin-16 gene mutation. *Clin. Nephrol. Case Stud.* **2019**, *7*, 27–34. [CrossRef]

32. Brochard, K.; Boyer, O.; Blanchard, A.; Loirat, C.; Niaudet, P.; Macher, M.A.; Deschenes, G.; Bensman, A.; Decramer, S.; Cochat, P.; et al. Phenotype-genotype correlation in antenatal and neonatal variants of Bartter syndrome. *Nephrol. Dial. Transplant.* **2008**, *24*, 1455–1464. [CrossRef]

33. Gollasch, B.; Anistan, Y.M.; Canaan-Kühl, S.; Gollasch, M. Late-onset Bartter syndrome type II. *Clin. Kidney J.* **2017**, *10*, 594–599. [CrossRef]

34. Walsh, P.R.; Tse, Y.; Ashton, E.; Iancu, D.; Jenkins, L.; Bienias, M.; Kleta, R.; van't Hoff, W.; Bockenhauer, D. Clinical and diagnostic features of Bartter and Gitelman syndromes. *Clin. Kidney J.* **2017**, *11*, 302–309. [CrossRef]

35. Huang, L.; Luiken, G.P.M.; van Riemsdijk, I.C.; Petrij, F.; Zandbergen, A.A.M.; Dees, A. Nephrocalcinosis as adult presentation of Bartter syndrome type II. *Neth. J. Med.* **2014**, *72*, 91–93. [PubMed]

36. Jeck, N.; Reinalter, S.C.; Henne, T.; Marg, W.; Mallmann, R.; Pasel, K.; Vollmer, M.; Klaus, G.; Leonhardt, A.; Seyberth, H.W.; et al. Hypokalemic Salt-Losing Tubulopathy With Chronic Renal Failure and Sensorineural Deafness. *Pediatrics* **2001**, *108*, e5. [CrossRef] [PubMed]

37. Online Mendelian Inheritance in Man, OMIM. OMIM Entry-#300971. Available online: https://www.omin.org/entry/300971#editHistory (accessed on 29 December 2019).

38. Pidasheva, S.; D'Souza-Li, L.; Canaff, L.; Cole, D.E.C.; Hendy, G.N. CASRdb: Calcium-sensing receptor locus-specific database for mutations causing familial (benign) hypocalciuric hypercalcemia, neonatal severe hyperparathyroidism, and autosomal dominant hypocalcemia. *Hum. Mutat.* **2004**, *24*, 107–111. [CrossRef] [PubMed]

39. Vargas-Poussou, R.; Huang, C.; Hulin, P.; Houillier, P.; Jeunemaître, X.; Paillard, M.; Planelles, G.; Déchaux, M.; Miller, R.T.; Antignac, C. Functional Characterization of a Calcium-Sensing Receptor Mutation in Severe Autosomal Dominant Hypocalcemia with a Bartter-Like Syndrome. *J. Am. Soc. Nephrol.* **2002**, *13*, 2259–2266. [CrossRef] [PubMed]

40. Pearce, S.H.S.; Williamson, C.; Kifor, O.; Bai, M.; Coulthard, M.G.; Davies, M.; Lewis-Barned, N.; McCredie, D.; Powell, H.; Kendall-Taylor, P.; et al. A Familial Syndrome of Hypocalcemia with Hypercalciuria Due to Mutations in the Calcium-Sensing Receptor. *N. Engl. J. Med.* **1996**, *335*, 1115–1122. [CrossRef]

41. Vezzoli, G.; Arcidiacono, T.; Paloschi, V.; Terranegra, A.; Biasion, R.; Weber, G.; Mora, S.; Syren, M.L.; Coviello, D.; Cusi, D.; et al. Autosomal dominant hypocalcemia with mild type 5 Bartter syndrome. *J. Nephrol.* **2006**, *19*, 525–528.

42. Hannan, F.M.; Thakker, R.V. Calcium-sensing receptor (CaSR) mutations and disorders of calcium, electrolyte and water metabolism. *Best Pract. Res. Clin. Endocrinol. Metab.* **2013**, *27*, 359–371. [CrossRef]

43. Online Mendelian Inheritance in Man, OMIM. OMIM Entry-#143870. Available online: https://www.omim. org/entry/143870#8 (accessed on 29 December 2019).

44. Reed, B.Y.; Heller, H.J.; Gitomer, W.L.; Pak, C.Y.C. Mapping a Gene Defect in Absorptive Hypercalciuria to Chromosome 1q23.3–q241. *J. Clin. Endocrinol. Metab.* **1999**, *84*, 3907–3913. [CrossRef]

45. Watanabe, T. Improving outcomes for patients with distal renal tubular acidosis: Recent advances and challenges ahead. *Pediatr Heal Med Ther.* **2018**, *9*, 181–190. [CrossRef]

46. Enerbäck, S.; Nilsson, D.; Edwards, N.; Heglind, M.; Alkanderi, S.; Ashton, E.; Deeb, A.; Kokash, F.E.; Bakhsh, A.R.; van't Hoff, W.; et al. Acidosis and Deafness in Patients with Recessive Mutations in FOXI1. *J. Am. Soc. Nephrol.* **2018**, *29*, 1041–1048. [CrossRef]

47. Rungroj, N.; Nettuwakul, C.; Sawasdee, N.; Sangnual, S.; Deejai, N.; Misgar, R.A.; Pasena, A.; Khositseth, S.; Kirdpon, S.; Sritippayawan, S.; et al. Distal renal tubular acidosis caused by tryptophan-aspartate repeat domain 72 (WDR72) mutations. *Clin. Genet.* **2018**, *94*, 409–418. [CrossRef] [PubMed]

48. Park, E.; Cho, M.H.; Hyun, H.S.; Shin, J.I.; Lee, J.H.; Park, Y.S.; Choi, H.J.; Kang, H.G.; Cheong, H.I. Genotype-Phenotype Analysis in Pediatric Patients with Distal Renal Tubular Acidosis. *Kidney Blood Press. Res.* **2018**, *43*, 513–521. [CrossRef] [PubMed]

49. Strauss, S.B.; Waltuch, T.; Bivin, W.; Kaskel, F.; Levin, T.L. Primary hyperoxaluria: Spectrum of clinical and imaging findings. *Pediatr. Radiol.* **2017**, *47*, 96–103. [CrossRef] [PubMed]

50. Milliner, D.; Hoppe, B.; Groothoff, J. A randomised Phase II/III study to evaluate the efficacy and safety of orally administered Oxalobacter formigenes to treat primary hyperoxaluria. *Urolithiasis* **2018**, *46*, 313–323. [CrossRef]

51. Cochat, P.; Basmaison, O. Current approaches to the management of primary hyperoxaluria. *Arch. Dis. Child.* **2000**, *82*, 470–473. [CrossRef]

52. Sas, D.J.; Harris, P.C.; Milliner, D.S. Recent advances in the identification and management of inherited hyperoxalurias. *Urolithiasis* **2019**, *47*, 79–89. [CrossRef]

53. Grujic, D.; Salido, E.C.; Shenoy, B.C.; Langman, C.B.; McGrath, M.E.; Patel, R.J.; Rashid, A.; Mandapati, S.; Jung, C.W.; Margolin, A.L. Hyperoxaluria Is Reduced and Nephrocalcinosis Prevented with an Oxalate-Degrading Enzyme in Mice with Hyperoxaluria. *Am. J. Nephrol.* **2009**, *29*, 86–93. [CrossRef]

54. Matthew, L.; Victoria, B.; Meekah, C.; Ming, Y.; Qing-Shan, L.; Haifeng, L. MP03-06 Oxalate decarboxylase enzyme reduces hyperoxaluria in an animal model that mimics primary hyperoxaluria. *J. Urol.* **2019**, *201*, e22.

55. National Kidney Foundation. Medullary Sponge Kidney. Available online: https://www.kidney.org/atoz/ content/medullary-sponge-kidney (accessed on 29 December 2019).

56. Fabris, A.; Anglani, F.; Lupo, A.; Gambaro, G. Medullary sponge kidney: State of the art. *Nephrol. Dial. Transplant.* **2012**, *28*, 1111–1119. [CrossRef]

57. Torregrossa, R.; Anglani, F.; Fabris, A.; Gozzini, A.; Tanini, A.; Del Prete, D.; Cristofaro, R.; Artifoni, L.; Abaterusso, C.; Marchionna, N.; et al. Identification of GDNF gene sequence variations in patients with medullary sponge kidney disease. *Clin. J. Am. Soc. Nephrol.* **2010**, *5*, 1205–1210. [CrossRef]

58. Azizi, E.; Eshel, G.; Aladjem, M. Hypercalciuria and nephrolithiasis as a presenting sign in Wilson disease. *Eur. J. Pediatr.* **1989**, *148*, 548–549. [CrossRef] [PubMed]

59. Di Stefano, V.; Lionetti, E.; Rotolo, N.; La Rosa, M.; Leonardi, S. Hypercalciuria and nephrocalcinosis as early feature of Wilson disease onset: Description of a pediatric case and literature review. *Hepat. Mon.* **2012**, *12*, e6233. [CrossRef] [PubMed]

60. Sindhar, S.; Lugo, M.; Levin, M.D.; Danback, J.R.; Brink, B.D.; Yu, E.; Dietzen, D.J.; Clark, A.L.; Purgert, C.A.; Waxler, J.L.; et al. Hypercalcemia in Patients with Williams-Beuren Syndrome. *J. Pediatr.* **2016**, *178*, 254–260. [CrossRef]

61. Katz, S.M.; Krueger, L.J.; Falkner, B. Microscopic Nephrocalcinosis in Cystic Fibrosis. *N. Engl. J. Med.* **1988**, *319*, 263–266. [CrossRef]

62. Elizabeth, J.; Lakshmi Priya, E.; Umadevi, K.M.R.; Ranganathan, K. Amelogenesis imperfecta with renal disease—A report of two cases. *J. Oral Pathol. Med.* **2007**, *36*, 625–628. [CrossRef] [PubMed]

14

The Incidence of Chronic Kidney Disease Three Years after Non-Severe Acute Kidney Injury in Critically Ill Patients

Sébastien Rubin [1,*]**, Arthur Orieux** [1]**, Benjamin Clouzeau** [2]**, Claire Rigothier** [1]**, Christian Combe** [1]**, Didier Gruson** [2] **and Alexandre Boyer** [2]

[1] Service de Néphrologie, Transplantation, Dialyse, Aphérèses, Hôpital Pellegrin, Centre Hospitalier Universitaire de Bordeaux, 33076 Bordeaux CEDEX, France; arthur.orieux@chu-bordeaux.fr (A.O.); claire.rigothier@chu-bordeaux.fr (C.R.); christian.combe@chu-bordeaux.fr (C.C.)

[2] Service de Médecine Intensive Réanimation, Hôpital Pellegrin, Centre Hospitalier Universitaire de Bordeaux, 33076 Bordeaux Cedex, France; benjamin.clouzeau@chu-bordeaux.fr (B.C.); didier.gruson@chu-bordeaux.fr (D.G.); alexandre.boyer@chu-bordeaux.fr (A.B.)

* Correspondence: sebastien.rubin@chu-bordeaux.fr

Abstract: The risk of chronic kidney disease (CKD) following severe acute kidney injury (AKI) in critically ill patients is well documented, but not after less severe AKI. The main objective of this study was to evaluate the long-term incidence of CKD after non-severe AKI in critically ill patients. This prospective single-center observational three-years follow-up study was conducted in the medical intensive care unit in Bordeaux's hospital (France). From 2013 to 2015, all patients with severe (kidney disease improving global outcomes (KDIGO) stage 3) and non-severe AKI (KDIGO stages 1, 2) were enrolled. Patients with prior eGFR < 90 mL/min/1.73 m^2 were excluded. Primary outcome was the three-year incidence of CKD stages 3 to 5 in the non-severe AKI group. We enrolled 232 patients. Non-severe AKI was observed in 112 and severe AKI in 120. In the non-severe AKI group, 71 (63%) were male, age was 62 ± 16 years. The reason for admission was sepsis for 56/112 (50%). Sixty-two (55%) patients died and nine (8%) were lost to follow-up. At the end of the follow-up the incidence of CKD was 22% (9/41); Confidence Interval (CI) $_{95\%}$ (9.3–33.60)% in the non-severe AKI group, tending to be significantly lower than in the severe AKI group (44% (14/30); CI $_{95\%}$ (28.8–64.5)%; $p = 0.052$). The development of CKD three years after non-severe AKI, despite it being lower than after severe AKI, appears to be a frequent event highlighting the need for prolonged follow-up.

Keywords: acute kidney injury; critically ill patients; renal recovery; chronic kidney disease; end stage renal disease

1. Introduction

Acute kidney injury (AKI) is very common in Intensive Care Unit (ICU) patients since it is estimated to develop in up to 50% of them [1]. The short-term implications have been studied extensively and include an increase in mortality [2], hospitalization length, rehospitalizations [3], and impaired quality of life [4]. The long-term implications in critically-ill patients are still not well known, except for severe AKI (defined most of the time by AKI-requiring renal replacement therapy (RRT)). In that category of patients, Schiffl et al. (2008) found that five years after RRT, 14% of them developed chronic kidney disease (CKD) [5]. Gammelager et al. (2013) demonstrated that among surviving patients requiring RRT, the incidence of end-stage renal disease (ESRD) at five years was 4% [6].

To date, non-severe AKI outcomes were predominantly studied in non-critically ill patients, using large administrative data sets [7], e.g., veterans' health administration data [8]. These analyses are known to have low sensibility [9] and to underestimate the less severe form of AKI [10]. Another big cohort including non-severe AKI in non-critically ill patients is the 5-year prospective case-control 'AKI Risk in Derby' study. Patients were divided into two groups according to the kidney disease improving global outcomes (KDIGO) classification (severe AKI corresponding to KDIGO 3 and non-severe AKI corresponding to KDIGO 1 or 2) [11]. Preliminary results after a 12-month follow-up showed that patients with severe AKI had worse kidney function than patients with non-severe AKI, but kidney function declined in both groups compared to control patients [12]. These studies did not enroll many critically ill patients who typically present with a different spectrum of AKI etiologies [13]. These patients are often exposed to multiple nephrotoxic agents (antibiotics, iodine contrast products, etc.), severe hemodynamic variations, and inflammatory state ("sepsis"), each being able to worsen the long-term renal prognosis.

To date, it is difficult to determine the real risk of developing CKD in critically ill patients with non-severe AKI. The incidence of CKD many years after a non-severe AKI in ICU could be thus underestimated. The main objective of this study was to evaluate the long-term incidence of CKD after non-severe AKI in critically ill patients. This would be the first study to address this issue. Secondary objectives were to compare CKD incidence after non-severe vs. severe AKI episodes, to evaluate risk factors for developing CKD, and to identify the proportion among CKD patients followed by a nephrologist.

2. Materials and Methods

2.1. Study Design

This prospective three-year follow-up observational study was carried out in Bordeaux, France, from September 2013 to May 2015. Our center participated in the artificial kidney initiation in kidney injury (AKIKI) study [14], during which all patients with AKI from stage 1 of the KDIGO classification were prospectively and carefully screened. Data were collected during the period of hospitalization. After discharge, the follow-up was carried out three years after enrollment. A direct contact with the general practitioner (GP) and/or the patient was achieved. According to French law, the database was declared to the French data protection authority (declaration number 2168624). The study obtained the approval of the ethics commission of the French society of intensive care medicine and was assigned as CE SRLF 18-20.

2.2. Participants

Patients were enrolled if they were 18 years of age or older, received invasive mechanical ventilation, catecholamine infusion, or both, and developed AKI assessed by an increase of serum creatinine (SCr) of >26.5 μmol/L within 48 h or an increase of >1.5 times the baseline value, according to KDIGO guidelines [11]. Patients with an estimated glomerular filtration rate (eGFR) < 90 mL/min/1.73 m^2 prior to ICU admission, using the chronic kidney disease epidemiology collaboration (CKD-EPI) formula, were excluded. Serum creatinine assays were standardized (IDMS calibration). Enrollment and collection of hospitalization data were recorded prospectively. Follow-up outcomes were collected prospectively three years after enrollment for each patient, in order to limit memorization bias or loss of data, using medical records and phone calls with GPs and patients.

2.3. Acute Kidney Injury Classification

The KDIGO staging of AKI was used to define non-severe AKI (AKI stages 1 and 2) and severe AKI (AKI stage 3) [11]. Only SCr was considered because of inconsistent urine output data. Baseline SCr were SCr at admission in the case of normal renal function or SCr less than 1 year in the case of abnormal SCr at admission. All baseline SCr were obtained by previous blood tests.

2.4. Exposure Variables

Information relative to smoker status, past medical history of hypertension, diabetes, chronic heart failure, ischemic heart disease (IHD), stroke, peripheral arterial disease (PAD), prior CKD, reason of admission, simplified acute physiology score II (SAPS II), length of hospitalization, catecholamine, aminoglycoside, contrast agent use, or death were collected using prospectively recorded data and patient questioning if applicable.

Because some patients were treated both with continuous veno-venous hemodialysis (CVVHD) and intermittent hemodialysis (IHD), we only recorded the first RRT modality that was used during the ICU stay.

2.5. Long-Term Incidence of CKD at Three Years

We defined CKD as eGFR <60 mL/min/1.73 m^2, using the chronic kidney disease epidemiology collaboration (CKD-EPI) corresponding to CKD stage 3 or more according to the KDIGO classification. Creatinine level were collected by family calls or GP calls. In the case of abnormal creatinine level, absence of AKI was checked using an anteriority blood test.

2.6. Other Outcomes

Recovery from AKI was determined at ICU discharge. It was defined as a return of SCr to <26.5 μmol/L (<0.3 mg/dL) above baseline for alive and non-dependent RRT patients. These data were collected using hospital records or using data from blood tests performed outside the hospital, with prior consent of the patient. We called CKD patients to ask if they were followed by a nephrologist. The survival state and date of death if applicable were collected using hospital records, GP, and family phone calls.

2.7. Statistical Analysis

Statistical analysis was carried out using JMP® Version 14, SAS Institute Inc., Cary, NC, USA, 1989–2007. Descriptive statistics included mean ± standard deviation (SD) or median (Quartile 1-Quartile 3). Quantitative variables were compared using a t-test, and qualitative variables using Chi^2 Pearson test. The multivariate analysis was carried out using logistic regression. To choose independent variables included in the model, we allowed one independent variable for every 20 patients analyzed. Interactions between independent variables were checked using the Pearson correlation test for quantitative variables and the Chi^2 test for ordinal or binomial variables using Yates' correction if the sample size was <10. Quantitative variables were stratified into a range when a constant magnitude of association was not consistent. Renal survival was studied using the Kaplan–Meier curve. Survival curves were compared using a log-rank test. A value of $p < 0.05$ was considered statistically significant (double-sided).

3. Results

3.1. Participants

From 2013–2015, 304 patients with AKI were admitted to the ICU (Figure 1). Among them, 72 had prior CKD and were excluded and 232 patients were enrolled. No patients had missing baseline creatinine value. Non-severe AKI was present in 112 (AKI stage 1, 62; stage 2, 50) and severe AKI in 120 (AKI stage 3). In the non-severe AKI group, 71/112 (63%) were male with a mean age of 62 ± 16 years. In 56/112 (50%), the reason for admission was sepsis, 89/112 (79%) required catecholamines, and 92/112 (79%) were intubated. The simplified acute physiology score II (SAPS II) was 59 ± 17. The duration of hospitalization was 9 ± 10 days. All descriptive characteristics and the comparison between non-severe AKI vs. severe AKI are presented in Table 1. In severe AKI, patients had a higher SAPS II (65 ± 20 vs. 59 ± 17; $p = 0.01$). The ICU mortality rate was also higher in the severe patients group (57/120 (48%) vs. 34/112 (30%); $p = 0.01$). Renal replacement therapy was performed in 73/120 (61%) of patients with severe AKI, and CVVHD was used in 57/73 (78%) of these patients. One hundred and seven patients died in hospital (40 in the non-severe group and 67 in the severe group). Cause of death was multiple organ failure (35 patients), withholding or withdrawing of life-prolonging therapy (16), neurologic disorder (15), septic shock (11), acute respiratory distress syndrome (10), hemorrhagic shock (3), cardiac arrest (4), or others (13). Among the 78/112 (69%) patients with non-severe AKI who survived at ICU discharge, renal recovery was observed in 68/78 (87%) patients compared to 22/63 (35%) patients with severe AKI ($p < 0.001$).

Table 1. Descriptive characteristics of patients enrolled in the cohort and comparative descriptive characteristics of patients with non-severe AKI and severe AKI.

Characteristics of Patients	Patients Enrolled $n = 232$ (%)	Non-Severe AKI $n = 112$ (%)	Severe AKI $n = 120$ (%)	p Value
Males	142 (63)	71 (63)	71 (59)	0.5
Age	62 ± 16	62 ± 16	62 ± 16	0.8
Smoker	97 (42)	50 (45)	47 (39)	0.4
Hypertension	115 (50)	62 (55)	53 (44)	0.1
Diabetes	55 (24)	31 (28)	24 (20)	0.2
Heart failure	42 (18)	20 (18)	22 (18)	0.9
Stroke	21 (9)	12 (11)	9 (8)	0.4
PAD	17 (7)	6 (5)	11 (9)	0.3
IHD	33 (14)	19 (17)	14 (11)	0.2
Basal SCr	78 ± 18	78 ± 19	77 ± 17	0.6
Sepsis	118 (51)	56 (50)	62 (52)	0.8
Contrast agent	55 (24)	26 (23)	29 (24)	0.9
Aminosid use	84 (36)	43 (38)	42 (35)	0.6
NIV or HFNC	192 (83)	6 (5)	5 (4)	0.7
Orotracheal intubation	192 (83)	92 (82)	100 (83)	0.8
Catecholamine use	191 (82)	89 (79)	102 (85)	0.3
SAPS II	62 ± 19	59 ± 17	65 ± 20	0.01
Maximal SCr (μmol/L)	266 ± 181	153 ± 56	371 ± 195	<0.001
AKI stage:				
1	62 (27)	62 (55)	0 (0)	
2	50 (21)	50 (45)	0 (0)	
3	120 (52)		120 (100)	
RRT		0	73 (61)	
CVVHD		0	57 (48)	
IHH		0	16 (13)	
Renal recovery	90/141 (64)	68/78 (87)	22/63 (35)	<0.001
ICU length of stay (days)	9 ± 10	9 ± 10	9 ± 11	0.9
Intra-ICU deaths	91 (39)	34 (30)	57 (48)	0.01
Hospital length of stay (days)	36 ± 100	37 ± 109	34 ± 91	0.8

PAD: Peripheral arterial disease; IHD: Ischemic heart disease; HFNC: High-flow nasal cannula; NIV: Non-invasive ventilation; AKI: Acute kidney injury; SAPS II: Simplified acute physiology score II; SCr: Serum creatinine; ICU: Intensive care unit; RRT: renal replacement therapy; CVVHD: Continuous venovenous hemodialysis; IH: Intermittent hemodialysis.

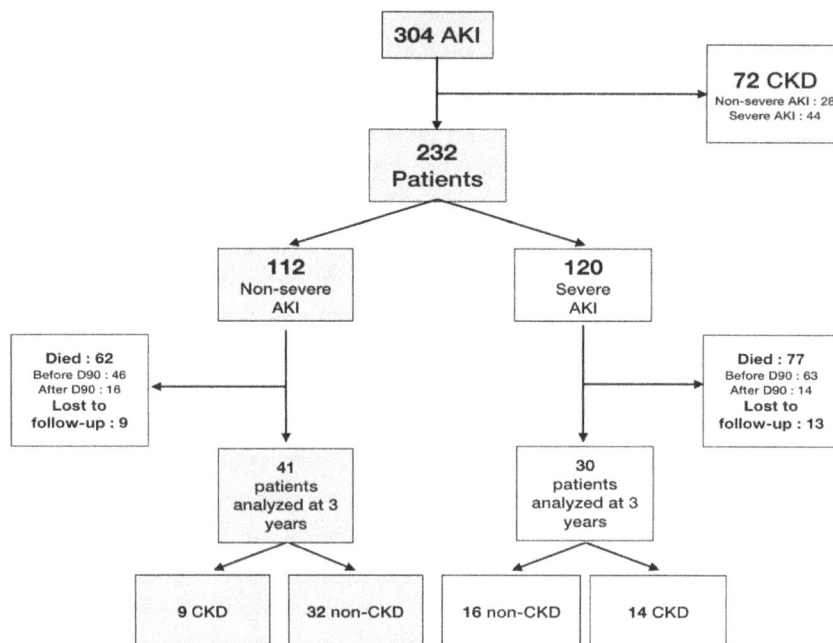

Figure 1. Flow chart. CKD: chronic kidney disease; AKI: acute kidney injury.

Descriptive characteristics of all patients enrolled (patients enrolled) and comparative descriptive characteristics between non-severe AKI and severe AKI. Statistical analysis was carried out to compare these two subgroups.

3.2. Follow-Up

A flow diagram is presented in Figure 1. In non-severe AKI, 34/112 (30%) died in the ICU and 28/112 (25%) during the follow-up. We lost 9/112 (8%) patients to follow-up. In this group, 41 patients completed the study.

3.3. Primary Outcome: Long-Term Incidence of CKD at Three Years

In non-severe AKI, the incidence of CKD during a three years follow-up amongst patients who survived was 9/41 (22% CI $_{95\%}$ (9.3–33.6)). It tended to be lower than in in the severe AKI group (14/30 (44% CI $_{95\%}$ (28.8–64.5)) $p = 0.052$. Among the 23 patients who developed CKD, whatever the group, 8 had recovered from AKI (6 in the non-severe group) and 9 had eGFR < 60 mL/min/1.73 m^2 (4 in the non-severe group) at ICU discharge. CKD stages at three years are summarized in Table 2.

Table 2. Chronic kidney disease stage at three years follow-up (eGFR (mL/min/1.73 m^2)).

CKD Stages At 3 Years	Non-Severe AKI at Inclusion $n = 41$ (%)	Severe AKI at Inclusion $n = 30$ (%)	Total $n = 71$ (%)
CKD3 (60 < eGFR < 30)	7 (17)	10 (33)	17 (24)
CKD4 (30 < eGFR < 15)	2 (5)	1 (3)	3 (4)
CKD5 (eGFR < 15))	0	3 (10)	3 (4)

AKI: acute kidney injury; CKD: chronic kidney disease.

3.4. Secondary Outcomes

3.4.1. Risk Factors for CKD at Three Years

In the univariate analysis, hypertension (Odd Ratio (OR) = 3.5 (1.2–10.5)), diabetes (OR = 3.6 (1.2–10.3)), SCr (OR = 1.007 (1.002–1.011)), and severe AKI (OR = 3 (1.1–8.5)) were significantly associated with CKD at three years.

In the multivariate analysis, hypertension and diabetes presented interactions (Chi^2 p = 0.004), as well as Scr and severe AKI. Diabetes and severe AKI were the variables maintained in the analysis. In this model, only diabetes (OR = 3.3 (1.3–8.3)) was significantly associated with CKD at three years. Conversely, the severity of AKI was not associated with CKD (severe vs. non-severe) (OR = 1.96 (0.8–5)) (Table 3).

Table 3. Risk factors for developing CKD at three years.

	Univariate Analysis		Multivariate Analysis	
	Odds Ratio eGFR < 60 (mL/min/1.73 m^2)	Confidence Interval 5%	Odds Ratio eGFR < 60 (mL/min/1.73 m^2)	Confidence Interval 5%
Male	0.5	(0.2–1.4)		
Age	1.1	(0.99–1.2)		
Smoker	1.8	(0.6–4.8)		
Hypertension	3.5	(1.2–10.5)		
Diabetes	3.6	(1.2–10.3)	3.3	(1.3–8.3)
Heart failure	2.3	(0.6–9.1)		
Stroke	0.3	(0.04–2.7)		
PAD	2.1	(0.3–16.3)		
IHD	1.8	(0.4–7.3)		
Sepsis	1.7	(0.6–4.6)		
Contrast agent	1.3	(0.4–3.8)		
Aminosid use	2.1	(0.8 5.8)		
Orotracheal intubation	0.7	(0.2–2.1)		
Vasopressor	1.6	(0.4–6.5)		
SAPS II	1.5	(0.2–12.9)		
Length of hospitalization in ICU (days)	0.97	(0.94–1.04)		
Hospital length of stay (days)	0.99	(0.98–1.01)		
Maximum SCr	1.007	(1.002–1.01)		
Non-severe AKI	1		1	
Severe AKI	3	(1.1–8.5)	1.96	(0.8–5)
AKI stage 1	0.2	(0.05–0.4)		
AKI stage 2	0.5	(0.2–1.5)		
AKI stage 3	1			
RRT	2.7	(0.9–8.2)		
CVVHD	0.8	(0.2–3.1)		
Readmission at hospital during follow-up	1.5	(0.5–4.3)		

Multivariate analysis was proceeded using logistic regression. PAD: Peripheral arterial disease; IHD: Ischemic heart disease; HFNC: High-flow nasal cannula; NIV: Non-invasive ventilation; AKI: Acute kidney injury; SAPS II: Simplified Acute physiology score; SCr: Serum creatinine; CVVHD: Continuous veno-venous hemodialysis; RRT: Renal replacement therapy; ICU: Intensive care unit.

3.4.2. Patients Survival

Patients survival was assessed in the set of 232 included patients. At three years, survival was 38% in our series. The three years survival was 43% in the non-severe AKI group and 32% in the severe AKI group with statistical difference (p = 0.02) (Figure 2).

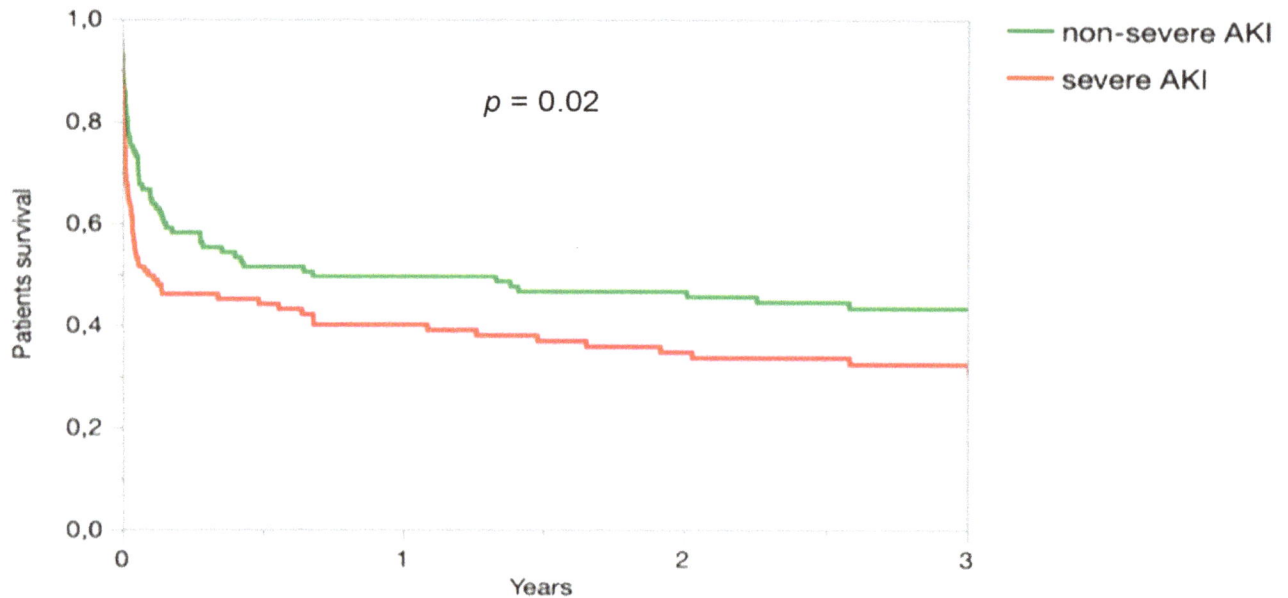

Figure 2. Patients' survival rate. Renal survival was assessed in 232 patients. The three years renal survival was 43% in the non-severe AKI group and 32% in the severe AKI group with statistical difference. Comparison of renal survival rate using log-rank test.

Time	0	90 days	1 year	2 years	3 years
Non-severe AKI	n = 112	63	52	46	27
Severe AKI	n = 120	49	41	33	21

3.4.3. Renal Specialist Following

Eleven out of twenty-three (48%) patients who developed CKD were followed by a nephrologist.

4. Discussion

This study is the first in the literature to estimate the incidence of CKD three years after non-severe AKI in critically ill patients. At three years, an eGFR of <60 mL/min1.73 m^2 (defining CKD) was present in 22% CI $_{95\%}$ (9.3–33.6) in the non-severe AKI group, half of whom were not followed by a nephrologist.

Our study is original. The incidence of CKD only three years after non-severe AKI is high (22%). No study has focused on stage 1 and 2 AKI in critically ill patients while only a few studies have studied stage 1 and 2 AKI in non-critically ill patients. In the recent analysis of U.S. veterans' health administration data, incidence of CKD (eGFR < 60 mL/min/1.73 m^2) at 1 year was 31% in AKI stage 1-patients and 27% in AKI stage 2-patients [15]. However, patients had more risk factor to develop CKD than ours; they were male (95%), older than ours, and basal eGFR was 84 mL/min/1.73 m^2. We excluded patients with an eGFR of <90 mL/min/1.73 m^2 prior to AKI Many similar studies excluded patients with prior eGFR < 60 mL/min/1.73 m^2. Indeed, patients with an eGFR of 60–90 mL/min/1.73 m^2 do not have normal renal function and it has been very well demonstrated that even a slight degree of chronic renal failure promotes future alteration of eGFR [16]. By excluding patients with DFG < 90 mL/min/1.73 m^2 at inclusion, we ensure a decrease of 30 mL/min in three years, which is clinically very significant.

Nevertheless, many factors may influence CKD development three years after an AKI in ICU and we cannot conclude whether non-severe AKI itself was independently implicated in the high CKD incidence at three years. First, AKI itself: in vitro studies have highlighted different mechanisms linking AKI and CKD, such as persistent interstitial inflammation or tubular's vascular damages [16]. Secondly, individual factor can lead to the development of CKD at long-term. For example, diabetes is associated with a decrease in kidney function in many studies. In the multivariate analysis, diabetes was a risk factor for a decline in kidney function in AKI patients without prior CKD. These results were already demonstrated in non-critically ill patients. However, many other clinical conditions are associated with the risk of developing CKD such as age, sex, diabetes, hypertension, albuminuria, initial eGFR, high triglyceride levels, and low HDL cholesterol levels [17,18]. In a future study, the Kidneyfailurerisk.com Canadian score, which estimates the risk to develop CKD at 2 or 5 years and is well validated in a variety of populations [19], could be used to compare the expected incidence assessed by this score with the observed increased incidence of CKD.

One third of surviving patients had apparent complete renal recovery at ICU discharge but later developed CKD. However, for the other patients, we could not determine if they recovered later or if they kept low eGFR over the three years. These findings are in accordance with studies performed in non-critically ill patients, which found an increased risk of CKD following non-dialysis-dependent AKI, even after biological renal recovery [20,21]. Absence of renal recovery at ICU discharge remains common in our study (about a third of the cases). Kellum et al. studied 17,000 ICU patients with stage 2–3 AKI and showed that early relapse of AKI occurred in 37% of cases. Late sustained reversal (after 7 days and sustained through hospital discharge) and relapse were two risk factors for a decreased age-adjusted one-year renal survival [22].

One of the strength of our study comes from the recording of anterior SCr rather than MDRD estimated SCr. The main limitation of our study is its single-center characteristic with a consecutive low number of surviving patients at three years, which favors a risk of type 2 error. We have screened more than 300 patients in three years. The enrollment was exhaustive because it was integrated in a clinical trial in which the medical team was very involved. Only 22 patients were lost to follow-up (<10%), a satisfactory proportion for this type of study. Despite this, because of CKD occurring before AKI accounted for many exclusions but also because of many deaths, few patients (23%) could be analyzed at the three-year follow-up. This lack of power probably explains the absence of significant association between AKI severity and CKD. This association was already suggested by many studies showing that severe AKI remains the main prognostic factor of CKD after a long follow-up period. We could not determine whether CKD developed before death in the patients who died. However, 109/139 patients (78%) died before day 90, which is the time limit after which CKD can be defined. Our hypothesis is that less severe patients with a longer outcome need a specific follow-up to detect and to prevent CKD. This pragmatic view led us to identify incidence of CKD only in patients who survived at three years.

It is clear that AKI survivors require a long-term follow-up [23]. First, they are at high risk of developing CKD even in cases of non-severe AKI, including if their kidney function has recovered at ICU discharge. Second, this risk is probably underestimated both by the patient and the general practitioner because less than 50% of patients with CKD were followed by a nephrologist in our study. Third, it was already shown that the risk of mortality and cardiovascular complications is very high in patients with an eGFR of <60 mL/min/1.73 m^2 and the long-term consequences concern other organs and persist despite renal recovery [24,25].

The risk of developing CKD at three years after non-severe AKI, despite it being lower than after a severe AKI, remains high. These findings have to be confirmed by larger studies. A long-term follow up is required and all physicians involved in the patient's follow-up, including intensivists, should pay attention to that phenomenon.

Author Contributions: S.R. conceived and designed the study analyzed the data and drafted the manuscript. A.O. collected the data and helped to draft the manuscript, B.C. and D.G. helped to conduct the study. C.R. and C.C. helped to analyze the data and to draft the manuscript. A.B. supervised the conduct of the trial, helped to provide statistical advice and to draft the manuscript. All authors read and approved the final manuscript.

Acknowledgments: We thank Michaela LaPlante, a native American speaker, for an English check.

References

1. Hoste, E.A.J.; Bagshaw, S.M.; Bellomo, R.; Cely, C.M.; Colman, R.; Cruz, D.N.; Edipidis, K.; Forni, L.G.; Gomersall, C.D.; Govil, D.; et al. Epidemiology of acute kidney injury in critically ill patients: The multinational AKI-EPI study. *Intensive Care Med.* **2015**, *41*, 1411–1423. [CrossRef] [PubMed]

2. Uchino, S.; Kellum, J.A.; Bellomo, R.; Doig, G.S.; Morimatsu, H.; Morgera, S.; Schetz, M.; Tan, I.; Bouman, C.; Macedo, E.; et al. Beginning and Ending Supportive Therapy for the Kidney, I. Acute renal failure in critically ill patients: A multinational, multicenter study. *JAMA J. Am. Med Assoc.* **2005**, *294*, 813–818. [CrossRef] [PubMed]

3. Horkan, C.M.; Purtle, S.W.; Mendu, M.L.; Moromizato, T.; Gibbons, F.K.; Christopher, K.B. The Association of Acute Kidney Injury in the Critically Ill and Postdischarge Outcomes. *Crit. Care Med.* **2015**, *43*, 354–364. [CrossRef] [PubMed]

4. Delannoy, B.; Floccard, B.; Thiolliere, F.; Kaaki, M.; Badet, M.; Rosselli, S.; Ber, C.E.; Saez, A.; Flandreau, G.; Guérin, C. Six-month outcome in acute kidney injury requiring renal replacement therapy in the ICU: A multicentre prospective study. *Intensive Care Med.* **2009**, *35*, 1907–1915. [CrossRef]

5. Schiffl, H.; Fischer, R. Five-year outcomes of severe acute kidney injury requiring renal replacement therapy. *Nephrol. Dial. Transplant. Off. Publ. Eur. Dial. Transpl. Assoc. Eur. Ren. Assoc.* **2008**, *23*, 2235–2241. [CrossRef]

6. Gammelager, H.; Christiansen, C.F.; Johansen, M.B.; Tønnesen, E.; Jespersen, B.; Sørensen, H.T. Five-year risk of end-stage renal disease among intensive care patients surviving dialysis-requiring acute kidney injury: A nationwide cohort study. *Crit. Care* **2013**, *17*, R145. [CrossRef]

7. Lafrance, J.-P.; Miller, D.R. Acute kidney injury associates with increased long-term mortality. *J. Am. Soc. Nephrol. JASN* **2010**, *21*, 345–352. [CrossRef]

8. Heung, M.; Steffick, D.E.; Zivin, K.; Gillespie, B.W.; Banerjee, T.; Hsu, C.-Y.; Powe, N.R.; Pavkov, M.E.; Williams, D.E.; Saran, R.; et al. Centers for Disease Control and Prevention CKD Surveillance Team Acute Kidney Injury Recovery Pattern and Subsequent Risk of CKD: An Analysis of Veterans Health Administration Data. *Am. J. Kidney Dis. Off. J. Natl. Kidney Found.* **2016**, *67*, 742–752. [CrossRef]

9. Tomlinson, L.A.; Riding, A.M.; Payne, R.A.; Abel, G.A.; Tomson, C.R.; Wilkinson, I.B.; Roland, M.O.; Chaudhry, A.N. The accuracy of diagnostic coding for acute kidney injury in England—A single centre study. *BMC Nephrol.* **2013**, *14*, 58. [CrossRef]

10. Sawhney, S.; Fraser, S.D. Epidemiology of AKI: Utilizing Large Databases to Determine the Burden of AKI. *Adv. Chronic Kidney Dis.* **2017**, *24*, 194–204. [CrossRef]

11. Palevsky, P.M.; Liu, K.D.; Brophy, P.D.; Chawla, L.S.; Parikh, C.R.; Thakar, C.V.; Tolwani, A.J.; Waikar, S.S.; Weisbord, S.D. KDOQI US commentary on the 2012 KDIGO clinical practice guideline for acute kidney injury. *Am. J. Kidney Dis. Off. J. Natl. Kidney Found.* **2013**, *61*, 649–672. [CrossRef] [PubMed]

12. Horne, K.L.; Shardlow, A.; Taal, M.W.; Selby, N.M. Long Term Outcomes after Acute Kidney Injury: Lessons from the ARID Study. *Nephron* **2015**, *131*, 102–106. [CrossRef] [PubMed]

13. Rewa, O.; Bagshaw, S.M. Acute kidney injury-epidemiology, outcomes and economics. *Nat. Publ. Group* **2014**, *10*, 193–207. [CrossRef] [PubMed]

14. Gaudry, S.; Hajage, D.; Schortgen, F.; Martin-Lefevre, L.; Pons, B.; Boulet, E.; Boyer, A.; Chevrel, G.; Lerolle, N.; Carpentier, D.; et al. AKIKI Study Group Initiation Strategies for Renal-Replacement Therapy in the Intensive Care Unit. *N. Engl. J. Med.* **2016**, *375*, 122–133. [CrossRef] [PubMed]

15. Gansevoort, R.T.; Matsushita, K.; van der Velde, M.; Astor, B.C.; Woodward, M.; Levey, A.S.; de Jong, P.E.; Coresh, J. Chronic Kidney Disease Prognosis Consortium Lower estimated GFR and higher albuminuria are associated with adverse kidney outcomes. A collaborative meta-analysis of general and high-risk population cohorts. *Kidney Int.* **2011**, *80*, 93–104. [CrossRef]

16. Heung, M.; Chawla, L.S. Acute kidney injury: Gateway to chronic kidney disease. *Nephron Clin. Pract.* **2014**, *127*, 30–34. [CrossRef]

17. O'Seaghdha, C.M.; Lyass, A.; Massaro, J.M.; Meigs, J.B.; Coresh, J.; D'Agostino, R.B.; Astor, B.C.; Fox, C.S. A risk score for chronic kidney disease in the general population. *Am. J. Med.* **2012**, *125*, 270–277. [CrossRef]

18. McMahon, G.M.; Preis, S.R.; Hwang, S.-J.; Fox, C.S. Mid-adulthood risk factor profiles for CKD. *J. Am. Soc. Nephrol. JASN* **2014**, *25*, 2633–2641. [CrossRef]

19. Tangri, N.; Grams, M.E.; Levey, A.S.; Coresh, J.; Appel, L.J.; Astor, B.C.; Chodick, G.; Collins, A.J.; Djurdjev, O.; Elley, C.R.; et al. CKD Prognosis Consortium Multinational Assessment of Accuracy of Equations for Predicting Risk of Kidney Failure: A Meta-analysis. *JAMA J. Am. Med Assoc.* **2016**, *315*, 164–174. [CrossRef]

20. Jones, J.; Holmen, J.; De Graauw, J.; Jovanovich, A.; Thornton, S.; Chonchol, M. Association of complete recovery from acute kidney injury with incident CKD stage 3 and all-cause mortality. *Am. J. Kidney Dis. Off. J. Natl. Kidney Found.* **2012**, *60*, 402–408. [CrossRef]

21. Bucaloiu, I.D.; Kirchner, H.L.; Norfolk, E.R.; Hartle, J.E.; Perkins, R.M. Increased risk of death and de novo chronic kidney disease following reversible acute kidney injury. *Kidney Int.* **2012**, *81*, 477–485. [CrossRef] [PubMed]

22. Kellum, J.A.; Sileanu, F.E.; Bihorac, A.; Hoste, E.A.J.; Chawla, L.S. Recovery after Acute Kidney Injury. *Am. J. Respir. Crit. Care Med.* **2017**, *195*, 784–791. [CrossRef] [PubMed]

23. Vandenberghe, W.; Hoste, E.A.J. Acute kidney injury survivors should have long-term follow-up. *Crit. Care* **2014**, *18*, 703. [CrossRef] [PubMed]

24. Tonelli, M.; Muntner, P.; Lloyd, A.; Manns, B.J.; Klarenbach, S.; Pannu, N.; James, M.T.; Hemmelgarn, B.R. Alberta Kidney Disease Network Risk of coronary events in people with chronic kidney disease compared with those with diabetes: A population-level cohort study. *Lancet* **2012**, *380*, 807–814. [CrossRef]

25. Shiao, C.-C.; Wu, P.-C.; Huang, T.-M.; Lai, T.-S.; Yang, W.-S.; Wu, C.-H.; Lai, C.-F.; Wu, V.-C.; Chu, T.-S.; Wu, K.-D. National Taiwan University Hospital Study Group on Acute Renal Failure (NSARF) and the Taiwan Consortium for Acute Kidney Injury and Renal Diseases (CAKs) Long-term remote organ consequences following acute kidney injury. *Crit. Care* **2015**, *19*, 438. [CrossRef]

15

Incidence and Impact of Acute Kidney Injury in Patients Receiving Extracorporeal Membrane Oxygenation

Charat Thongprayoon [1], Wisit Cheungpasitporn [2], Ploypin Lertjitbanjong [3], Narothama Reddy Aeddula [4], Tarun Bathini [5], Kanramon Watthanasuntorn [3], Narat Srivali [6], Michael A. Mao [7] and Kianoush Kashani [1,8,*]

[1] Division of Nephrology and Hypertension, Mayo Clinic, Rochester, MN 55905, USA
[2] Division of Nephrology, Department of Medicine, University of Mississippi Medical Center, Jackson, MS 39216, USA
[3] Department of Internal Medicine, Bassett Medical Center, Cooperstown, NY 13326, USA
[4] Division of Nephrology, Department of Medicine, Deaconess Health System, Evansville, IN 47747, USA
[5] Department of Internal Medicine, University of Arizona, Tucson, AZ 85721, USA
[6] Division of Pulmonary and Critical Care Medicine, St. Agnes Hospital, Baltimore, MD 21229, USA
[7] Division of Nephrology and Hypertension, Mayo Clinic, Jacksonville, FL 32224, USA
[8] Division of Pulmonary and Critical Care Medicine, Department of Medicine, Mayo Clinic, Rochester, MN 55905, USA
*   Correspondence: Kashani.Kianoush@mayo.edu

Abstract: Background: Although acute kidney injury (AKI) is a frequent complication in patients receiving extracorporeal membrane oxygenation (ECMO), the incidence and impact of AKI on mortality among patients on ECMO remain unclear. We conducted this systematic review to summarize the incidence and impact of AKI on mortality risk among adult patients on ECMO. Methods: A literature search was performed using EMBASE, Ovid MEDLINE, and Cochrane Databases from inception until March 2019 to identify studies assessing the incidence of AKI (using a standard AKI definition), severe AKI requiring renal replacement therapy (RRT), and the impact of AKI among adult patients on ECMO. Effect estimates from the individual studies were obtained and combined utilizing random-effects, generic inverse variance method of DerSimonian-Laird. The protocol for this systematic review is registered with PROSPERO (no. CRD42018103527). Results: 41 cohort studies with a total of 10,282 adult patients receiving ECMO were enrolled. Overall, the pooled estimated incidence of AKI and severe AKI requiring RRT were 62.8% (95%CI: 52.1%–72.4%) and 44.9% (95%CI: 40.8%–49.0%), respectively. Meta-regression showed that the year of study did not significantly affect the incidence of AKI ($p = 0.67$) or AKI requiring RRT ($p = 0.83$). The pooled odds ratio (OR) of hospital mortality among patients receiving ECMO with AKI on RRT was 3.73 (95% CI, 2.87–4.85). When the analysis was limited to studies with confounder-adjusted analysis, increased hospital mortality remained significant among patients receiving ECMO with AKI requiring RRT with pooled OR of 3.32 (95% CI, 2.21–4.99). There was no publication bias as evaluated by the funnel plot and Egger's regression asymmetry test with $p = 0.62$ and $p = 0.17$ for the incidence of AKI and severe AKI requiring RRT, respectively. Conclusion: Among patients receiving ECMO, the incidence rates of AKI and severe AKI requiring RRT are high, which has not changed over time. Patients who develop AKI requiring RRT while on ECMO carry 3.7-fold higher hospital mortality.

Keywords: acute kidney injury; AKI; extracorporeal membrane oxygenation; ECMO; epidemiology; meta-analysis

1. Introduction

Extracorporeal membrane oxygenation (ECMO), as a mechanical circulatory support system, is utilized as a treatment for cardiovascular or respiratory failure [1–3]. There are two main types of ECMO, including venovenous (VV)-ECMO for patients with isolated respiratory failure and venoarterial (VA)-ECMO for combined severe cardiac and respiratory failure [4]. Over the past 40 years, the clinical applications and feasibility of ECMO have expanded in patients with refractory cardiorespiratory failure, and there has been an exponential increase in the number of centers utilizing ECMO globally [3,5–9]. Studies have demonstrated survival benefits of ECMO ranging from 20% to 50% in patients with cardiac arrest, severe adult respiratory distress syndrome (ARDS), and refractory cardiogenic shock [5,10–16].

Despite these benefits, there have been a number of reports to highlight the concomitant occurrence of organ failures and complications including acute kidney injury (AKI), infections, thrombosis, bleeding and coagulopathy, and neurological events [17,18]. The underlying mechanisms for AKI among patients requiring ECMO appear to be complex and include hemodynamic instabilities, inflammatory responses, coagulation-platelet abnormalities, and immune-mediated injury that arise from the primary underlying disease, premorbid conditions and the ECMO circuit [18–28]. Due to previously non-uniform definitions of AKI, the reported incidences of AKI among patients requiring ECMO therapy ranged widely from 8% up to 85% [4,7,15,18–70]. In addition, the incidence and mortality associated with AKI in patients requiring ECMO and their trends remain unclear.

This systematic review was conducted with the aim to summarize the incidence (using standard AKI definitions) and the impact of AKI on mortality risk among adult patients on ECMO.

2. Methods

2.1. Information Sources and Search Strategy

The protocol for this systematic review and meta-analysis is registered with International Prospective Register of Systematic Reviews (PROSPERO no. CRD42018103527). A systematic literature review of EMBASE, Ovid MEDLINE, and the Cochrane Database of Systematic Reviews from database inception through March 2019 was conducted to summarize the incidence and impact of AKI on mortality risk among adult patients on ECMO. Two authors (C.T. and W.C.) independently performed a systematic literature search utilizing a search approach that consolidated the search terms "extracorporeal membrane oxygenation" OR "ECMO" AND "acute kidney injury" OR "acute renal failure." Further details regarding the search strategy utilized for each database are provided in Online Supplementary Data 1. No language restriction was implemented. A manual search for conceivably related articles utilizing references of the included studies was additionally performed. This systematic review was performed following the PRISMA (Preferred Reporting Items for Systematic Reviews and Meta-Analysis) statement [71].

2.2. Study Selection

Studies were included in this systematic review if they were clinical trials or observational studies that reported the incidence of AKI (using standard AKI definitions including RIFLE (Risk, Injury, Failure, Loss of kidney function, and End-stage kidney disease) [72], AKIN (Acute Kidney Injury Network) [73], and KDIGO (Kidney Disease: Improving Global Outcomes) classifications) [74], severe AKI requiring renal replacement therapy (RRT), and mortality risk of AKI among adult patients (age $\geq$ 18 years old) on ECMO. Eligible studies needed to provide the data to evaluate the incidence or mortality rate of AKI with 95% confidence intervals (CI). Retrieved articles were independently examined for eligibility by the two authors (C.T. and W.C.). Inconsistencies were discussed and resolved by shared agreement. The size of the study did not limit inclusion.

2.3. Data Collection Process

A structured data collecting form was adopted to gather the following data from individual study including title, name of authors, publication year, year of the study, country where the study was conveyed, type of ECMO, AKI definition, incidence of AKI, incidence of severe AKI requiring RRT, and mortality risk of AKI among patients on ECMO.

2.4. Statistical Analysis

We used the Comprehensive Meta-Analysis software version 3.3.070 (Biostat Inc, Englewood, NJ, USA) to conduct the meta-analysis. Adjusted point estimates of included studies were consolidated by the generic inverse variance method of DerSimonian-Laird, which assigned the weight of individual study based on its variance [75]. Due to the probability of between-study variance, we applied a random-effects model to pool outcomes of interest, including the incidence of AKI and mortality risk. Statistical heterogeneity of studies was assessed by the Cochran's Q test ($p < 0.05$ for a statistical significance) and the I^2 statistic ($\leq$25%: insignificant heterogeneity, 26%–50%: low heterogeneity, 51%–75%: moderate heterogeneity and $\geq$75%: high heterogeneity) [76]. The presence of publication bias was evaluated by both the funnel plot and the Egger test [77].

3. Results

A total of 1,632 potentially eligible articles were identified with our search approach. After excluding 644 articles that were either in-vitro studies, focused on pediatric patient population, animal studies, case reports, correspondences, or review articles, and 831 articles due to being duplicates, 157 articles remained for full-length article review. Seventy-three articles were subsequently excluded as they did not provide data on the incidence of AKI or mortality of AKI, while 33 articles were excluded because they were not clinical trials or observational studies. Ten studies [19–28] were additionally excluded because they did not use a standard AKI definition or did not report the incidence of severe AKI requiring RRT. Therefore, 41 cohort studies [7,15,29–67] with a total of 10,282 adult patients receiving ECMO were enrolled. The systematic review of the literature flowchart is demonstrated in Figure 1. The characteristics of the included studies are shown in Table 1.

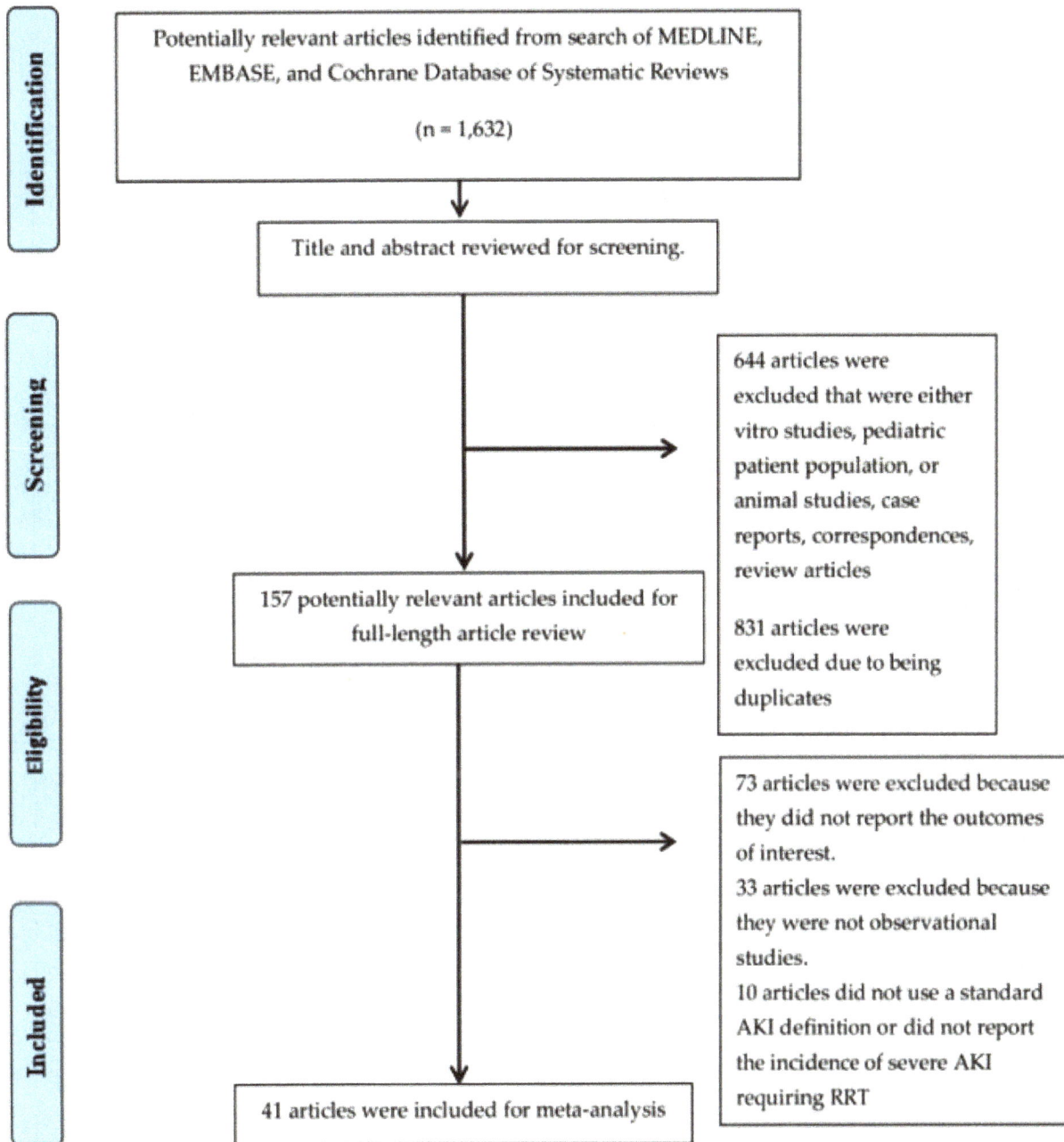

Figure 1. The flowchart for the systematic review.

Table 1. Main characteristic of studies included in this meta-analysis of AKI incidence and mortality among patients requiring ECMO [7,15,29–67].

Study	Year	Country	Patients	Number	AKI Definition	AKI Incidence	Mortality
Pagani et al. [15]	2001	USA	ECMO for cardiogenic shock or arrest	33	RRT	RRT 10/33 (30.3%)	Hospital mortality 9/10 (90%)
Yap et al. [29]	2003	Taiwan	ECMO for cardiogenic shock	10	RRT	RRT 5/10 (50%)	Mortality 5/5 (100%)
Lin et al. [30]	2006	Taiwan	ECMO	46	AKI; RIFLE criteria	AKI 36/46 (78.3%) CRRT 16/46 (34.8%)	AKI: Hospital mortality 28/36 (78%) CRRT: Hospital mortality 16/16 (100%)
Tsai et al. [31]	2008	Taiwan	ECMO	288	CRRT	CRRT 104/288 (36.1%)	Hospital mortality 79/104 (76%)
Bakhtiary et al. [32]	2008	Germany	VA-ECMO for refractory cardiogenic shock	45	CRRT	CRRT 39/45 (86.7%)	N/A
Luo et al. [33]	2009	China	VA-ECMO in severe heart failure	45	CRRT	CRRT 12/45 (26.6%)	Hospital mortality 7/9 (78%)
Brogan et al. [34]	2009	USA	ECMO in severe respiratory failure	1473	RRT	RRT 648/1473 (44%)	Hospital mortality RRT 390/648 (60%)
Wang et al. [35]	2009	China	VA ECMO for refractory cardiogenic shock after cardiac surgery	62	CRRT	CRRT 23/62 (37.0%)	N/A
Yan et al. [36]	2010	China	ECMO after cardiac surgery	67	AKI; RIFLE and AKIN criteria	RIFLE AKI 54/67 (80.6%) AKIN AKI 57/67 (85.1%) RRT 30/67 (44.8%)	Hospital mortality RIFLE AKI 32/54 (59%) AKIN AKI 33/57 (58%) RRT 22/30 (73%)
Elsharkawy et al. [37]	2010	USA	VA-ECMO after cardiac surgery	233	RRT	RRT 101/233 (43.3%)	Hospital mortality 79/101 (78%)
Hsu et al. [38]	2010	Taiwan	VA-ECMO for cardiogenic shock after cardiac surgery	51	CRRT	CRRT 38/51 (74.5%)	N/A

Table 1. *Cont.*

Study	Year	Country	Patients	Number	AKI Definition	AKI Incidence	Mortality
Lan et al. [39]	2010	Taiwan	ECMO	607	RRT	RRT 301/607 (49.6%)	Hospital mortality 259/301 (86%)
Rastan et al. [40]	2010	Germany	VA-ECMO for cardiogenic shock after cardiac surgery	517	RRT	RRT 336/517 (65.0%)	N/A
Wu et al. [41]	2010	Taiwan	ECMO	346	RRT	RRT 187/346 (54%)	RRT 72/102 (71%)
Chen et al. [42]	2011	Taiwan	ECMO	102	AKI; AKIN criteria	AKI 62/102 (60.8%) CRRT 26/102 (25.5%)	Hospital mortality AKI 51/62 (82%) CRRT 22/26 (85%)
Bermudez et al. [43]	2011	USA	ECMO for refractory cardiogenic shock; VA (88%)	42	RRT	RRT 17/42 (40.5%)	N/A
Chang et al. [44]	2012	Taiwan	Successfully weaned from ECMO	113	AKI; AKIN criteria at 48 h post-ECMO removal	AKI 51/113 (45.1%)	Hospital mortality AKI 23/51 (45%)
Kim et al. [45]	2012	Korea	ECMO; VA-ECMO (85%), VV-ECMO (15%)	26	AKI; AKIN criteria	AKI 10/26 (38.5%)	N/A
Lee et al. [46]	2012	Korea	ECMO; VA-ECMO (74%), VV-ECMO (26%)	185	CRRT	CRRT 76/185 (41.1%)	N/A
Loforte et al. [47]	2012	Italy	VA-ECMO	73	CRRT	CRRT 38/73 (52.1%)	N/A
Wu et al. [48]	2012	Taiwan	ECMO for non-post cardiotomy cardiogenic shock or cardiac arrest	60	RRT	RRT 19/60 (31.7%)	Hospital mortality 13/19 (68%)

Table 1. *Cont.*

Study	Year	Country	Patients	Number	AKI Definition	AKI Incidence	Mortality
Aubron et al. [49]	2013	Australia	ECMO; VA-ECMO (67%), VV-ECMO (33%)	158	RRT	VA-ECMO RRT 61/105 (58.1%) VV-ECMO RRT 27/53 (50.9%)	Hospital mortality VA-ECMO RRT 27/61 (44%) VV-ECMO RRT 13/27 (48%)
Kielstein et al. [50]	2013	Germany	ECMO; VA-ECMO (45%), VV-ECMO (55%)	200	RRT	RRT 117/200 (58.5%) RRT after ECMO 92/175 (52.6%)	90-day mortality 97/117 (83%)
Wu et al. [51]	2013	Taiwan	ECMO for acute myocardial infarction-induced cardiac arrest	35	RRT	RRT 16/35 (45.7%)	Hospital mortality 14/16 (88%)
Lazzeri et al. [52]	2013	Italy	ECMO for refractory cardiac arrest	25	RRT	RRT 16/24 (66.7%)	Mortality 9/16 (56%)
Unosawa et al. [53]	2013	Japan	VA-ECMO for refractory cardiogenic shock after cardiac surgery	47	RRT	RRT 15/47 (31.9%)	Mortality on ECMO 7/15 (46.7%)
Xue et al. [54]	2014	China	ECMO in lung transplantation	45	AKI; AKIN criteria	AKI 17/45 (37.8%)	N/A
Schmidt et al. [7]	2014	Australia	ECMO for refractory cardiogenic shock or acute respiratory failure	172	AKI; RIFLE criteria	AKI at ECMO day 1 98/172 (57.0%) CRRT during ECMO 103/172 (59.9%)	90-day mortality CRRT 34/103 (33%)
Hsiao et al. [55]	2014	Taiwan	ECMO for ARDS	81	CRRT	CRRT 33/81 (40.7%)	Hospital mortality CRRT 22/33 (67%)
Lee et al. [56]	2015	Korea	ECMO; VA-ECMO (71%), VV-ECMO (29%)	322	AKI; KDIGO criteria	AKI 265/322 (82.3%)	Hospital mortality 151/265 (57%)
Haneya [57]	2015	Germany	VV-ECMO for ARDS	262	AKI; KDIGO criteria	AKI 109/262 (41.6%) RRT during ECMO 52/262 (19.8%)	Mortality AKI 56/109 (51%) RRT during ECMO 23/52 (44%)

Table 1. *Cont.*

Study	Year	Country	Patients	Number	AKI Definition	AKI Incidence	Mortality
Huang et al. [58]	2016	China	ECMO for acute respiratory distress syndrome; VA-ECMO (17%), VV-ECMO (83%)	23	AKI; AKIN criteria	AKI 13/23 (56.5%)	Mortality 9/13 (69%)
Antonucci et al. [59]	2016	Belgium	ECMO; VA-ECMO (59%), VV-ECMO (41%)	135	AKI; AKIN criteria	AKI 95/135 (70.4%) CRRT 63/135 (46.7%)	ICU mortality AKI 55/95 (58%) CRRT 38/63 (60%)
Tsai et al. [60]	2017	Taiwan	ECMO	167	AKI; RIFLE, AKIN and KDIGO on ECMO day 1	RIFLE AKI 126/167 (75.4%) AKIN AKI 141/167 (84.4%) KDIGO AKI 142/167 (85.0%)	Hospital mortality RIFLE AKI 85/126 (67%) AKIN AKI 90/126 (71%) RIFLE AKI 90/126 (71%)
Panholzer et al. [61]	2017	Germany	VV-ECMO for ARDS	46	RRT	RRT 31/46 (67.4%)	Mortality RRT 23/31 (74%)
Chong et al. [62]	2018	Taiwan	VA-ECMO for acute fulminant myocarditis and cardiogenic shock	35	AKI; not specified	AKI 26/35 (74.3%) RRT 15/35 (42.9%)	Hospital mortality AKI 14/26 (54%) RRT 11/15 (73%)
Devasagayaraj et al. [63]	2018	USA	VV-ECMO for ARDS	54	CRRT	CRRT 16/54 (29.6%)	Hospital mortality 9/16 (56%)
Liao et al. [64]	2018	China	ECMO; VA-ECMO (93%), VV-ECMO (7%)	170	AKI; KDIGO criteria	AKI 91/170 (53.5%)	N/A
Paek et al. [65]	2018	Korea	ECMO	538	CRRT	CRRT 296/838 (35.3%)	30-day mortality 195/296 (66%)
He et al. [66]	2018	China	ECMO	92	CRRT	CRRT 32/92 (34.8%)	Hospital mortality 19/32 (59%)
Chen et al. [67]	2019	Taiwan	ECMO	3251	RRT	RRT 1759/3251 (54.1%)	Hospital mortality 1298/1759 (74%)

Abbreviations: AKI, acute kidney injury.; ARDS, acute respiratory distress syndrome; AKIN, Acute Kidney Injury Network; CRRT, continuous renal replacement therapy; ECMO, Extracorporeal membrane oxygenation; ICU, intensive care unit; KDIGO, Kidney Disease Improving Global Outcomes; N/A, not available; RIFLE, Risk, Injury, Failure, Loss of kidney function, and End-stage kidney disease; RRT, Renal replacement therapy; USA, United States of America; VA-ECMO, venoarterial extracorporeal membrane oxygenation; VV-ECMO, venovenous extracorporeal membrane oxygenation.

3.1. Incidence of AKI in Patients Requiring ECMO

Overall, the pooled estimated incidence of AKI and severe AKI requiring RRT while on ECMO were 62.8% (95%CI: 52.1%–72.4%, I^2 = 94%, Figure 2A) and 44.9% (95%CI: 40.8%-49.0%, I^2 = 91%, Figure 2B), respectively. Subgroup analyses were performed according to AKI definitions. The pooled estimated incidence rates of AKI by RIFLE, AKIN, and KDIGO criteria were 67.5% (95%CI: 43.9%–84.6%, I^2 = 85%), 57.8% (95%CI: 44.6%–70.0%, I^2 = 86%), and 68.2% (95%CI: 43.8%–85.55%, I^2 = 98%), respectively.

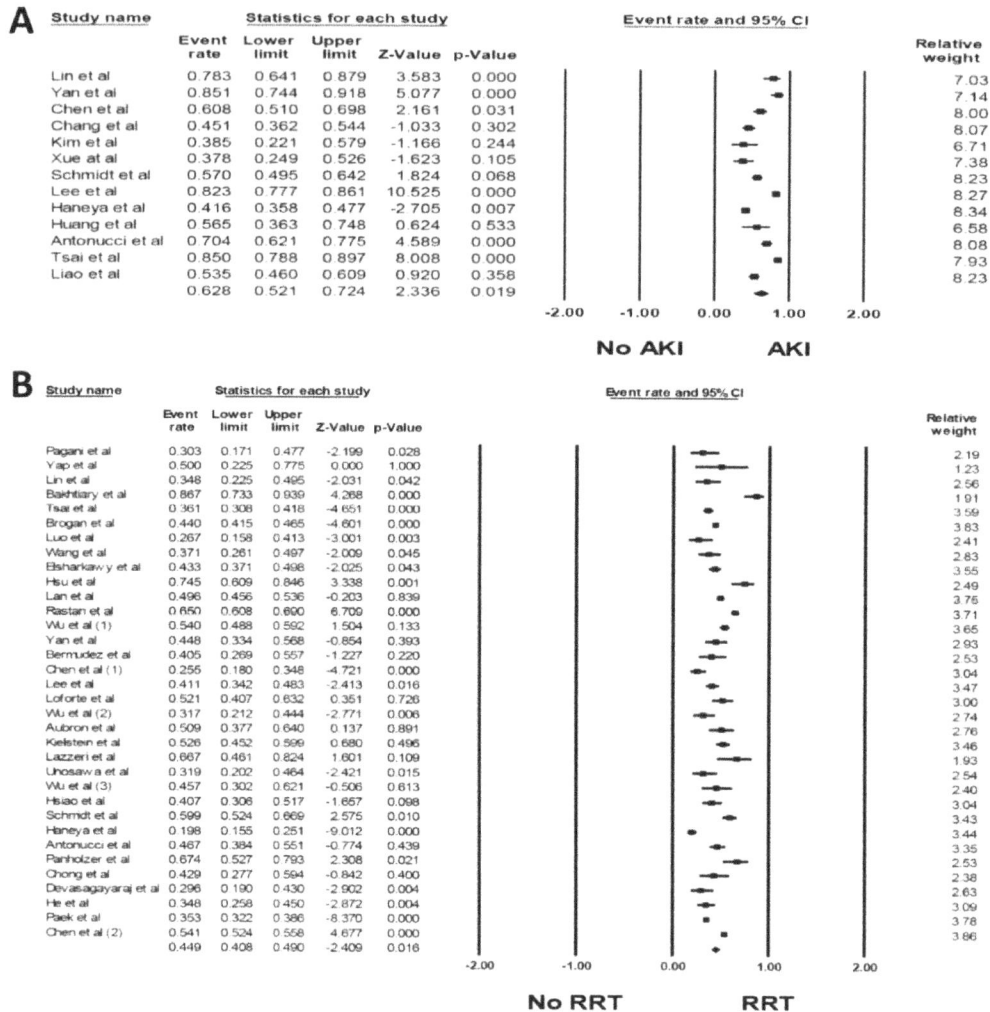

A

Study name	Event rate	Lower limit	Upper limit	Z-Value	p-Value	Relative weight
Lin et al	0.783	0.641	0.879	3.583	0.000	7.03
Yan et al	0.851	0.744	0.918	5.077	0.000	7.14
Chen et al	0.608	0.510	0.698	2.161	0.031	8.00
Chang et al	0.451	0.362	0.544	-1.033	0.302	8.07
Kim et al	0.385	0.221	0.579	-1.166	0.244	6.71
Xue at al	0.378	0.249	0.526	-1.623	0.105	7.38
Schmidt et al	0.570	0.495	0.642	1.824	0.068	8.23
Lee et al	0.823	0.777	0.861	10.525	0.000	8.27
Haneya et al	0.416	0.358	0.477	-2.705	0.007	8.34
Huang et al	0.565	0.363	0.748	0.624	0.533	6.58
Antonucci et al	0.704	0.621	0.775	4.589	0.000	8.08
Tsai et al	0.850	0.788	0.897	8.008	0.000	7.93
Liao et al	0.535	0.460	0.609	0.920	0.358	8.23
	0.628	0.521	0.724	2.336	0.019	

Event rate and 95% CI — No AKI / AKI (-2.00, -1.00, 0.00, 1.00, 2.00)

B

Study name	Event rate	Lower limit	Upper limit	Z-Value	p-Value	Relative weight
Pagani et al	0.303	0.171	0.477	-2.199	0.028	2.19
Yap et al	0.500	0.225	0.775	0.000	1.000	1.23
Lin et al	0.348	0.225	0.495	-2.031	0.042	2.56
Bakhtiary et al	0.867	0.733	0.939	4.268	0.000	1.91
Tsai et al	0.361	0.308	0.418	-4.651	0.000	3.59
Brogan et al	0.440	0.415	0.465	-4.601	0.000	3.83
Luo et al	0.267	0.158	0.413	-3.001	0.003	2.41
Wang et al	0.371	0.261	0.497	-2.009	0.045	2.83
Elsharkawy et al	0.433	0.371	0.498	-2.025	0.043	3.55
Hsu et al	0.745	0.609	0.846	3.338	0.001	2.49
Lan et al	0.496	0.456	0.536	-0.203	0.839	3.75
Rastan et al	0.650	0.608	0.690	6.709	0.000	3.71
Wu et al (1)	0.540	0.488	0.592	1.504	0.133	3.65
Yan et al	0.448	0.334	0.568	-0.854	0.393	2.93
Bermudez et al	0.405	0.269	0.557	-1.227	0.220	2.53
Chen et al (1)	0.255	0.180	0.348	-4.721	0.000	3.04
Lee et al	0.411	0.342	0.483	-2.413	0.016	3.47
Loforte et al	0.521	0.407	0.632	0.351	0.726	3.00
Wu et al (2)	0.317	0.212	0.444	-2.771	0.006	2.74
Aubron et al	0.509	0.377	0.640	0.137	0.891	2.76
Kielstein et al	0.526	0.452	0.599	0.680	0.496	3.46
Lazzeri et al	0.667	0.461	0.824	1.601	0.109	1.93
Unosawa et al	0.319	0.202	0.464	-2.421	0.015	2.54
Wu et al (3)	0.457	0.302	0.621	-0.506	0.613	2.40
Hsiao et al	0.407	0.306	0.517	-1.657	0.098	3.04
Schmidt et al	0.599	0.524	0.669	2.575	0.010	3.43
Haneya et al	0.198	0.155	0.251	-9.012	0.000	3.44
Antonucci et al	0.467	0.384	0.551	-0.774	0.439	3.35
Panholzer et al	0.674	0.527	0.793	2.308	0.021	2.53
Chong et al	0.429	0.277	0.594	-0.842	0.400	2.38
Devasagayaraj et al	0.296	0.190	0.430	-2.902	0.004	2.63
He et al	0.348	0.258	0.450	-2.872	0.004	3.09
Paek et al	0.353	0.322	0.386	-8.370	0.000	3.78
Chen et al (2)	0.541	0.524	0.558	4.677	0.000	3.86
	0.449	0.408	0.490	-2.409	0.016	

Event rate and 95% CI — No RRT / RRT (-2.00, -1.00, 0.00, 1.00, 2.00)

Figure 2. Forest plots of the included studies assessing (**A**) incidence rates of AKI while on ECMO and (**B**) incidence rate of severe AKI requiring RRT while on ECMO. A diamond data marker depicts the overall rate from each included study (square data marker) and 95%CI.

Subgroup analysis based on the type of ECMO was also performed. Pooled estimated incidence of AKI and severe AKI requiring RRT while on venoarterial (VA)-ECMO were 60.8% (95%CI: 32.9%–83.1%, I^2 = 96%) and 49.5% (95%CI: 39.6%–59.4%, I^2 = 90%), respectively. Pooled estimated incidence of AKI and severe AKI requiring RRT while on venovenous (VV)-ECMO were 45.7% (95%CI: 33.2%–58.8%, I^2 = 47%) and 37.0% (95%CI: 14.8%–66.5%, I^2 = 95%), respectively. Meta-regression showed that year of the study did not significantly affect the incidence of AKI (p = 0.67) or AKI requiring RRT (p = 0.83), as shown in Figure 3.

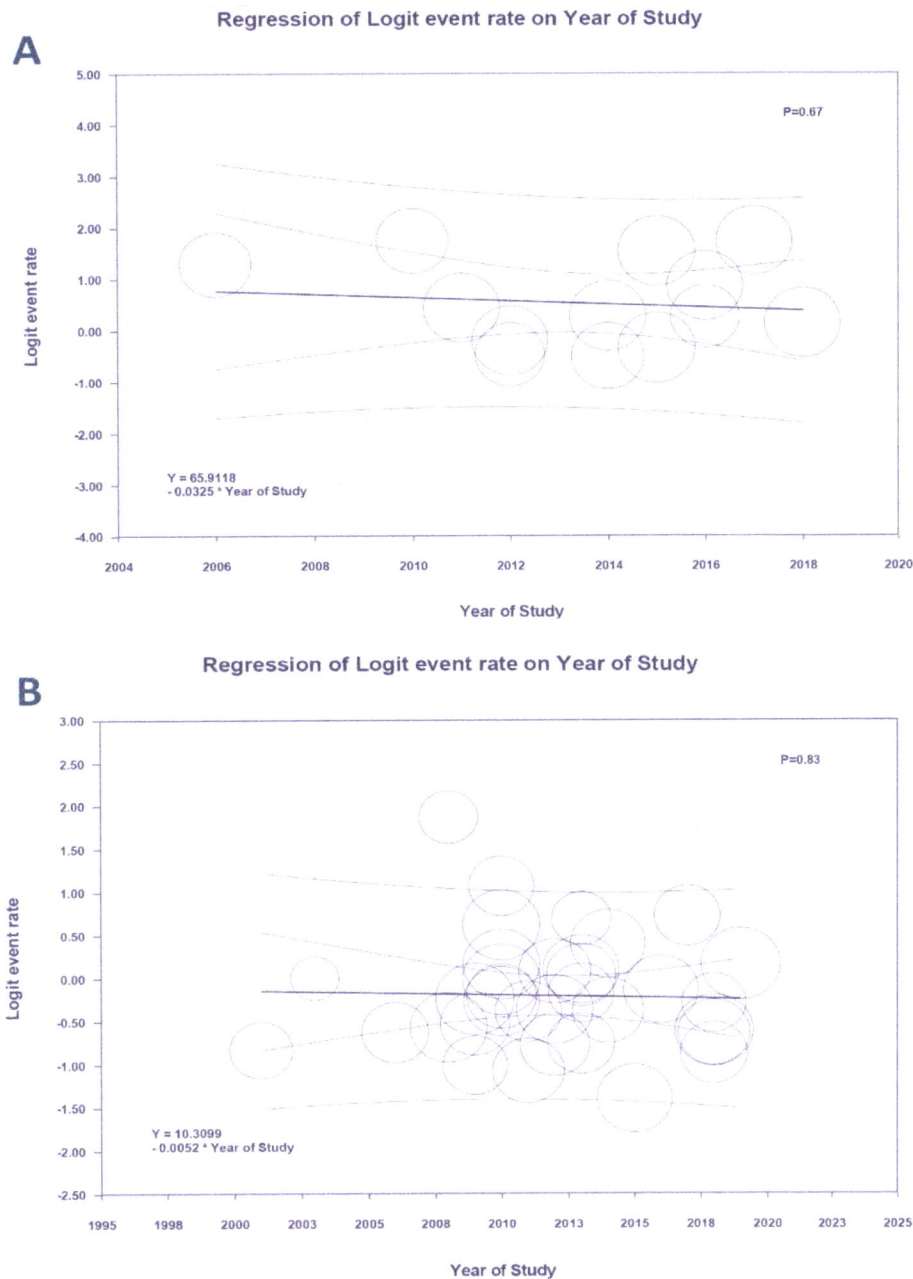

Figure 3. Meta-regression analyses showed that year of the study did not significantly affect (**A**) the incidence of AKI ($p = 0.67$) or (**B**) AKI requiring RRT ($p = 0.83$). The solid black line depicts the weighted regression line based on variance-weighted least squares. The inner and outer lines represent the 95%CI and prediction interval encompassing the regression line. The circles indicate log event rates in individual study.

3.2. AKI associated Mortality in Patients Requiring ECMO

Mortality rate and mortality risk associated with AKI in patients requiring ECMO are demonstrated in Tables 1 and 2, respectively. The pooled estimated hospital and/or 90-day mortality rates of patients with AKI and severe AKI requiring RRT while on ECMO were 62.0% (95%CI: 54.7%–68.8%, $I^2 = 73\%$, Figure 4A) and 68.4% (95%CI: 62.6%–73.6%, $I^2 = 87\%$, Figure 4B), respectively.

Table 2. Characteristics of studies included in this meta-analysis of AKI associated mortality risk among patients requiring ECMO.

Study.	Year	Number	Outcomes	Confounder Adjustment
Pagani et al. [15]	2001	33	Hospital mortality 8.25 (0.89–76.12)	None
Lin et al. [30]	2006	46	Hospital mortality AKI: 14.0 (2.46–79.55) CRRT: 16/16 vs. 14/30	None
Luo et al. [33]	2009	45	Hospital mortality CRRT: 7.0 (1.26–38.99)	None
Brogan et al. [34]	2009	1473	Hospital mortality Renal insufficiency/failure: 2.13 (1.69–2.72) RRT: 2.13 (1.73–2.63)	Age, duration of mechanical ventilation, weight, pre-ECMO pH, race, diagnosis, ECMO mode, post-ECMO complication
Elsharkawy et al. [37]	2010	233	Hospital mortality RRT: 3.18 (1.77–5.70)	None
Yan et al. [36]	2010	67	Hospital mortality RIFLE AKI: 8.0 (1.61–39.68) AKIN AKI: 12.38 (1.47–104.33) CRRT: 5.73 (1.98–16.58)	None
Lan et al. [39]	2010	607	Hospital mortality RRT: 6.49 (4.12–10.23)	Age, stroke, pre-ECMO infection, hypoglycemia, alkalosis
Chen et al. [67]	2011	102	Hospital mortality AKI: 4.32 (1.65–11.30) CRRT: 5.80 (1.82–18.43)	Age, GCS
Chang et al. [44]	2012	113	Hospital mortality AKI: 2.1 (1.48–3.00)	None
Wu et al. [48]	2012	60	Hospital mortality RRT: 3.76 (1.18–11.95)	None
Kielstein et al. [50]	2013	200	90-day mortality RRT: 5.47(2.87–10.44)	None

Table 2. *Cont.*

Study.	Year	Number	Outcomes	Confounder Adjustment
Aubron et al. [49]	2013	158	VA ECMO RRT: 2.12 (0.92–4.88) VV ECMO RRT: 2.52 (0.80–7.95)	None
Wu et al. [51]	2013	35	Hospital mortality RRT: 12 (2.08–69.09)	None
Slottosch et al. [23]	2013	77	30-day mortality Renal failure: 2.20 (0.78–6.12)	None
Unosawa et al. [53]	2013	47	Mortality during ECMO RRT: 1.67 (0.48–5.83)	None
Lazzeri et al. [52]	2013	25	Mortality RRT: 2.14 (0.38–12.20)	None
Hsiao et al. [55]	2014	81	Hospital mortality CRRT: 2.17 (0.87–5.45)	None
Schmidt et al. [7]	2014	172	Hospital mortality CRRT at ECMO day 1–3: 4.1 (1.71–9.82) 90-day mortality CRRT at ECMO day 1–3: 3.17 (1.32–7.61)	APACHE, fluid balance, major bleeding, propensity score
Lee et al. [56]	2015	322	Hospital mortality AKI: 3.71 (1.96–7.02)	None
Haneya et al. [57]	2015	262	Mortality AKI: 2.18 (1.31–3.61) RRT during ECMO: 1.72 (0.53–5.59)	Age, SOFA score, minute volume, pH, lactate, RRT prior to ECMO, RBC, and FFP transfusion
Huang et al. [58]	2016	23	Mortality AKI: 20.25 (1.88–218.39)	None

Table 2. *Cont.*

Study.	Year	Number	Outcomes	Confounder Adjustment
Lyu et al. [27]	2016	84	Mortality ARF: 23.90 (7.00–81.60)	None
Antonucci et al. [59]	2016	135	ICU mortality AKI: 1.86 (0.88–3.93) CRRT: 1.70 (0.85–3.37)	None
Tsai et al. [60]	2017	167	Hospital mortality RIFLE AKI: 8.55 (3.63–20.16) AKIN AKI: 13.53 (3.87–47.28) KDIGO AKI: 12.69 (3.62–44.46)	None
Panholzer et al. [61]	2017	46	Mortality RRT: 40.25 (4.54–356.93)	None
Martucci et al. [28]	2017	82	Mortality on ECMO AKI stage 3: 4.55 (1.37–15.17)	None
Chong et al. [62]	2018	35	Hospital mortality AKI: 9.33 (1.02–85.70) RRT: 11.0 (2.26–53.64)	None
Devasagayaraj et al. [63]	2018	54	Hospital mortality RRT: 5.69 (1.58–20.56)	None
Chen et al. [67]	2019	3,251	Hospital mortality RRT: 3.92 (3.36–4.57)	Age, sex, ECMO indication, comorbid conditions, hospital level, study year

Abbreviations: AKI, acute kidney injury; ARDS, acute respiratory distress syndrome; AKIN, Acute Kidney Injury Network; APACHE, Acute Physiology and Chronic Health Evaluation; CRRT, continuous renal replacement therapy; ECMO, Extracorporeal membrane oxygenation; FFP, fresh frozen plasma; GCS, Glasgow Coma Scale/Score; ICU, intensive care unit; KDIGO, Kidney Disease Improving Global Outcomes; N/A, not available; RIFLE, Risk, Injury, Failure, Loss of kidney function, and End-stage kidney disease; RBC, red blood cells; RRT, Renal replacement therapy; pH, potential hydrogen; SOFA, Sequential Organ Failure Assessment; VA-ECMO, venoarterial extracorporeal membrane oxygenation; VV-ECMO, venovenous extracorporeal membrane oxygenation.

A

Study name	Event rate	Lower limit	Upper limit	Z-Value	p-Value	Event rate and 95% CI	Relative weight
Lin et al	0.778	0.615	0.885	3.125	0.002		7.49
Yan et al	0.579	0.448	0.699	1.187	0.235		10.47
Chen et al	0.823	0.707	0.899	4.614	0.000		8.93
Chang et al	0.451	0.321	0.588	-0.699	0.485		10.14
Lee et al	0.570	0.509	0.628	2.265	0.023		14.03
Haneya et al	0.514	0.421	0.606	0.287	0.774		12.43
Huang et al	0.692	0.409	0.880	1.349	0.177		4.56
Antonucci et al	0.579	0.478	0.674	1.532	0.125		12.02
Tsai et al	0.714	0.629	0.786	4.646	0.000		12.29
Chong et al	0.538	0.350	0.716	0.392	0.695		7.64
	0.620	0.547	0.688	3.207	0.001		

-2.00   -1.00   0.00   1.00   2.00

No Mortality   Mortality

B

Study name	Event rate	Lower limit	Upper limit	Z-Value	p-Value	Event rate and 95% CI	Relative weight
Pagani et al	0.900	0.533	0.986	2.084	0.037		1.20
Yap et al	0.917	0.378	0.995	1.623	0.105		0.68
Lin et al	0.971	0.664	0.998	2.436	0.015		0.72
Tsai et al	0.760	0.668	0.832	5.014	0.000		4.87
Luo et al	0.778	0.421	0.944	1.562	0.118		1.80
Brogan et al	0.602	0.564	0.639	5.149	0.000		5.62
Yan et al	0.733	0.550	0.861	2.450	0.014		3.64
Elsharkawy et al	0.782	0.691	0.852	5.303	0.000		4.80
Lan et al	0.860	0.817	0.895	10.936	0.000		5.25
Wu et al (1)	0.706	0.611	0.786	4.029	0.000		4.95
Chen et al (1)	0.846	0.655	0.941	3.136	0.002		2.86
Wu et al (2)	0.684	0.452	0.851	1.567	0.117		3.14
Aubron et al	0.455	0.354	0.559	-0.852	0.394		4.97
Kielstein et al	0.829	0.750	0.887	6.430	0.000		4.77
Wu et al (3)	0.875	0.614	0.969	2.574	0.010		1.95
Lazzeri et al	0.563	0.324	0.775	0.499	0.618		3.08
Unosawa et al	0.467	0.241	0.707	-0.258	0.796		3.00
Schmidt et al	0.330	0.246	0.426	-3.378	0.001		5.00
Hsiao et al	0.667	0.492	0.805	1.877	0.061		3.92
Haneya et al	0.442	0.315	0.578	-0.830	0.406		4.54
Antonucci et al	0.603	0.479	0.716	1.626	0.104		4.69
Panholzer et al	0.742	0.563	0.865	2.573	0.010		3.65
Chong et al	0.733	0.467	0.896	1.733	0.083		2.66
Devasagayaraj et al	0.563	0.324	0.775	0.499	0.618		3.08
Paek et al	0.659	0.603	0.711	5.366	0.000		5.47
He et al	0.594	0.419	0.747	1.054	0.292		3.99
Chen et al (2)	0.738	0.717	0.758	19.093	0.000		5.69
	0.684	0.626	0.736	5.943	0.000		

-2.00   -1.00   0.00   1.00   2.00

No Mortality   Mortality

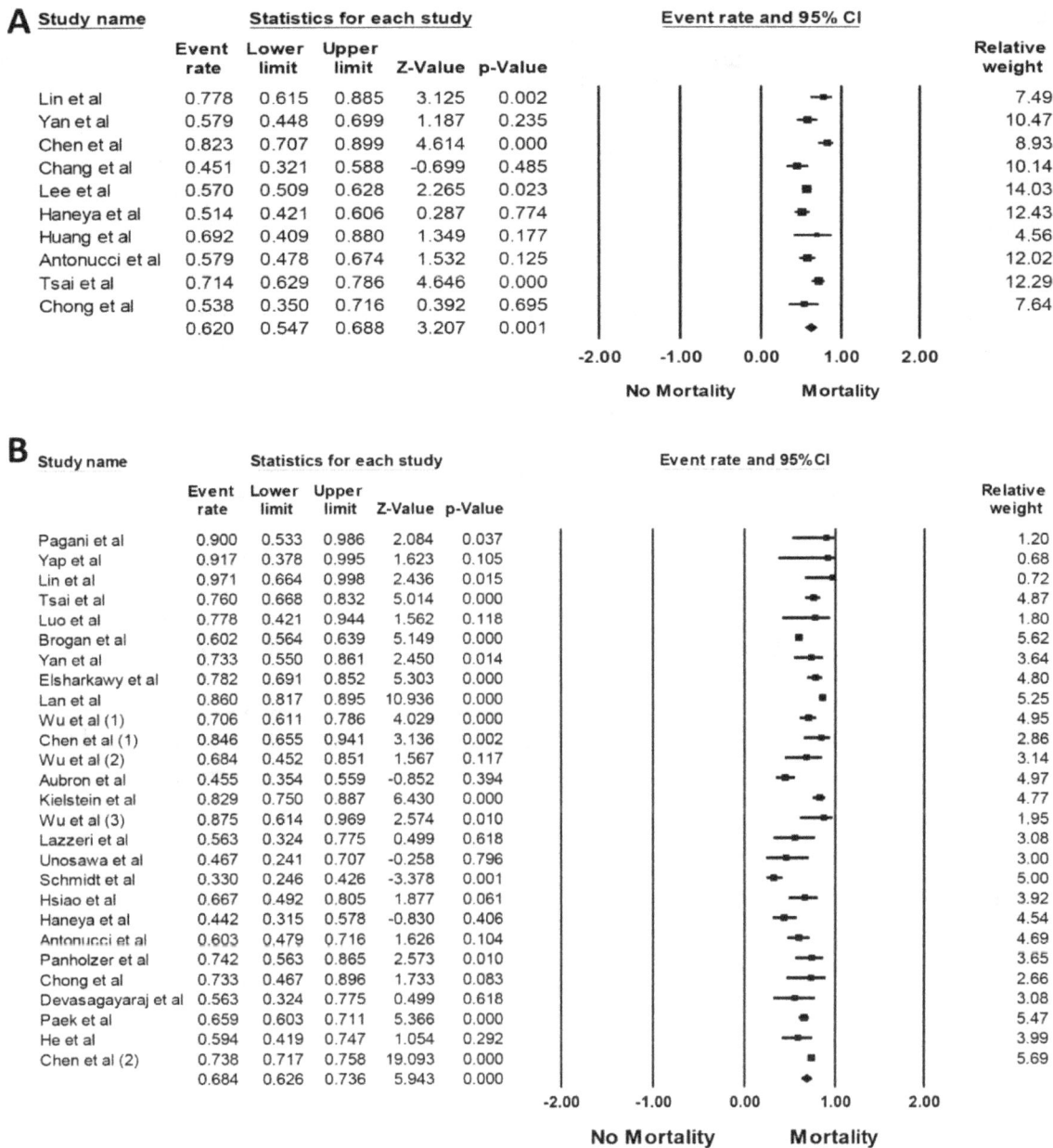

Figure 4. Forest plots of the included studies assessing (**A**) mortality rate of patients with AKI while on ECMO and (**B**) mortality rate of patients with severe AKI requiring RRT while on ECMO. A diamond data label serves as the overall rate from each study (square data marker) and 95%CI.

The pooled OR of hospital mortality among patients receiving ECMO with AKI on RRT was 3.73 (95% CI, 2.87–4.85, $I^2 = 62\%$, Figure 5A). When the analysis was limited to studies with confounder-adjusted analysis, the increased hospital mortality remained significant among patients receiving ECMO with AKI requiring RRT with pooled OR of 3.32 (95% CI, 2.21–4.99, $I^2 = 82\%$, Figure 5B).

A Study name | Statistics for each study | Odds ratio and 95% CI

Study name	Odds ratio	Lower limit	Upper limit	Z-Value	p-Value	Relative weight
Pagani et al	8.250	0.892	76.297	1.859	0.063	1.26
Luo et al	7.000	1.258	38.939	2.222	0.026	1.98
Yan et al	5.730	1.980	16.581	3.220	0.001	4.11
Chen et al (1)	5.800	1.823	18.457	2.976	0.003	3.65
Kielstein et al	5.470	2.868	10.433	5.158	0.000	7.11
Wu et al (1)	12.000	2.082	69.160	2.781	0.005	1.91
Lazzeri et al	2.140	0.378	12.126	0.860	0.390	1.94
Schmidt et al	4.100	1.711	9.825	3.164	0.002	5.24
Antonucci et al	1.700	0.854	3.385	1.510	0.131	6.72
Chong et al	11.000	2.258	53.590	2.968	0.003	2.26
Devasagayaraj et al	5.690	1.577	20.526	2.656	0.008	3.14
Aubron et al	2.520	0.799	7.944	1.578	0.115	3.69
Brogan et al	2.130	1.728	2.626	7.076	0.000	11.54
Elsahrkawy et al	3.180	1.772	5.707	3.878	0.000	7.71
Hsaio et al	2.170	0.867	5.431	1.655	0.098	4.95
Lan et al	6.490	4.119	10.227	8.061	0.000	9.07
Unosawa et al	1.670	0.479	5.820	0.805	0.421	3.27
Wu et al (2)	3.760	1.182	11.965	2.242	0.025	3.65
Panholzer et al	40.250	4.539	356.886	3.319	0.001	1.30
Haneya et al	1.720	0.530	5.586	0.902	0.367	3.56
Chen (2)	3.920	3.361	4.572	17.410	0.000	11.94
	3.730	2.868	4.852	9.812	0.000	

0.01   0.1   1   10   100
Lower Mortality   Higher Mortality

B Study name | Statistics for each study | Odds ratio and 95% CI

Study name	Odds ratio	Lower limit	Upper limit	Z-Value	p-Value	Relative weight
Brogan et al	2.130	1.728	2.626	7.076	0.000	22.40
Lan et al	6.490	4.119	10.227	8.061	0.000	18.34
Chen et al (1)	5.800	1.823	18.457	2.976	0.003	8.11
Schmidt et al	4.100	1.711	9.825	3.164	0.002	11.32
Haneya et al	1.720	0.530	5.586	0.902	0.367	7.92
Antonucci et al	1.380	0.470	4.056	0.586	0.558	8.89
Chen et al (2)	3.920	3.361	4.572	17.410	0.000	23.03
	3.323	2.214	4.986	5.797	0.000	

0.01   0.1   1   10   100
Lower Mortality   Higher Mortality

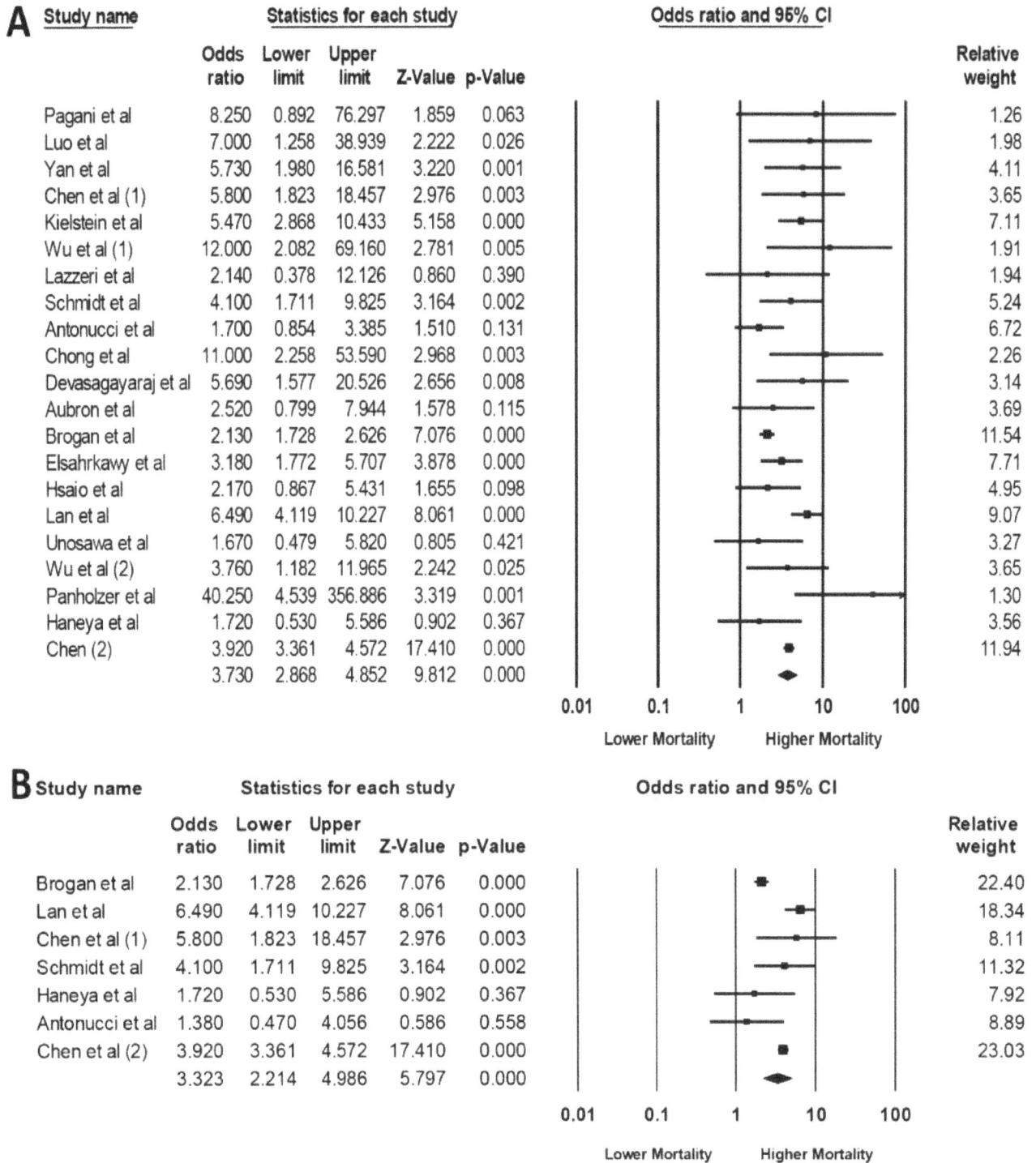

Figure 5. Forest plots of the included studies assessing (**A**) hospital mortality among patients receiving ECMO with AKI on RRT and (**B**) hospital mortality among patients receiving ECMO with AKI on RRT limited to studies with confounder-adjusted analysis. A diamond data label serves as the overall rate from each included study (square data marker) and 95%CI.

Meta-regression showed that year of the study did not significantly affect hospital mortality among patients receiving ECMO with AKI requiring RRT ($p = 0.86$), as shown in Figure 6.

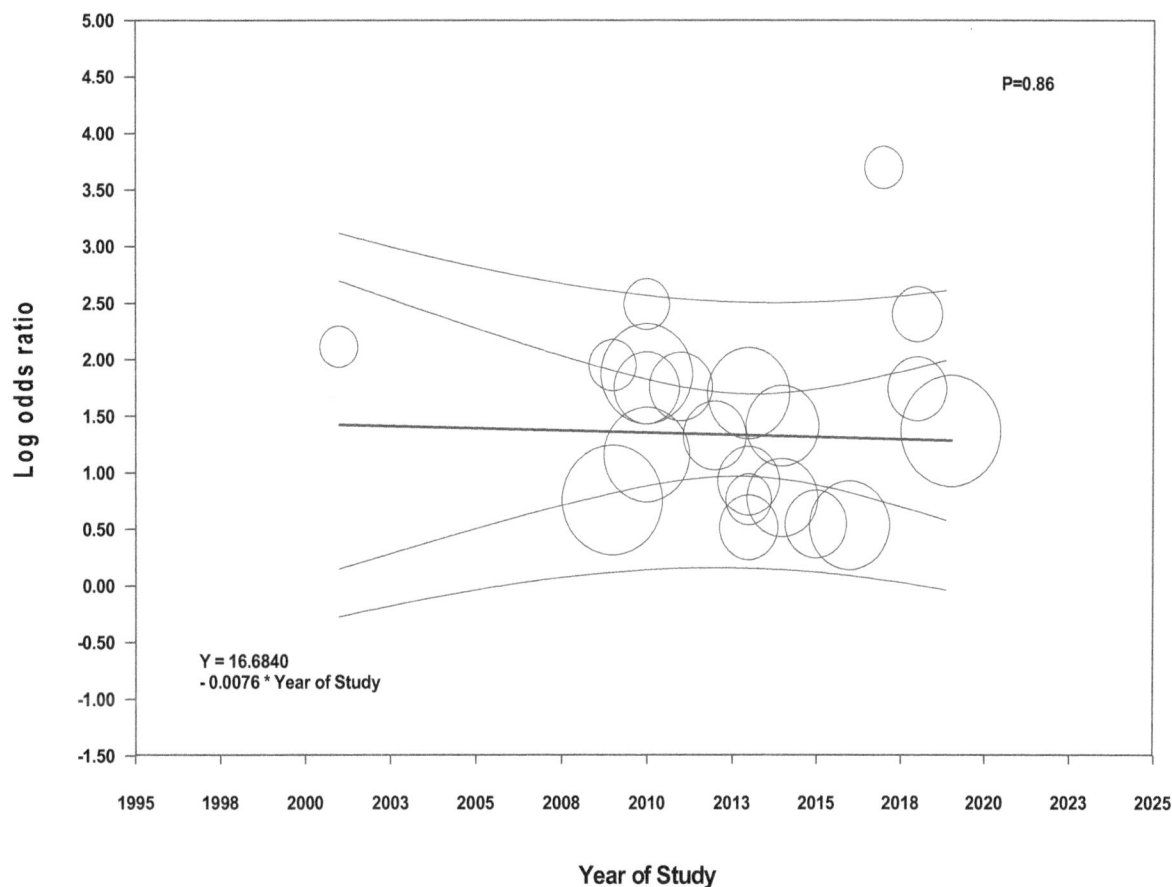

Regression of Log odds ratio on Year of Study

Figure 6. Meta-regression analyses showed that year of the study did not significantly affect hospital mortality among patients receiving ECMO with AKI requiring RRT ($p = 0.86$). The solid black line depicts the weighted regression line based on variance-weighted least squares. The inner and outer lines represent the 95%CI and prediction interval encompassing the regression line. The circles indicate log event rates in an individual study.

3.3. Evaluation for Publication Bias

Funnel plots (Figure 7) and Egger's regression asymmetry tests were utilized to assess for publication bias in our meta-analyses evaluating the incidence of AKI and severe AKI requiring RRT while on ECMO. There was no publication bias as determined by the funnel plot and Egger's regression asymmetry test with $p = 0.62$ and $p = 0.17$ for the incidence of AKI and severe AKI requiring RRT, respectively.

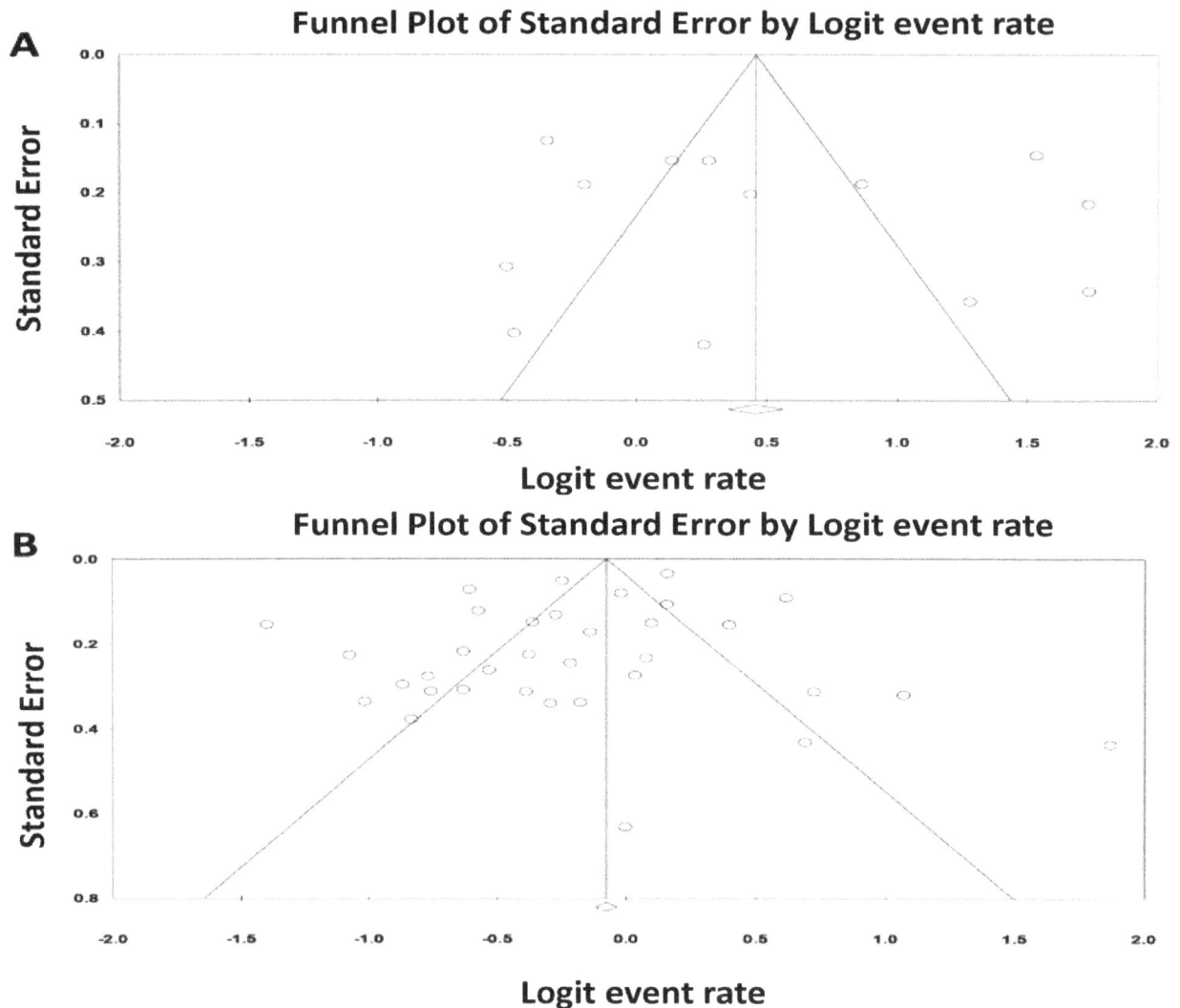

Figure 7. Funnel plot demonstrated no publication bias in analyses evaluating (**A**) incidence of AKI in patients requiring ECMO and (**B**) severe AKI requiring RRT.

4. Discussion

The findings of our meta-analysis demonstrate that patients who required ECMO had incidence rates of AKI (using standard AKI definitions) and severe AKI requiring RRT of 62.8% and 44.9%, respectively. Moreover, patients with AKI and severe AKI requiring RRT had high associated mortality rates of 62.0% and 68.4%, respectively.

Although the mechanisms underlying ECMO associated-AKI remains unclear, it is likely complex and multifactorial, including contributing factors such as primary disease progression, altered hemodynamics, low cardiac output syndrome, exposure to nephrotoxic agents (for management of underlying diseases), new-onset sepsis, high intrathoracic pressures, fluid overload, ischemia-reperfusion injury, release of proinflammatory mediators and oxidative stress, hemolysis and iron-mediated (hemoglobin-induced) renal injury, and hypercoagulable state resulting in renal microembolisms [4,8,68,78,79]. Studies have demonstrated the activation of proinflammatory mediators such as tumor necrosis factor-alpha (TNF-α), interleukins (e.g., IL-1β, IL-6, IL-8) and other cytokine signaling cascades due to the continuous exposure of blood to non-biological and non-endothelialized ECMO interface [68,80,81]. Activation of the inflammatory cascades can result in hyperdynamic vasodilated hypotensive states, leading to AKI [68,78].

Following the initiation of ECMO treatment, there are improvements in oxygenation and oxygen consumption as well as hemodynamics [3,5–9]. However, ischemia-reperfusion injury can also occur after the restoration of circulation to previously hypoxic cells and hypoperfused organs, leading to the production of reactive oxygen species (ROS) and oxidative stress-mediated injury [68,78]. In addition, ECMO-associated complications or adverse effects such as hemolysis, hemorrhage or thrombosis also can play important roles in the development of AKI [29,68,82–84]. Despite the advance of a new miniaturized ECMO system, hemolysis due to shear stress from the ECMO circuit has been reported among ECMO patients with incidences between 5% and 18% [17,85–87]. This can contribute to heme pigment-induced AKI [83,84]. Although improvements in the ECMO technology have led to less thrombus development in its circuit with an improved capacity of the circuit to remove large emboli [68,82], smaller thrombi can still develop and result in renal microembolism [68,82], particularly with VA-ECMO [82].

The type of ECMO may also differently affect AKI risk. Our study demonstrated a higher incidence of AKI among patients requiring VA-ECMO (60.8%) than those requiring VV-ECMO (45.7%). While VV-ECMO is typically utilized for patients with isolated respiratory failure, VA-ECMO is used for combined severe cardiac and respiratory failure [4]. In VA-ECMO, there is a mixture of pulsatile arterial flow from the native heart and non-pulsatile arterial flow from the ECMO pump. Conversely, VV-ECMO maintains pulsatile cardiac output, and alterations in renal perfusion may conceivably be smaller [4]. Recent studies have shown that pulsatile flow may provide beneficial effects over non-pulsatile flow, especially protective effects on microcirculation and renal perfusion [88–90]. The differences in patient population and pulsatility between the two types of ECMO are likely explanations underlying the higher AKI incidence among patients requiring VA-ECMO.

As there is no treatment available for AKI, management of AKI is limited to appropriate secondary preventive measures and supportive strategies [91–96]. RRT in the form of continuous renal replacement therapy (CRRT) is often required among patients requiring ECMO with severe AKI [42,55,97]. Our study demonstrated no significant correlation between the year of study and the incidence of AKI and/or severe AKI requiring RRT despite considerable changes in technology and practice of ECMO among adult patients. Furthermore, we showed a 3.7-fold increased risk of hospital mortality among ECMO patients with severe AKI requiring RRT. Thus, prevention and early identification of AKI among patients at-risk of ECMO-associated AKI could potentially play a crucial role in improved survival. Studies have shown several important AKI risk factors among patients requiring ECMO including older age, elevated lactate levels before ECMO initiation, high dose of inotropic drugs, severely reduced left ventricular ejection fraction, cirrhosis, postcardiotomy shock as an indication for ECMO, and finally ECMO pump speed and its duration [56,64,67]. Lee et al. recently observed a lower AKI association with a higher ECMO pump speed [56]. Although the underlying pathophysiology remains unclear, excessive ECMO pump speed has been shown to induce hemolysis and complement activation in vitro and animal model [98,99]. In pediatric patients receiving ECMO, Lou et al. also demonstrated higher pump speeds are associated with hemolysis and a number of other adverse clinical outcomes [100]. To prevent hemolysis-mediated kidney injury, it is suggested to limit pump revolutions/min (RPM) to safe levels (i.e., 3000 to 3500 RPM) in order to avoid excessive negative pressures generated within the pump [101]. Future prospective studies are required to assess the effects of ECMO pump speed on AKI risk in ECMO patients. In addition, future studies creating risk prediction models for ECMO-associated AKI are needed to assist with the prevention of AKI in a timely manner, which could potentially lead to an improvement in patient survival.

Our study has several limitations. Firstly, there are statistical heterogeneities in our meta-analysis. Potential sources for heterogeneities were the variations in patient characteristics among the included studies. However, we performed subgroup analysis to assess the AKI incidence based on types of ECMO and a separate meta-analysis that only included studies with confounder-adjusted analysis for mortality risk. Another limitation was that AKI diagnosis was mainly based on serum creatinine [102–104] while the data on urine output and novel biomarkers for AKI [105–108] were limited. Lastly, this systematic review is primarily based on observational studies, as the data from clinical trials or population-based studies were limited. Therefore, it can at best, demonstrate an association but not a causal relationship.

5. Conclusions

In conclusion, there is an overall high incidence of AKI and severe AKI requiring RRT in ECMO patients of 62.8% and 44.9%, respectively. The incidence of ECMO-associated AKI has not changed over time. AKI requiring RRT while on ECMO is associated with 3.7-fold increased risk of hospital mortality. Future studies should focus on strategies for prediction, detection, and prevention of AKI among patients who receive ECMO.

Author Contributions: Conceptualization, C.T., W.C., M.A.M. and K.K.; Data curation, C.T., W.C. and P.L.; Formal analysis, C.T., W.C.; Funding acquisition, K.K.; Investigation, C.T., W.C., P.L. and K.K.; Methodology, C.T., W.C. and K.K.; Project administration, P.L., K.W. and N.S.; Resources, P.L., T.B. and K.W.; Software, K.W.; Supervision, M.A.M. and K.K.; Validation, W.C. and P.L.; Visualization, W.C., T.B. and K.K.; Writing – original draft, C.T. and N.R.A; Writing – review & editing, C.T., W.C., P.L., N.R.A., T.B., K.W., N.S., M.A.M. and K.K.

References

1. Guru, P.K.; Singh, T.D.; Passe, M.; Kashani, K.B.; Schears, G.J.; Kashyap, R. Derivation and Validation of a Search Algorithm to Retrospectively Identify CRRT Initiation in the ECMO Patients. *Appl. Clin. Inform.* **2016**, *7*, 596–603. [CrossRef] [PubMed]
2. Hill, J.D.; O'Brien, T.G.; Murray, J.J.; Dontigny, L.; Bramson, M.L.; Osborn, J.J.; Gerbode, F. Prolonged extracorporeal oxygenation for acute post-traumatic respiratory failure (shock-lung syndrome). Use of the Bramson membrane lung. *N. Engl. J. Med.* **1972**, *286*, 629–634. [CrossRef] [PubMed]
3. Peek, G.J.; Mugford, M.; Tiruvoipati, R.; Wilson, A.; Allen, E.; Thalanany, M.M.; Hibbert, C.L.; Truesdale, A.; Clemens, F.; Cooper, N.; et al. Efficacy and economic assessment of conventional ventilatory support versus extracorporeal membrane oxygenation for severe adult respiratory failure (CESAR): A multicentre randomised controlled trial. *Lancet* **2009**, *374*, 1351–1363. [CrossRef]
4. Chen, Y.C.; Tsai, F.C.; Fang, J.T.; Yang, C.W. Acute kidney injury in adults receiving extracorporeal membrane oxygenation. *J. Formos. Med. Assoc.* **2014**, *113*, 778–785. [CrossRef] [PubMed]
5. Thiagarajan, R.R.; Barbaro, R.P.; Rycus, P.T.; Mcmullan, D.M.; Conrad, S.A.; Fortenberry, J.D.; Paden, M.L. Extracorporeal Life Support Organization Registry International Report 2016. *ASAIO J.* **2017**, *63*, 60–67. [CrossRef] [PubMed]
6. Paden, M.L.; Conrad, S.A.; Rycus, P.T.; Thiagarajan, R.R. Extracorporeal Life Support Organization Registry Report 2012. *ASAIO J.* **2013**, *59*, 202–210. [CrossRef]
7. Schmidt, M.; Bailey, M.; Kelly, J.; Hodgson, C.; Cooper, D.J.; Scheinkestel, C.; Pellegrino, V.; Bellomo, R.; Pilcher, D. Impact of fluid balance on outcome of adult patients treated with extracorporeal membrane oxygenation. *Intensive Care Med.* **2014**, *40*, 1256–1266. [CrossRef]
8. Hamdi, T.; Palmer, B.F. Review of Extracorporeal Membrane Oxygenation and Dialysis-Based Liver Support Devices for the Use of Nephrologists. *Am. J. Nephrol.* **2017**, *46*, 139–149. [CrossRef]
9. Husain-Syed, F.; Ricci, Z.; Brodie, D.; Vincent, J.L.; Ranieri, V.M.; Slutsky, A.S.; Taccone, F.S.; Gattinoni, L.; Ronco, C. Extracorporeal organ support (ECOS) in critical illness and acute kidney injury: From native to artificial organ crosstalk. *Intensive Care Med.* **2018**, *44*, 1447–1459. [CrossRef]
10. Bosarge, P.L.; Raff, L.A.; McGwin, G., Jr.; Carroll, S.L.; Bellot, S.C.; Diaz-Guzman, E.; Kerby, J.D. Early initiation of extracorporeal membrane oxygenation improves survival in adult trauma patients with severe adult respiratory distress syndrome. *J. Trauma Acute Care Surg.* **2016**, *81*, 236–243. [CrossRef]
11. Combes, A.; Leprince, P.; Luyt, C.E.; Bonnet, N.; Trouillet, J.L.; Léger, P.; Pavie, A.; Chastre, J. Outcomes and long-term quality-of-life of patients supported by extracorporeal membrane oxygenation for refractory cardiogenic shock. *Crit. Care Med.* **2008**, *36*, 1404–1411. [CrossRef] [PubMed]

12. Massetti, M.; Tasle, M.; Le Page, O.; Deredec, R.; Babatasi, G.; Buklas, D.; Thuaudet, S.; Charbonneau, P.; Hamon, M.; Grollier, G.; et al. Back from irreversibility: Extracorporeal life support for prolonged cardiac arrest. *Ann. Thorac. Surg.* **2005**, *79*, 178–183. [CrossRef] [PubMed]

13. Shin, T.G.; Choi, J.H.; Jo, I.J.; Sim, M.S.; Song, H.G.; Jeong, Y.K.; Song, Y.B.; Hahn, J.Y.; Choi, S.H.; Gwon, H.C.; et al. Extracorporeal cardiopulmonary resuscitation in patients with inhospital cardiac arrest: A comparison with conventional cardiopulmonary resuscitation. *Crit. Care Med.* **2011**, *39*, 1–7. [CrossRef] [PubMed]

14. Bednarczyk, J.M.; White, C.W.; Ducas, R.A.; Golian, M.; Nepomuceno, R.; Hiebert, B.; Bueddefeld, D.; Manji, R.A.; Singal, R.K.; Hussain, F.; et al. Resuscitative extracorporeal membrane oxygenation for in hospital cardiac arrest: A Canadian observational experience. *Resuscitation* **2014**, *85*, 1713–1719. [CrossRef] [PubMed]

15. Pagani, F.D.; Aaronson, K.D.; Swaniker, F.; Bartlett, R.H. The use of extracorporeal life support in adult patients with primary cardiac failure as a bridge to implantable left ventricular assist device. *Ann. Thorac. Surg.* **2001**, *71* (Suppl. 3), S77–S81. [CrossRef]

16. Kagawa, E.; Dote, K.; Kato, M.; Sasaki, S.; Nakano, Y.; Kajikawa, M.; Higashi, A.; Itakura, K.; Sera, A.; Inoue, I.; et al. Should we emergently revascularize occluded coronaries for cardiac arrest?: Rapid-response extracorporeal membrane oxygenation and intra-arrest percutaneous coronary intervention. *Circulation* **2012**, *126*, 1605–1613. [CrossRef]

17. Zangrillo, A.; Landoni, G.; Biondi-Zoccai, G.; Greco, M.; Greco, T.; Frati, G.; Patroniti, N.; Antonelli, M.; Pesenti, A.; Pappalardo, F. A meta-analysis of complications and mortality of extracorporeal membrane oxygenation. *Crit. Care Resusc.* **2013**, *15*, 172–178.

18. Ostermann, M.; Connor, M.; Jr Kashani, K. Continuous renal replacement therapy during extracorporeal membrane oxygenation: Why, when and how? *Curr. Opin. Crit. Care* **2018**, *24*, 493–503. [CrossRef]

19. Kagawa, E.; Inoue, I.; Kawagoe, T.; Ishihara, M.; Shimatani, Y.; Kurisu, S.; Nakama, Y.; Dai, K.; Takayuki, O.; Ikenaga, H.; et al. Assessment of outcomes and differences between in- and out-of-hospital cardiac arrest patients treated with cardiopulmonary resuscitation using extracorporeal life support. *Resuscitation* **2010**, *81*, 968–973. [CrossRef]

20. Hei, F.; Lou, S.; Li, J.; Yu, K.; Liu, J.; Feng, Z.; Zhao, J.; Hu, S.; Xu, J.; Chang, Q.; et al. Five-year results of 121 consecutive patients treated with extracorporeal membrane oxygenation at Fu Wai Hospital. *Artif. Organs* **2011**, *35*, 572–578. [CrossRef]

21. Tsai, T.Y.; Tsai, F.C.; Chang, C.H.; Jenq, C.C.; Hsu, H.H.; Chang, M.Y.; Tian, Y.C.; Hung, C.C.; Fang, J.T.; Yang, C.W.; et al. Prognosis of patients on extracorporeal membrane oxygenation plus continuous arteriovenous hemofiltration. *Chang. Gung Med. J.* **2011**, *34*, 636–643. [PubMed]

22. Belle, L.; Mangin, L.; Bonnet, H.; Fol, S.; Santre, C.; Delavenat, L.; Savary, D.; Bougon, D.; Vialle, E.; Dompnier, A.; et al. Emergency extracorporeal membrane oxygenation in a hospital without on-site cardiac surgical facilities. *EuroIntervention* **2012**, *8*, 375–382. [CrossRef] [PubMed]

23. Slottosch, I.; Liakopoulos, O.; Kuhn, E.; Deppe, A.C.; Scherner, M.; Madershahian, N.; Choi, Y.H.; Wahlers, T. Outcomes after peripheral extracorporeal membrane oxygenation therapy for postcardiotomy cardiogenic shock: A single-center experience. *J. Surg. Res.* **2013**, *181*, e47–e55. [CrossRef] [PubMed]

24. Seco, M.; Forrest, P.; Jackson, S.A.; Martinez, G.; Andvik, S.; Bannon, P.G.; Ng, M.; Fraser, J.F.; Wilson, M.K.; Vallely, M.P. Extracorporeal membrane oxygenation for very high-risk transcatheter aortic valve implantation. *Heart Lung Circ.* **2014**, *23*, 957–962. [CrossRef] [PubMed]

25. Saxena, P.; Neal, J.; Joyce, L.D.; Greason, K.L.; Schaff, H.V.; Guru, P.; Shi, W.Y.; Burkhart, H.; Li, Z.; Oliver, W.C.; et al. Extracorporeal Membrane Oxygenation Support in Postcardiotomy Elderly Patients: The Mayo Clinic Experience. *Ann. Thorac. Surg.* **2015**, *99*, 2053–2060. [CrossRef] [PubMed]

26. Thajudeen, B.; Kamel, M.; Arumugam, C.; Ali, S.A.; John, S.G.; Meister, E.E.; Mosier, J.M.; Raz, Y.; Madhrira, M.; Thompson, J.; et al. Outcome of patients on combined extracorporeal membrane oxygenation and continuous renal replacement therapy: A retrospective study. *Int. J. Artif. Organs* **2015**, *38*, 133–137. [CrossRef] [PubMed]

27. Lyu, L.; Long, C.; Hei, F.; Ji, B.; Liu, J.; Yu, K.; Chen, L.; Yao, J.; Hu, Q.; Hu, J.; et al. Plasma Free Hemoglobin Is a Predictor of Acute Renal Failure During Adult Venous-Arterial Extracorporeal Membrane Oxygenation Support. *J. Cardiothorac. Vasc. Anesth.* **2016**, *30*, 891–895. [CrossRef]

28. Martucci, G.; Panarello, G.; Occhipinti, G. Anticoagulation and Transfusions Management in Veno-Venous Extracorporeal Membrane Oxygenation for Acute Respiratory Distress Syndrome: Assessment of Factors Associated With Transfusion Requirements and Mortality. *J. Intensive Care Med.* **2017**, *34*, 630–639. [CrossRef]

29. Yap, H.J.; Chen, Y.C.; Fang, J.T.; Huang, C.C. Combination of continuous renal replacement therapies (CRRT) and extracorporeal membrane oxygenation (ECMO) for advanced cardiac patients. *Ren. Fail.* **2003**, *25*, 183–193. [CrossRef]

30. Lin, C.Y.; Chen, Y.C.; Tsai, F.C.; Tian, Y.C.; Jenq, C.C.; Fang, J.T.; Yang, C.W. RIFLE classification is predictive of short-term prognosis in critically ill patients with acute renal failure supported by extracorporeal membrane oxygenation. *Nephrol. Dial. Transplant.* **2006**, *21*, 2867–2873. [CrossRef]

31. Tsai, C.W.; Lin, Y.F.; Wu, V.C.; Chu, T.S.; Chen, Y.M.; Hu, F.C.; Wu, K.D.; Ko, W.J. SAPS 3 at dialysis commencement is predictive of hospital mortality in patients supported by extracorporeal membrane oxygenation and acute dialysis. *Eur. J. Cardiothorac. Surg.* **2008**, *34*, 1158–1164. [CrossRef]

32. Bakhtiary, F.; Keller, H.; Dogan, S.; Dzemali, O.; Oezaslan, F.; Meininger, D.; Ackermann, H.; Zwissler, B.; Kleine, P.; Moritz, A. Venoarterial extracorporeal membrane oxygenation for treatment of cardiogenic shock: Clinical experiences in 45 adult patients. *J. Thorac. Cardiovasc. Surg.* **2008**, *135*, 382–388. [CrossRef] [PubMed]

33. Luo, X.J.; Wang, W.; Hu, S.S.; Sun, H.S.; Gao, H.W.; Long, C.; Song, Y.H.; Xu, J.P. Extracorporeal membrane oxygenation for treatment of cardiac failure in adult patients. *Interact. Cardiovasc. Thorac. Surg.* **2009**, *9*, 296–300. [CrossRef] [PubMed]

34. Brogan, T.V.; Thiagarajan, R.R.; Rycus, P.T.; Bartlett, R.H.; Bratton, S.L. Extracorporeal membrane oxygenation in adults with severe respiratory failure: A multi-center database. *Intensive Care Med.* **2009**, *35*, 2105–2114. [CrossRef]

35. Wang, J.; Han, J.; Jia, Y.; Zeng, W.; Shi, J.; Hou, X.; Meng, X. Early and intermediate results of rescue extracorporeal membrane oxygenation in adult cardiogenic shock. *Ann. Thorac. Surg.* **2009**, *88*, 1897–1903. [CrossRef] [PubMed]

36. Yan, X.; Jia, S.; Meng, X.; Dong, P.; Jia, M.; Wan, J.; Hou, X. Acute kidney injury in adult postcardiotomy patients with extracorporeal membrane oxygenation: Evaluation of the RIFLE classification and the Acute Kidney Injury Network criteria. *Eur. J. Cardiothorac. Surg.* **2010**, *37*, 334–338. [CrossRef]

37. Elsharkawy, H.A.; Li, L.; Esa, W.A.; Sessler, D.I.; Bashour, C.A. Outcome in patients who require venoarterial extracorporeal membrane oxygenation support after cardiac surgery. *J. Cardiothorac. Vasc. Anesth.* **2010**, *24*, 946–951. [CrossRef]

38. Hsu, P.S.; Chen, J.L.; Hong, G.J.; Tsai, Y.T.; Lin, C.Y.; Lee, C.Y.; Chen, Y.G.; Tsai, C.S. Extracorporeal membrane oxygenation for refractory cardiogenic shock after cardiac surgery: Predictors of early mortality and outcome from 51 adult patients. *Eur. J. Cardiothorac. Surg.* **2010**, *37*, 328–333. [CrossRef]

39. Lan, C.; Tsai, P.R.; Chen, Y.S.; Ko, W.J. Prognostic factors for adult patients receiving extracorporeal membrane oxygenation as mechanical circulatory support—A 14-year experience at a medical center. *Artif. Organs* **2010**, *34*, E59–E64. [CrossRef]

40. Rastan, A.J.; Dege, A.; Mohr, M.; Doll, N.; Falk, V.; Walther, T.; Mohr, F.W. Early and late outcomes of 517 consecutive adult patients treated with extracorporeal membrane oxygenation for refractory postcardiotomy cardiogenic shock. *J. Thorac. Cardiovasc. Surg.* **2010**, *139*, 302–311. [CrossRef]

41. Wu, V.C.; Tsai, H.B.; Yeh, Y.C.; Huang, T.M.; Lin, Y.F.; Chou, N.K.; Chen, Y.S.; Han, Y.Y.; Chou, A.; Lin, Y.H.; et al. Patients supported by extracorporeal membrane oxygenation and acute dialysis: Acute physiology and chronic health evaluation score in predicting hospital mortality. *Artif. Organs* **2010**, *34*, 828–835. [CrossRef] [PubMed]

42. Chen, Y.C.; Tsai, F.C.; Chang, C.H.; Lin, C.Y.; Jenq, C.C.; Juan, K.C.; Hsu, H.H.; Chang, M.Y.; Tian, Y.C.; Hung, C.C.; et al. Prognosis of patients on extracorporeal membrane oxygenation: The impact of acute kidney injury on mortality. *Ann. Thorac. Surg.* **2011**, *91*, 137–142. [CrossRef] [PubMed]

43. Bermudez, C.A.; Rocha, R.V.; Toyoda, Y.; Zaldonis, D.; Sappington, P.L.; Mulukutla, S.; Marroquin, O.C.; Toma, C.; Bhama, J.K.; Kormos, R.L. Extracorporeal membrane oxygenation for advanced refractory shock in acute and chronic cardiomyopathy. *Ann. Thorac. Surg.* **2011**, *92*, 2125–2131. [CrossRef] [PubMed]

44. Chang, W.W.; Tsai, F.C.; Tsai, T.Y.; Chang, C.H.; Jenq, C.C.; Chang, M.Y.; Tian, Y.C.; Hung, C.C.; Fang, J.T.; Yang, C.W.; et al. Predictors of mortality in patients successfully weaned from extracorporeal membrane oxygenation. *PLoS ONE* **2012**, *7*, e42687. [CrossRef] [PubMed]

45. Kim, T.H.; Lim, C.; Park, I.; Kim, D.J.; Jung, Y.; Park, K.H. Prognosis in the patients with prolonged extracorporeal membrane oxygenation. *Korea J. Thorac. Cardiovasc. Surg.* **2012**, *45*, 236–241. [CrossRef] [PubMed]

46. Lee, S.H.; Chung, C.H.; Won Lee, J.; Ho Jung, S.; Choo, S.J. Factors predicting early- and long-term survival in patients undergoing extracorporeal membrane oxygenation (ECMO). *J. Card. Surg.* **2012**, *27*, 255–263. [CrossRef] [PubMed]

47. Loforte, A.; Montalto, A.; Ranocchi, F.; Della Monica, P.L.; Casali, G.; Lappa, A.; Menichetti, A.; Contento, C.; Musumeci, F. Peripheral extracorporeal membrane oxygenation system as salvage treatment of patients with refractory cardiogenic shock: Preliminary outcome evaluation. *Artif. Organs* **2012**, *36*, E53–E61. [CrossRef] [PubMed]

48. Wu, M.Y.; Lee, M.Y.; Lin, C.C.; Chang, Y.S.; Tsai, F.C.; Lin, P.J. Resuscitation of non-postcardiotomy cardiogenic shock or cardiac arrest with extracorporeal life support: The role of bridging to intervention. *Resuscitation* **2012**, *83*, 976–981. [CrossRef]

49. Aubron, C.; Cheng, A.C.; Pilcher, D.; Leong, T.; Magrin, G.; Cooper, D.J.; Scheinkestel, C.; Pellegrino, V. Factors associated with outcomes of patients on extracorporeal membrane oxygenation support: A 5-year cohort study. *Crit. Care* **2013**, *17*, R73. [CrossRef]

50. Kielstein, J.T.; Heiden, A.M.; Beutel, G.; Gottlieb, J.; Wiesner, O.; Hafer, C.; Hadem, J.; Reising, A.; Haverich, A.; Kühn, C.; et al. Renal function and survival in 200 patients undergoing ECMO therapy. *Nephrol. Dial. Transplant.* **2013**, *28*, 86–90. [CrossRef]

51. Wu, M.Y.; Tseng, Y.H.; Chang, Y.S.; Tsai, F.C.; Lin, P.J. Using extracorporeal membrane oxygenation to rescue acute myocardial infarction with cardiopulmonary collapse: The impact of early coronary revascularization. *Resuscitation* **2013**, *84*, 940–945. [CrossRef] [PubMed]

52. Lazzeri, C.; Bernardo, P.; Sori, A.; Innocenti, L.; Passantino, S.; Chiostri, M.; Gensini, G.F.; Valente, S. Renal replacement therapy in patients with refractory cardiac arrest undergoing extracorporeal membrane oxygenation. *Resuscitation* **2013**, *84*, e121–e122. [CrossRef] [PubMed]

53. Unosawa, S.; Sezai, A.; Hata, M.; Nakata, K.; Yoshitake, I.; Wakui, S.; Kimura, H.; Takahashi, K.; Hata, H.; Shiono, M. Long-term outcomes of patients undergoing extracorporeal membrane oxygenation for refractory postcardiotomy cardiogenic shock. *Surg. Today* **2013**, *43*, 264–270. [CrossRef] [PubMed]

54. Xue, J.; Wang, L.; Chen, C.M.; Chen, J.Y.; Sun, Z.X. Acute kidney injury influences mortality in lung transplantation. *Ren. Fail.* **2014**, *36*, 541–545. [CrossRef] [PubMed]

55. Hsiao, C.C.; Chang, C.H.; Fan, P.C.; Ho, H.T.; Jenq, C.C.; Kao, K.C.; Chiu, L.C.; Lee, S.Y.; Hsu, H.H.; Tian, Y.C.; et al. Prognosis of patients with acute respiratory distress syndrome on extracorporeal membrane oxygenation: The impact of urine output on mortality *Ann. Thorac. Surg.* **2014**, *97*, 1939–1944. [CrossRef] [PubMed]

56. Lee, S.W.; Yu, M.Y.; Lee, H.; Ahn, S.Y.; Kim, S.; Chin, H.J.; Na, K.Y. Risk Factors for Acute Kidney Injury and In-Hospital Mortality in Patients Receiving Extracorporeal Membrane Oxygenation. *PLoS ONE* **2015**, *10*, e0140674. [CrossRef] [PubMed]

57. Haneya, A.; Diez, C.; Philipp, A.; Bein, T.; Mueller, T.; Schmid, C.; Lubnow, M. Impact of Acute Kidney Injury on Outcome in Patients With Severe Acute Respiratory Failure Receiving Extracorporeal Membrane Oxygenation. *Crit. Care Med.* **2015**, *43*, 1898–1906. [CrossRef]

58. Huang, L.; Li, T.; Xu, L.; Hu, X.M.; Duan, D.W.; Li, Z.B.; Gao, X.J.; Li, J.; Wu, P.; Liu, Y.W. Extracorporeal Membrane Oxygenation Outcomes in Acute Respiratory Distress Treatment: Case Study in a Chinese Referral Center. *Med. Sci. Monit.* **2017**, *23*, 741–750. [CrossRef]

59. Antonucci, E.; Lamanna, I.; Fagnoul, D.; Vincent, J.L.; De Backer, D.; Silvio Taccone, F. The Impact of Renal Failure and Renal Replacement Therapy on Outcome During Extracorporeal Membrane Oxygenation Therapy. *Artif. Organs* **2016**, *40*, 746–754. [CrossRef]

60. Tsai, T.Y.; Chien, H.; Tsai, F.C.; Pan, H.C.; Yang, H.Y.; Lee, S.Y.; Hsu, H.H.; Fang, J.T.; Yang, C.W.; Chen, Y.C. Comparison of, R.I.F.L.E.; AKIN, and KDIGO classifications for assessing prognosis of patients on extracorporeal membrane oxygenation. *J. Formos. Med. Assoc.* **2017**, *116*, 844–851. [CrossRef]

61. Panholzer, B.; Meckelburg, K.; Huenges, K.; Hoffmann, G.; von der Brelie, M.; Haake, N.; Pilarczyk, K.; Cremer, J.; Haneya, A. Extracorporeal membrane oxygenation for acute respiratory distress syndrome in adults: An analysis of differences between survivors and non-survivors. *Perfusion* **2017**, *32*, 495–500. [CrossRef] [PubMed]

62. Chong, S.Z.; Fang, C.Y.; Fang, H.Y.; Chen, H.C.; Chen, C.J.; Yang, C.H.; Hang, C.L.; Yip, H.K.; Wu, C.J.; Lee, W.C. Associations with the In-Hospital Survival Following Extracorporeal Membrane Oxygenation in Adult Acute Fulminant Myocarditis. *J. Clin. Med.* **2018**, *7*, 452. [CrossRef] [PubMed]

63. Devasagayaraj, R.; Cavarocchi, N.C.; Hirose, H. Does acute kidney injury affect survival in adults with acute respiratory distress syndrome requiring extracorporeal membrane oxygenation? *Perfusion* **2018**, *33*, 375–382. [CrossRef] [PubMed]

64. Liao, X.; Cheng, Z.; Wang, L.; Li, B. Analysis of the risk factors of acute kidney injury in patients receiving extracorporeal membrane oxygenation. *Clin. Nephrol.* **2018**, *90*, 270–275. [CrossRef] [PubMed]

65. Paek, J.H.; Park, S.; Lee, A.; Park, S.; Chin, H.J.; Na, K.Y.; Lee, H.; Park, J.T.; Kim, S. Timing for initiation of sequential continuous renal replacement therapy in patients on extracorporeal membrane oxygenation. *Kidney Res. Clin. Pract.* **2018**, *37*, 239–247. [CrossRef]

66. He, P.; Zhang, S.; Hu, B.; Wu, W. Retrospective study on the effects of the prognosis of patients treated with extracorporeal membrane oxygenation combined with continuous renal replacement therapy. *Ann. Transl. Med.* **2018**, *6*, 455. [CrossRef] [PubMed]

67. Zhang, H.; Wu, J.; Zou, D.; Xiao, X.; Yan, H.; Li, X.C.; Chen, W. Ablation of interferon regulatory factor 4 in T cells induces "memory" of transplant tolerance that is irreversible by immune checkpoint blockade. *Am. J. Transplant.* **2019**, *19*, 884–893. [CrossRef]

68. Kilburn, D.J.; Shekar, K.; Fraser, J.F. The Complex Relationship of Extracorporeal Membrane Oxygenation and Acute Kidney Injury: Causation or Association? *BioMed Res. Int.* **2016**, *2016*, 1094296. [CrossRef]

69. Cheng, R.; Hachamovitch, R.; Kittleson, M.; Patel, J.; Arabia, F.; Moriguchi, J.; Esmailian, F.; Azarbal, B. Complications of extracorporeal membrane oxygenation for treatment of cardiogenic shock and cardiac arrest: A meta-analysis of 1,866 adult patients. *Ann. Thorac.Surg.* **2014**, *97*, 610–616. [CrossRef]

70. Lin, C.Y.; Tsai, F.C.; Tian, Y.C.; Jenq, C.C.; Chen, Y.C.; Fang, J.T.; Yang, C.W. Evaluation of outcome scoring systems for patients on extracorporeal membrane oxygenation. *Ann. Thorac. Surg.* **2007**, *84*, 1256–1262. [CrossRef]

71. Moher, D.; Liberati, A.; Tetzlaff JAltman, D.G. Preferred reporting items for systematic reviews and meta-analyses: The PRISMA statement. *PLoS Med.* **2009**, *6*, e1000097. [CrossRef] [PubMed]

72. Bellomo, R.; Ronco, C.; Kellum, J.A.; Mehta, R.L. Palevsky PAcute renal failure—Definition outcome measures animal, m.o.d.e.l.s., fluid therapy and information technology needs: The Second International Consensus Conference of the Acute Dialysis Quality Initiative (ADQI) Group. *Crit. Care* **2004**, *8*, R204–R212. [CrossRef] [PubMed]

73. Mehta, R.L.; Kellum, J.A.; Shah, S.V.; Molitoris, B.A.; Ronco, C.; Warnock, D.G.; Levin, A. Acute Kidney Injury Network: Report of an initiative to improve outcomes in acute kidney injury. *Crit. Care* **2007**, *11*, R31. [CrossRef] [PubMed]

74. Section 2: AKI Definition. *Kidney Int.* **2012**, *2*, 19–36. [CrossRef] [PubMed]

75. DerSimonian, R.; Laird, N. Meta-analysis in clinical trials. *Control. Clin. Trials* **1986**, *7*, 177–188. [CrossRef]

76. Higgins, J.P.; Thompson, S.G.; Deeks, J.J.; Altman, D.G. Measuring inconsistency in meta-analyses. *BMJ* **2003**, *327*, 557–560. [CrossRef] [PubMed]

77. Easterbrook, P.J.; Gopalan, R.; Berlin, J.A.; Matthews, D.R. Publication bias in clinical research. *Lancet* **1991**, *337*, 867–872. [CrossRef]

78. McDonald, C.I.; Fraser, J.F.; Coombes, J.S.; Fung, Y.L. Oxidative stress during extracorporeal circulation. *Eur. J. Cardiothorac. Surg.* **2014**, *46*, 937–943. [CrossRef] [PubMed]

79. Ikeda, M.; Prachasilchai, W.; Burne-Taney, M.J.; Rabb, H.; Yokota-Ikeda, N. Ischemic acute tubular necrosis models and drug discovery: A focus on cellular inflammation. *Drug Discov. Today* **2006**, *11*, 364–370. [CrossRef] [PubMed]

80. Yimin, H.; Wenkui, Y.; Jialiang, S.; Qiyi, C.; Juanhong, S.; Zhiliang, L.; Changsheng, H.; Ning, L.; Jieshou, L. Effects of continuous renal replacement therapy on renal inflammatory cytokines during extracorporeal membrane oxygenation in a porcine model. *J. Cardiothorac. Surg.* **2013**, *8*, 113. [CrossRef] [PubMed]

81. McILwain, R.B.; Timpa, J.G.; Kurundkar, A.R.; Holt, D.W.; Kelly, D.R.; Hartman, Y.E.; Neel, M.L.; Karnatak, R.K.; Schelonka, R.L.; Anantharamaiah, G.M.; et al. Plasma concentrations of inflammatory cytokines rise rapidly during ECMO-related SIRS due to the release of preformed stores in the intestine. *Lab. Investig.* **2010**, *90*, 128–139. [CrossRef] [PubMed]

82. Reed, R.C.; Rutledge, J.C. Laboratory and clinical predictors of thrombosis and hemorrhage in 29 pediatric extracorporeal membrane oxygenation nonsurvivors. *Pediatr. Dev. Pathol.* **2010**, *13*, 385–392. [CrossRef] [PubMed]

83. Williams, D.C.; Turi, J.L.; Hornik, C.P.; Bonnadonna, D.K.; Williford, W.L.; Walczak, R.J.; Watt, K.M.; Cheifetz, I.M. Circuit oxygenator contributes to extracorporeal membrane oxygenation-induced hemolysis. *ASAIO J.* **2015**, *61*, 190–195. [CrossRef] [PubMed]

84. Askenazi, D.J.; Selewski, D.T.; Paden, M.L.; Cooper, D.S.; Bridges, B.C.; Zappitelli, M.; Fleming, G.M. Renal replacement therapy in critically ill patients receiving extracorporeal membrane oxygenation. *Clin. J. Am. Soc. Nephrol.* **2012**, *7*, 1328–1336. [CrossRef] [PubMed]

85. Lubnow, M.; Philipp, A.; Foltan, M.; Enger, T.B.; Lunz, D.; Bein, T.; Haneya, A.; Schmid, C.; Riegger, G.; Müller, T.; et al. Technical complications during veno-venous extracorporeal membrane oxygenation and their relevance predicting a system-exchange—Retrospective analysis of 265 cases. *PLoS ONE* **2014**, *9*, e112316. [CrossRef] [PubMed]

86. Murphy, D.A.; Hockings, L.E.; Andrews, R.K.; Aubron, C.; Gardiner, E.E.; Pellegrino, V.A.; Davis, A.K. Extracorporeal membrane oxygenation-hemostatic complications. *Transfus. Med. Rev.* **2015**, *29*, 90–101. [CrossRef]

87. Lehle, K.; Philipp, A.; Zeman, F.; Lunz, D.; Lubnow, M.; Wendel, H.P.; Göbölös, L.; Schmid, C.; Müller, T. Technical-Induced Hemolysis in Patients with Respiratory Failure Supported with Veno-Venous ECMO—Prevalence and Risk Factors. *PLoS ONE* **2015**, *10*, e0143527. [CrossRef] [PubMed]

88. Adademir, T.; Ak, K.; Aljodi, M.; Elçi, M.E.; Arsan, S.; Isbir, S. The effects of pulsatile cardiopulmonary bypass on acute kidney injury. *Int. J. Artif. Organs* **2012**, *35*, 511–519. [CrossRef]

89. Abu-Omar, Y.; Ratnatunga, C. Cardiopulmonary bypass and renal injury. *Perfusion* **2006**, *21*, 209–213. [CrossRef]

90. Santana-Santos, E.; Marcusso, M.E.; Rodrigues, A.O.; Queiroz, F.G.; Oliveira, L.B.; Rodrigues, A.R.; Palomo, J.D. Strategies for prevention of acute kidney injury in cardiac surgery: An integrative review. *Revista Brasileira Terpia Intensiva* **2014**, *26*, 183–192. [CrossRef]

91. Thongprayoon, C.; Kaewput, W.; Thamcharoen, N.; Bathini, T.; Watthanasuntorn, K.; Lertjitbanjong, P.; Sharma, K.; Salim, S.A.; Ungprasert, P.; Wijarnpreecha, K.; et al. Incidence and Impact of Acute Kidney Injury after Liver Transplantation: A Meta-Analysis. *J. Clin. Med.* **2019**, *8*, 372. [CrossRef] [PubMed]

92. Thongprayoon, C.; Kaewput, W.; Thamcharoen, N.; Bathini, T.; Watthanasuntorn, K.; Salim, S.A.; Ungprasert, P.; Lertjitbanjong, P.; Aeddula, N.R.; Torres-Ortiz, A.; et al. Acute Kidney Injury in Patients Undergoing Total Hip Arthroplasty: A Systematic Review and Meta-Analysis. *J. Clin. Med.* **2019**, *8*, 66. [CrossRef] [PubMed]

93. Thongprayoon, C.; Cheungpasitporn, W.; Mao, M.A.; Harrison, A.M.; Erickson, S.B. Elevated admission serum calcium phosphate product as an independent risk factor for acute kidney injury in hospitalized patients. *Hosp. Pract. (1995)* **2019**, *47*, 73–79. [CrossRef] [PubMed]

94. Thongprayoon, C.; Cheungpasitporn, W.; Mao, M.A.; Sakhuja, A.; Kashani, K. U-shape association of serum albumin level and acute kidney injury risk in hospitalized patients. *PLoS ONE* **2018**, *13*, e0199153. [CrossRef] [PubMed]

95. Thongprayoon, C.; Cheungpasitporn, W.; Mao, M.A.; Sakhuja, A.; Erickson, S.B. Admission calcium levels and risk of acute kidney injury in hospitalised patients. *Int. J. Clin. Pract.* **2018**, *72*, e13057. [CrossRef] [PubMed]

96. Thongprayoon, C.; Cheungpasitporn, W.; Mao, M.A.; Sakhuja, A.; Erickson, S.B. Admission hyperphosphatemia increases the risk of acute kidney injury in hospitalized patients. *J. Nephrol.* **2018**, *31*, 241–247. [CrossRef] [PubMed]

97. Razo-Vazquez, A.O.; Thornton, K. Extracorporeal Membrane Oxygenation-What the Nephrologist Needs to Know. *Adv. Chronic Kidney Dis.* **2016**, *23*, 146–151. [CrossRef]

98. Pedersen, T.H.; Videm, V.; Svennevig, J.L.; Karlsen, H.; Østbakk, R.W.; Jensen, Ø.; Mollnes, T.E. Extracorporeal membrane oxygenation using a centrifugal pump and a servo regulator to prevent negative inlet pressure. *Ann. Thorac. Surg.* **1997**, *63*, 1333–1339. [CrossRef]

99. Kress, D.C.; Cohen, D.J.; Swanson, D.K.; Hegge, J.O.; Young, J.W.; Watson, K.M.; Rasmussen, P.W.; Berkoff, H.A. Pump-induced hemolysis in a rabbit model of neonatal ECMO. *ASAIO Trans.* **1987**, *33*, 446–452.

100. Lou, S.; MacLaren, G.; Best, D.; Delzoppo, C.; Butt, W. Hemolysis in pediatric patients receiving centrifugal-pump extracorporeal membrane oxygenation: Prevalence, risk factors, and outcomes. *Crit. Care Med.* **2014**, *42*, 1213–1220. [CrossRef]

101. Toomasian, J.M.; Bartlett, R.H. Hemolysis and ECMO pumps in the 21st Century. *Perfusion* **2011**, *26*, 5–6. [CrossRef] [PubMed]

102. Thongprayoon, C.; Cheungpasitporn, W.; Kittanamongkolchai, W.; Harrison, A.M.; Kashani, K. Prognostic Importance of Low Admission Serum Creatinine Concentration for Mortality in Hospitalized Patients. *Am. J. Med.* **2017**, *130*, 545–554. [CrossRef] [PubMed]

103. Thongprayoon, C.; Cheungpasitporn, W.; Kashani, K. Serum creatinine level, a surrogate of muscle mass, predicts mortality in critically ill patients. *J. Thorac. Dis.* **2016**, *8*, E305–E311. [CrossRef] [PubMed]

104. Thongprayoon, C.; Cheungpasitporn, W.; Kittanamongkolchai, W.; Srivali, N.; Ungprasert, P.; Kashani, K. Optimum methodology for estimating baseline serum creatinine for the acute kidney injury classification. *Nephrology (Carlton)* **2015**, *20*, 881–886. [CrossRef] [PubMed]

105. Vaidya, V.S.; Ramirez, V.; Ichimura, T.; Bobadilla, N.A.; Bonventre, J.V. Urinary kidney injury molecule-1: A sensitive quantitative biomarker for early detection of kidney tubular injury. *Am. J. Physiol. Renal Physiol.* **2006**, *290*, F517–F529. [CrossRef]

106. Mishra, J.; Ma, Q.; Prada, A.; Mitsnefes, M.; Zahedi, K.; Yang, J.; Barasch, J.; Devarajan, P. Identification of neutrophil gelatinase-associated lipocalin as a novel early urinary biomarker for ischemic renal injury. *J. Am. Soc. Nephrol.* **2003**, *14*, 2534–2543. [CrossRef]

107. Hosohata, K.; Ando, H.; Fujimura, A. Urinary vanin-1 as a novel biomarker for early detection of drug-induced acute kidney injury. *J. Pharmacol. Exp. Ther.* **2012**, *341*, 656–662. [CrossRef]

108. Kashani, K.; Cheungpasitporn, W.; Ronco, C. Biomarkers of acute kidney injury: The pathway from discovery to clinical adoption. *Clin. Chem. Lab. Med.* **2017**, *55*, 1074–1089. [CrossRef]

16

Impact on Outcomes across KDIGO-2012 AKI Criteria According to Baseline Renal Function

Isabel Acosta-Ochoa [1,*], Juan Bustamante-Munguira [2], Alicia Mendiluce-Herrero [1], Jesús Bustamante-Bustamante [3] and Armando Coca-Rojo [1]

[1]   Department of Nephrology, Hospital Clinico Universitario, 47003 Valladolid, Spain
[2]   Department of Cardiac Surgery, Hospital Clinico Universitario, 47003 Valladolid, Spain
[3]   Department of Medicine, Dermatology and Toxicology, School of Medicine, University of Valladolid, 47005 Valladolid, Spain
*   Correspondence: susty21@hotmail.com

Abstract: Acute kidney injury (AKI) and Chronic Kidney Disease (CKD) are global health problems. The pathophysiology of acute-on-chronic kidney disease (AoCKD) is not well understood. We aimed to study clinical outcomes in patients with previous normal (pure acute kidney injury; P-AKI) or impaired kidney function (AoCKD) across the 2012 Kidney Disease Improving Global Outcomes (KDIGO) AKI classification. We performed a retrospective study of patients with AKI, divided into P-AKI and AoCKD groups, evaluating clinical and epidemiological features, distribution across KDIGO-2012 criteria, in-hospital mortality and need for dialysis. One thousand, two hundred and sixty-nine subjects were included. AoCKD individuals were older and had higher comorbidity. P-AKI individuals fulfilled more often the serum creatinine (SCr) $\geq 3.0\times$ criterion in AKI-Stage3, AoCKD subjects reached SCr ≥ 4.0 mg/dL criterion more frequently. AKI severity was associated with in-hospital mortality independently of baseline renal function. AoCKD subjects presented higher mortality when fulfilling AKI-Stage1 criteria or SCr $\geq 3.0\times$ criterion within AKI-Stage3. The relationship between mortality and associated risk factors, such as the net increase of SCr or AoCKD status, fluctuated depending on AKI stage and stage criteria sub-strata. AoCKD patients that fulfil SCr increment rate criteria may be exposed to more severe insults, possibly explaining the higher mortality. AoCKD may constitute a unique clinical syndrome. Adequate staging criteria may help prompt diagnosis and administration of appropriate therapy.

Keywords: acute kidney injury; chronic kidney disease; AKI staging

1. Introduction

Acute kidney injury (AKI) is a global public health problem [1]. Using the 2012 Kidney Disease: Improving Global Outcomes AKI definition (KDIGO-2012) [2], one in five adults and one in three children worldwide experience AKI during a hospital episode of care [3]. AKI implicates a great burden in morbidity and mortality, increases sanitary costs [4,5], and affects long-term outcomes, including cardiovascular events and survival [6–9]. It is a clinical syndrome with a variety of aetiologies [10], once instituted, the treatment is mostly supportive [11,12], and the best approach remains prevention [13–15]. Based on the KDIGO definition of Chronic Kidney Disease (CKD) [16] its prevalence approximates 8–16% worldwide [17], affecting one in nine Americans and more than 300 million persons globally [18]. AKI is more prevalent in (and a significant risk factor for) patients with impaired renal function [2]; AKI, in turn, may act as a promoter of progression of the underlying CKD [2,19–23].

This evidence has led to a renewed interest in an old clinical concept: Acute on chronic renal failure, coined by Lim et al. in 1969 [24] and currently referred to as acute on chronic kidney disease

(AoCKD) and its pathophysiology [23,25–29]. Few studies compare patients directly with prior normal (pure acute kidney injury [P-AKI]) and impaired renal function (AoCKD) during an AKI episode: Some conclude that patients with previous CKD bare worst clinical and renal outcomes [30–34], while others conclude that it could be protective against the negative consequences of AKI [35–38].

The most frequently used AKI classifications: RIFLE [39], AKIN [40] and KDIGO-2012 [2] do not discriminate patients with or without previous CKD, so the same criteria are used interchangeably in these individuals; therefore, a knowledge gap exists in the evaluation and staging of AoCKD. We hypothesized that AKI affects individuals with baseline normal and impaired renal function in a different way; in order to verify this theory we examined the distribution of patients in the strata defined by KDIGO-2012 criteria, and the relationship of AKI severity with short-term outcomes, such as in-hospital mortality and initiation of renal replacement therapy (RRT) between P-AKI and AoCKD subjects.

2. Experimental Section

All consecutive hospitalized patients treated by nephrologists in a 762-bed teaching institution, with a diagnosis of AKI by KDIGO-2012 criteria (Table 1), during a three-year period (June 2012 through May 2015) were reviewed.

Table 1. KDIGO-2012 acute kidney injury (AKI) classification and criteria.

Stage	Serum Creatinine	Urine Output
1	1.5–1.9 times baseline	<0.5 mL/kg/h for 6–12 h
	OR	
	≥0.3 mg/dL increase	
2	2.0–2.9 times baseline	<0.5 mL/kg/h for ≥ 12 h
3	3.0 times baseline	<0.3 mL/kg/h for ≥ 24 h
	OR	OR
	Increase in serum creatinine to ≥4.0 mg/dL	
	OR	Anuria for ≥ 12 h
	Initiation of renal replacement therapy	
	OR	
	In patients <18 years. Decrease in eGFR to <35 mL/min/1.73 m^2	

Inclusion criteria: Age ≥ 18 years, admission for >2 or and ≤91 days and rise in serum creatinine (SCr) sustained at least for 24 h. Exclusion criteria: History of solid organ transplantation, hospital readmission less than 3 months before or after index hospitalization, patients without baseline SCr, end-stage renal disease (previous RRT) or estimated glomerular filtration rate (eGFR) < 15 mL/min/1.73 m^2 calculated by the four item Modification of Diet in Renal Disease formula (MDRD-4) [41] and pregnant and puerperal women (Figure 1). Previous and later hospitalizations were searched even if a nephrologist was not consulted and included as a new index hospitalization if they met the inclusion criteria.

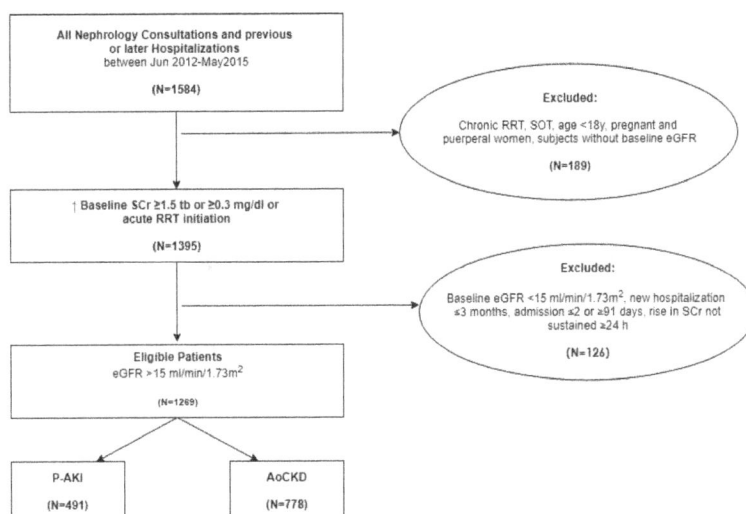

Figure 1. Study flow chart for inclusion and exclusion criteria. RRT: Renal replacement therapy; SOT: Solid organ transplantation; Tb: Times baseline. SCr: Serum creatinine; eGFR: Estimated glomerular filtration rate; P-AKI: Pure acute kidney injury; AoCKD: Acute on chronic kidney disease.

We designed a retrospective cohorts study. The study conforms to the STROBE statement for reporting observational studies. Patients were divided in two groups: P-AKI (baseline eGFR ≥ 60 mL/min/1.73 m^2) and AoCKD (baseline eGFR ≥ 15 and <60 mL/min/1.73 m^2 for more than three months) (16). We defined baseline SCr as the lowest value in the six months prior to hospitalization, and when it was not available, we searched the 12 previous months [42]. Community-acquired AKI was defined as a SCr $\geq 1.5\times$ increment at hospital admission [43]. We used the KDIGO-2012 stage associated with the peak SCr reached during hospitalization.

We registered several epidemiological and clinical features, intensive care unit (ICU) admission and hospitalization in medical or surgical units. The study was conducted in accordance with the Declaration of Helsinki, and the protocol was approved by the Ethics Committee of Área de Salud Valladolid Este (CINV 14–45); because of the anonymous and non-interventional nature of the study, they waived the need for informed consent.

Our primary objective was to compare the rate of in-hospital mortality across every criterion of the KDIGO-2012 AKI classification between groups. Our secondary objectives included comparing the rate of initiation of RRT, length of hospital stay (LOS), time to nephrology consultation, and dialysis-dependence at discharge in both groups.

Patient demographics are summarized using mean and standard deviations (SD) or median (25th–75th percentile) for continuous variables and counts with percentages for binary variables, as appropriate and according to data distribution. Normal distribution of data was analyzed using a Kolmogorov-Smirnov test. Continuous data was analyzed using Mann-Whitney U tests (between P-AKI and AoCKD) or Kruskal-Wallis tests among P-AKI and CKD stage 3a (CKD-3a), 3b (CKD-3b) and 4 (CKD-4). Binary data were analyzed using the Chi-square test. A two-sided p-value ≤ 0.05 was considered statistically significant.

We used a Cox proportional hazards model, unadjusted and adjusted for age and Charlson Index (modeled as continuous variables), gender, ICU admission and comorbidities: Hypertension, diabetes, coronary artery disease, chronic heart failure, peripheral artery disease and chronic hepatic disease to study in-hospital survival rates. We tested the proportionality assumption of the Cox models using Schoenfeld residual plots. Age and ICU admission were considered as time-dependent covariates.

No collinearity was found between the independent variables included in the model. The adjusted Cox model for in-hospital mortality according to AKI severity and baseline renal function was used to create survival curves.

Statistical analysis was carried out using the Statistical Package for Social Sciences software, version 20.0 (SPSS, IBM, Armonk, NY, USA), GraphPad Prism, version 7.04 for Windows (GraphPad Software, La Jolla California USA) and Microsoft Excel 2013 (Microsoft, Inc. Redmond, WA, USA).

3. Results

3.1. Demographic Characteristics of Patients

We revised all 1584 nephrology consultations and previous or later hospitalizations during the study period; 1269 cases met inclusion criteria (Figure 1), 491 in the P-AKI group and 778 in the AoCKD group.

Characteristics and comparison between groups are shown in Table 2. Individuals in the AoCKD group were older, had higher mean Charlson Index [44] and suffered hypertension, diabetes and cardiovascular disease at a significantly higher rate. Twenty-one patients of the AoCKD (3%) presented a baseline SCr $\geq$ 4.0 mg/dL. Patients in the P-AKI group were admitted to the ICU more frequently. The distribution across every KDIGO-2012 AKI stage and criterion between P-AKI and AoCKD patients, is shown in Table 2. The proportion of patients who developed AKI stage 1 (ST1) was higher among the AoCKD group; while AKI stage 2 (ST2) was more frequent in the P-AKI group. The criterion used to reach AKI stage 3 (ST3) differed between groups: Most P-AKI patients suffered a $\geq$ 3.0× increase in SCr from baseline, while the majority of AoCKD patients reached an SCr $\geq$ 4 mg/dL. The rate of initiation of RRT was similar between groups. In general, we found no statistically significant difference between groups in reaching ST3 (all criteria) (Table 2). We analyzed differences of peak value and SCr net increase (NI)—defined as the difference between peak and baseline SCr values-among P-AKI and AoCKD subjects that fulfilled a specific AKI criterion. Distribution of peak SCr and SCr NI values differed in P-AKI and AoCKD subjects when fulfilling the increment of SCr 1.5–1.9 times baseline criterion (Median peak SCr, P-AKI 1.45 mg/dL vs. AoCKD 2.81 mg/dL, U = 547.5, $p < 0.001$; Median SCr NI, P-AKI 0.57 mg/dL vs. AoCKD 1.2 mg/dL, U = 1045.5, $p < 0.001$), the ST2 criterion (Median peak SCr, P-AKI 2.24 mg/dL vs. AoCKD 3.32 mg/dL, U = 511, $p < 0.001$; Median SCr NI, P-AKI 1.28 mg/dL vs. AoCKD 1.87 mg/dL, U = 921.5, $p < 0.001$), the increment of SCr 3.0 times baseline criterion (Median peak SCr, P-AKI 4.66 mg/dL vs. AoCKD 6.8 mg/dL, U = 8161, $p < 0.001$; Median SCr NI, P-AKI 3.81 mg/dL vs. AoCKD 5.24 mg/dL, U = 10,090.5, $p < 0.001$) or the SCr $\geq$4.0 mg/dL criterion (Median peak SCr, P-AKI 6.05 mg/dL vs. AoCKD 5.64 mg/dL, U = 23,786, $p = 0.071$; Median SCr NI, P-AKI 5.13 mg/dL vs. AoCKD 3.26 mg/dL, U = 12,110, $p < 0.001$).

Table 2. Baseline Characteristics of AKI and AoCKD Groups and Distribution across KDIGO-2012 Criteria.

	ALL	P-AKI	AoCKD	p Value[1]	AoCKD			p Value[2]
					CKD-3A	CKD-3B	CKD-4	
N	1269	491	778		221	282	275	
Male sex—No. (%)	883 (70)	339 (69)	544 (70)	0.739	162 (73)	198 (70)	184 (67)	0.476
Age (years)—Median (IQR)	75 (65–81)	71 (61–79)	77 (69–83)	<0.001	76 (69–82)	78 (70–83)	77 (67–83)	<0.001
HTN—No. (%)	1125 (89)	395 (80)	730 (94)	<0.001	206 (93)	268 (95)	256 (93)	<0.001
DM—No. (%)	536 (42)	158 (32)	378 (49)	<0.001	96 (43)	145 (51)	137 (50)	<0.001
CAD—No. (%)	385 (30)	107 (22)	278 (36)	<0.001	73 (33)	105 (37)	100 (36)	<0.001
CHF—No. (%)	491 (39)	140 (29)	351 (45)	<0.001	94 (43)	146 (52)	111 (40)	<0.001
PAD—No. (%)	392 (31)	108 (22)	284 (37)	<0.001	89 (40)	112 (40)	83 (30)	<0.001
CHD—No. (%)	231 (18)	37 (8)	36 (5)	0.03	11 (5)	14 (5)	11 (4)	0.171
Charlson Comorbidity Index (SD)	4 (3–6)	4 (2–6)	5 (3–6)	<0.001	4 (3–6)	5 (3–6)	6 (4–7)	<0.001
Unit of Admission								
Medical Unit—No. (%)	808 (64)	180 (37)	281 (36)	0.845	91 (41)	110 (39)	80 (29)	0.025
ICU—No. (%)	241 (19)	117 (24)	124 (16)	<0.001	44 (20)	42 (15)	38 (14)	0.001
AKI Type								
Community Acquired—No. (%)	870 (69)	160 (33)	239 (31)	0.485	74 (34)	90 (32)	75 (27)	0.396
KDIGO-2012 AKI Stage 1 (global)—No. (%)	506 (40)	169 (34)	337 (43)	0.002	115 (53)	145 (51)	77 (28)	<0.001
≥0.3 mg/dL	506 (40)	169 (34)	337 (43)	0.002	115 (53)	145 (51)	77 (28)	<0.001
SCr 1.5-1.9×	264 (21)	115 (23)	149 (19)	0.068	59 (27)	70 (25)	20 (7)	<0.001
KDIGO-2012 AKI Stage 2 (SCr 2.0–2.9×)—No. (%)	158 (13)	88 (18)	70 (9)	<0.001	42 (19)	27 (10)	1 (0.4)	<0.001
KDIGO-2012 AKI Stage 3 (global)—No. (%)	605 (48)	234 (48)	371 (48)	0.992	60 (28)	112 (39)	199 (72)	<0.001
SCr ≥ 3.0×	354 (28)	229 (47)	125 (16)	<0.001	46 (21)	54 (19)	25 (9)	<0.001

Table 2. *Cont.*

	ALL	P-AKI	AoCKD	p Value[1]	AoCKD			p Value[2]
					CKD-3A	CKD-3B	CKD-4	
N	1269	491	778		221	282	275	
SCr ≥ 4.0 mg/dL	503 (40)	150 (31)	353 (45)	<0.001	48 (22)	108 (38)	197 (71)	<0.001
Initiation RRT	167 (13)	62 (13)	105 (14)	0.656	16 (7)	24 (9)	65 (24)	<0.001
Baseline SCr (mg/dL)	1.4 (1–2)	0.9 (0.7–1.1)	1.9 (1.5–2.5)	<0.001	1.4 (1.2–1.5)	1.8 (1.6–2)	2.7 (2.4–3.2)	<0.001
Peak SCr (mg/dL)	3.4 (2.2–5.2)	2.5 (1.5–4.5)	3.7 (2.6–5.5)	<0.001	2.6 (2–3.8)	3.4 (2.6–4.9)	5 (3.9–6.7)	<0.001
SCr Net Increase (mg/dL)	1.6 (0.7–3.3)	1.6 (0.6–3.6)	1.7 (0.9–3)	0.232	1.2 (0.7–2.4)	1.6 (0.8–3.2)	2.2 (1.2–3.5)	<0.001
Discharge SCr (mg/dL)	1.9 (1.3–2.9)	1.2 (0.9–1.7)	2.4 (1.7–3.5)	<0.001	1.7 (1.4–2.2)	2.3 (1.8–2.8)	3.6 (2.7–4.9)	<0.001

Data are expressed as mean ± standard deviation (SD), median and interquartilic range (IQR) or number (percentage). P-AKI, pure acute kidney injury; AoCKD, acute on chronic kidney disease; HTN, Hypertension; DM, diabetes mellitus; CAD, coronary artery disease; CHF, chronic heart failure; PAD, peripheral arterial disease; CHD, chronic hepatic disease; ICU, intensive care unit; AKI, acute kidney injury; SCr, serum creatinine; RRT, renal replacement therapy. p Value[1]: Comparison of P-AKI vs. AoCKD (all patients). p Value[2]: Comparison of P-AKI vs. AoCKD stages.

3.2. In-Hospital Mortality

279 (22%) patients died during hospitalization. We found no statistically significant difference in global mortality rates between groups. More patients died in the ST3 category in both groups compared to the other KDIGO-2012 AKI categories (Table 3).

Table 3. Primary and secondary endpoints. Mortality rates of subjects that met each KDIGO stage/criterion within P-AKI/AoCKD groups.

	ARF	AoCKD	p Value
N	491	778	
Primary Endpoint			
In-Hospital Mortality—No. (%)	100 (20.4)	179 (23)	0.15
Secondary Endpoints			
Initiation of RRT—No. (%)	62 (12.6)	105 (13.5)	0.36
Length of Hospital Stay (days)	12 (7–25)	12 (7–21)	0.08
Time to Nephrology Consultation (days)	4 (1–8)	3 (1–6)	<0.001
Dialysis Dependence at Discharge—No. (%)	7 (1.4)	40 (5.1)	<0.001
In-Hospital Mortality	**ARF**	**AoCKD**	**p Value**
KDIGO-2012 AKI Stage 1 (global)	10 (5.9)	44 (13.1)	0.014
≥0.3 mg/dL	10 (5.9)	44 (13.1)	0.014
SCr 1.5–1.9×	7 (6.1)	26 (17.4)	0.006
KDIGO-2012 AKI Stage 2	21 (23.9)	12 (17.1)	0.302
KDIGO-2012 AKI Stage 3 (global)	69 (29.5)	123 (33.2)	0.345
SCr 3.0×	67 (29.3)	50 (40)	0.04
SCr ≥ 4.0 mg/dL	41 (27.3)	116 (32.9)	0.221
Initiation RRT	24 (38.7)	39 (37.1)	0.84

Data are expressed as mean ± SD or number (percentage). P-AKI: Pure acute kidney injury; AoCKD: Acute on chronic kidney disease; RRT: Renal replacement therapy; AKI: Acute kidney injury; SCr: Serum creatinine.

We studied the distribution of all in-hospital deaths across each KDIGO-2012 AKI criterion in both groups (Table 3). AoCKD presented a higher death rate compared to P-AKI when fulfilling any ST1 criteria or the SCr ≥ 3.0× criterion within ST3 stage. Although the percentage of deaths associated with ST3 was similar between groups, its association with each criterion varied: RRT initiation was the ST3 criterion associated with the highest mortality rate among P-AKI patients, while SCr ≥ 3.0× was the criterion linked to the highest death rate in AoCKD subjects. The percentage of deaths associated with the SCr ≥ 4.0 mg/dL criterion in the P-AKI group was lower when compared to AoCKD subjects (Table 3).

The Cox proportional hazard model, using P-AKI ST1 individuals as the reference group, showed that AoCKD ST3 patients had significantly worse in-hospital survival, with an adjusted hazard ratio (HR) of 4.8 and 95% confidence interval (CI) of 2.5–9.2 ($p < 0.001$), followed by P-AKI ST3 subjects, P-AKI ST2 and AoCKD ST2 patients. In-hospital mortality of those with AoCKD ST1 did not significantly differ from that of P-AKI ST1 individuals (Figures 2 and 3). Other determinants that showed an association to in-hospital mortality were older age (HR: 1.001; 95% CI: 1–1.001; $p = 0.001$), Charlson Index (HR: 1.16; 95% CI: 1.1–1.23; $p < 0.001$), ICU admission (HR: 1.04; 95% CI: 1.03–1.05; $p < 0.001$) and CHF (HR: 1.5; 95% CI: 1.15–1.96; $p = 0.003$).

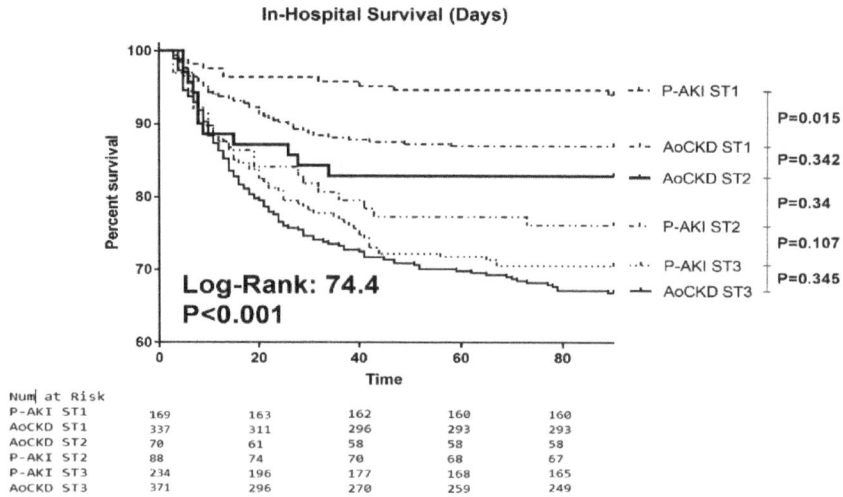

Figure 2. Kaplan-Meier curves. In-hospital survival curves stratified by baseline renal function and AKI severity. P-AKI: Pure Acute kidney injury. AoCKD: Acute-on-chronic kidney disease. AKI: Acute kidney injury. ST1: AKI stage 1. ST2: AKI stage 2. ST3: AKI stage 3.

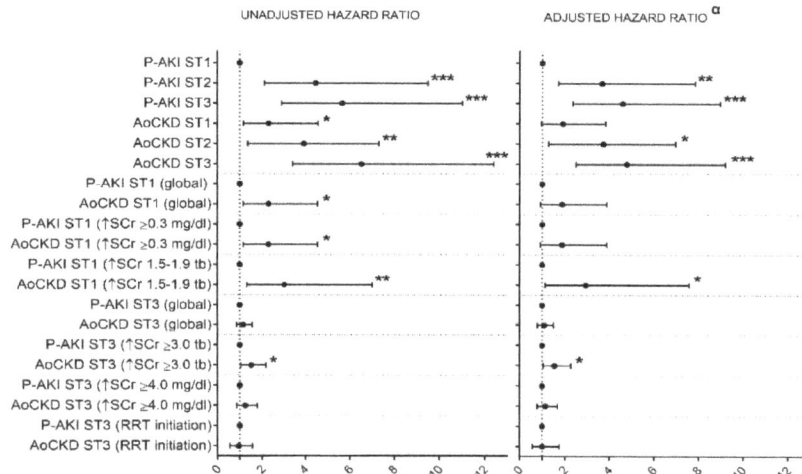

Figure 3. Unadjusted and adjusted hazard ratios (95% confidence interval) for death. P-AKI: Pure acute kidney injury. AoCKD: Acute-on-chronic kidney disease. AKI: Acute kidney injury. ST1: AKI stage 1. ST2: AKI stage 2. ST3: AKI stage 3. SCr: Serum creatinine. Tb: Times baseline. RRT: Renal replacement therapy. α: Models including P-AKI/AoCKD status, age, intensive care unit admission (considered as time-dependent variables), gender, Charlson Index, and comorbidity (hypertension, diabetes, coronary artery disease, chronic heart failure, peripheral arterial disease and chronic hepatic disease). * $p < 0.05$; ** $p < 0.01$; *** $p < 0.001$.

We also built Cox proportional hazards models to study the effect of fulfilling specific ST1 and ST3 criterion among groups. AoCKD patients presented significantly higher unadjusted mortality HR compared to P-AKI subjects when fulfilling any ST1 stage criterion or the ST3 SCr ≥ 3.0× criterion (Figure 3). After adjustment, only AoCKD individuals who reached ST1 through the SCr ≥ 1.5–1.9× criterion and those that attained ST3 fulfilling the SCr ≥3.0× criterion showed a significantly higher HR for death compared with P-AKI individuals. The AoCKD group showed a small, but not statistically significant, increase in the risk of in-hospital mortality when fulfilling the SCr ≥ 0.3 mg/dL criterion within ST1 or the SCr ≥ 4.0 mg/dL criterion within ST3 (Figure 3). To further investigate the effect of baseline kidney function and its modification during AKI on in-hospital mortality, we added related variables to the analysis. Peak SCr and SCr NI were, as expected, highly correlated variables ($r = 0.953$, $p < 0.001$). SCr NI and baseline eGFR were added to our model as independent variables. Models simultaneously, including baseline eGFR and P-AKI/AoCKD status, were not considered due to multicollinearity. In a global model, including all patients (Figure 4), SCr NI was an independent risk factor for in-hospital mortality, whereas baseline eGFR or P-AKI/AoCKD status were not. This approach was also tested in specific AKI strata that were associated with higher mortality rates among AoCKD patients, namely cases with SCr rise by 1.5–1.9 times or ≥ 3.0 times baseline (Figure 4). SCr NI proved to be independently associated with mortality among patients that reached an SCr rise 1.5–1.9 times baseline. Conversely, that association was not found among between subjects that suffered an SCr rise ≥ 3.0 times baseline, while in this group, AoCKD status was directly correlated with in-hospital death.

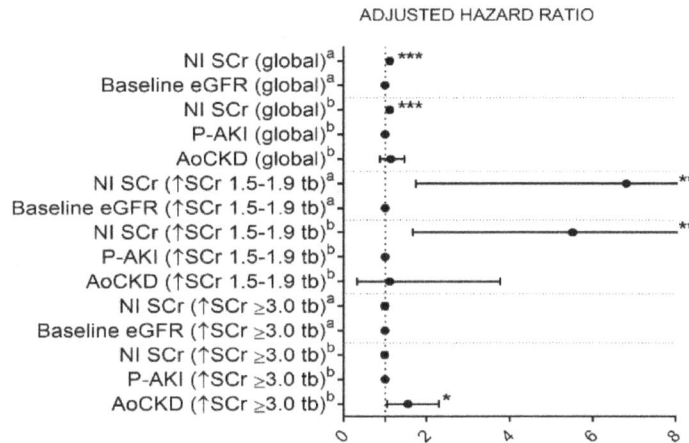

Figure 4. Adjusted hazard ratios (95% confidence interval) for death. NI: Net increase. SCr: Serum creatinine. eGFR: Estimated glomerular filtration rate. P-AKI: Pure acute kidney injury. AoCKD: Acute-on-chronic kidney disease. Tb: Times baseline. a: Models including SCr NI, baseline eGFR, age, Intensive care unit admission (considered as time-dependent variables), gender, Charlson Index, and comorbidity (hypertension, diabetes, coronary artery disease, chronic heart failure, peripheral arterial disease and chronic hepatic disease. b: Models including SCr NI, P-AKI/AoCKD status, age, intensive care unit admission (considered as time-dependent variables), gender, Charlson Index, and comorbidity (hypertension, diabetes, coronary artery disease, chronic heart failure, peripheral arterial disease and chronic hepatic disease. * $p < 0.05$; ** $p < 0.01$; *** $p < 001$.

Mean survival time was significantly higher among ST1 P-AKI individuals when compared to ST1 AoCKD subjects (86.2 ± 16.5 vs. 80.5 ± 24.9 days, $p < 0.01$). ST3 P-AKI patients with an SCr $\geq 3.0\times$ had a better in-hospital survival time compared to AoCKD individuals (69.9 ± 32.5 vs. 61.3 ± 37.1 days, $p < 0.05$) (Figure 5).

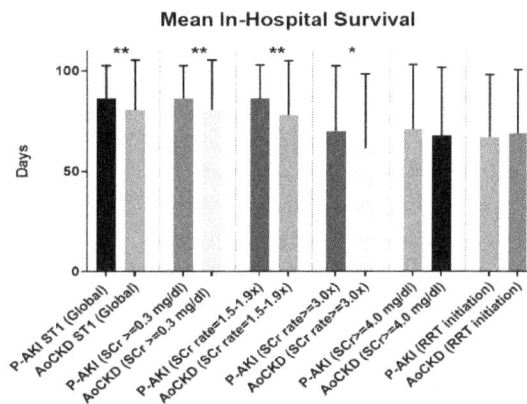

Figure 5. Mean in-hospital survival time (days) by baseline renal function and KDIGO AKI stage and criteria. P-AKI: Pure acute kidney injury. AoCKD: Acute-on-chronic kidney disease. AKI: Acute kidney injury. ST1: AKI stage 1. ST2: AKI stage 2. ST3: AKI stage 3. SCr: Serum creatinine. RRT: Renal replacement therapy. * $p < 0.05$; ** $p < 0.01$.

3.3. Secondary Outcomes

We found no statistically significant difference between groups in need of RRT. The severity of AKI was directly associated with LOS in both groups, but we found no differences in LOS between P-AKI and AoCKD patients. AoCKD group presented a significantly lower time to nephrology consultation compared to P-AKI and a higher dialysis-dependence at discharge (Table 3).

4. Discussion

We found that patients with previous impaired renal function were older and had a higher Charlson's Index, showing that AoCKD individuals differ in their baseline characteristics from the P-AKI group. In addition, we found that the distribution of patients across KDIGO-2012 criteria is different between groups; AKI severity is related with worse short-term outcomes, independently of baseline SCr, and that fulfilling a specific KDIGO-2012 AKI criterion, even within the same AKI stage, is associated with an increased risk of in-hospital death in patients with AoCKD.

In our sample, ST1 was the most common stage reached by CKD-3a and CKD-3b patients, while P-AKI and CKD-4 subjects most frequently reached ST3. The apparent predisposition of individuals with advanced CKD to suffer severe AKI could be due to the increasingly higher baseline SCr associated with CKD-4, which enables reaching the SCr $\geq$ 4 mg/dL criterion, and thus, ST3, even in the presence of mild insults. A recent study by Hatakeyama et al., [45] also described a higher incidence of ST3 among patients with P-AKI or advanced CKD stages compared to CKD-3a individuals. The percentage of patients in the ST2 stage was surprisingly low in both groups (Table 2). This is not a rare finding; an even lower percentage of patients in the ST2 category was found in individuals from a general (34) and cardiac surgery ICU [46]; the authors propose that this could be explained by the automatic classification of all patients that require RRT as ST3. The path followed by P-AKI and AoCKD individuals to reach a specific AKI stage was also different: Within ST3, the most common criterion fulfilled by AoCKD patients, regardless of CKD stage, was SCr $\geq$ 4.0 mg/dL, while P-AKI individuals fulfilled more frequently the SCr $\geq$ 3.0$\times$ criterion.

We observed no differences in overall in-hospital mortality rates between groups; but it was significantly higher among AoCKD/ST1 and AoCKD/ST3 subjects compared to P-AKI subjects within that same stage, although only if ST3 was attained through reaching an SCr $\geq$ 3.0$\times$ in the latter group. Peak SCr and SCr NI were significantly higher among AoCKD compared to P-AKI patients in these stages. Lack of differences in mortality between P-AKI and AoCKD individuals for ST2 may be due to the low prevalence of severe CKD among AoCKD subjects—defined as CKD-3b or CKD-4-in this specific stratum. However, within strata associated with higher mortality among AoCKD subjects, such as those with SCr rise by 1.5–1.9 times or $\geq$3 times vs. baseline, we observed no differences in severe CKD prevalence between AoCKD survivors and non-survivors (1.5–1.9 times baseline, survivors—56.1%, non-survivors—76.9%, p = 0.128; three times baseline, survivors—65.3%, non-survivors—56%, p = 0.336), indicating a complex relationship between mortality, CKD severity, SCr values and other risk factors among this subpopulation.

When compared with P-AKI/ST1 patients (reference group), patients with AoCKD/ST3 presented the highest adjusted HR for in-hospital death, followed by P-AKI/ST3, P-AKI/ST2 and AoCKD/ST2 patients. We found that AKI severity was associated with higher in-hospital mortality in a stepwise incremental fashion, regardless of baseline renal function; we found no significant differences in adjusted mortality HR within ST3 subjects among those that received RRT or not or those who fulfilled the SCr $\geq$ 4.0 mg/dL criterion or not. AoCKD patients that reached ST1 or ST3 while fulfilling the SCr $\geq$ 1.5–1.9$\times$ or SCr $\geq$ 3.0$\times$ criteria, respectively, presented a higher adjusted HR of death compared to P-AKI patients. This differential effect on mortality appears among those AoCKD individuals that fulfilled specific AKI criteria that require not a net increase in SCr values, but an increased rate of this parameter with respect to its baseline values. To further support the notion of a differential effect of risk factors, such as AoCKD status or a net increase of SCr in each AKI stratum, we found that SCr NI was closely associated with in-hospital mortality when studying the whole spectrum of AKI.

However, if we specifically analyzed the subset of patients that suffered a rise of SCr $\geq$ 3.0 times baseline, that relationship was no longer found while AoCKD status appeared as an independent risk factor for in-hospital death.

Our results are consistent with previous works: For example, Sawhney et al., [47] observed a higher mortality associated with AKI severity, regardless of baseline eGFR; Zhou et al., [31] reported that AKI severity in patients with decompensated heart failure, assessed using the RIFLE classification, was directly correlated with mortality rates both in P-AKI and AoCKD, but the latter group showed more comorbidities and higher risk of death than P-AKI individuals; Machado et al., [46] also described an increased risk of death associated with AKI severity in patients with preoperatively increased SCr who underwent cardiac surgery. Conversely, higher in-hospital mortality in P-AKI, but not in AoCKD patients, has been linked to AKI severity using the RIFLE and KDIGO-2012 classifications in other studies [35–38]. Some of these works are based on specific populations, such as the critically ill, describing similar mortality rates in both groups compared to our findings [34,36]. In these settings, the severity of illness could modify the course and outcomes of AKI, explaining the higher mortality observed in P-AKI subjects. Moreover, some of these studies included considerably younger patients in both groups, e.g., Prakash et al., [37]. Our population consists of elderly patients that suffer more frequently relevant comorbid conditions; this could explain the effect of AKI on the excess mortality in AoCKD individuals. We found a similar rate for need of RRT in both groups; irrespective of baseline renal function, these patients showed higher in-hospital mortality (Table 3). Dialysis-dependence at discharge was less frequent in the P-AKI group, regardless of AKI severity. Moreover, approximately 30% of AoCKD were dialysis-dependent at discharge, a lower percentage than that previously described in the literature [32,36], which may be linked to the higher in-hospital mortality observed in this group in our sample. P-AKI patients were admitted more frequently to the ICU; in both groups, AKI severity was directly correlated with admission to the ICU. AKI severity was associated with higher LOS in the P-AKI group, but not in the AoCKD group. This is probably due to AKI severity being intrinsically associated with severity of illness in P-AKI, but not in AoCKD patients.

The present study has several strengths: The study provides a novel approach regarding the influence of each KDIGO-2012 AKI criterion over outcomes in P-AKI and AoCKD patients. All patients have a baseline SCr value to calculate eGFR and the rate of SCr increments; data were obtained prior to the index hospitalization, thus, avoiding the use of surrogate values for calculating baseline renal function. Our cohort consists a heterogeneous sample of hospitalized patients with AKI, not restricted to critically ill or those with a specific condition, such as advanced heart failure, allowing a more reliable representation of a nephrologist day-to-day clinical activity; this increases the generalizability of results not limited to a specific clinical setting. We used standardized and updated definitions of AKI and CKD, following currently available KDIGO guidelines and recorded extensive data on comorbid conditions, which allowed us to adjust for these factors when considering outcomes.

We also acknowledge several important limitations: This is a retrospective single-center study of patients that were treated at least once by the nephrology department, which could lead to a selection bias toward higher AKI severity in both groups, but this circumstance could drive to increased specificity. Extensive efforts were undertaken to adjust for potential confounding, but residual confounding is still possible. Comorbid conditions, such as diabetes, hypertension or coronary artery disease, were considered as dichotomic variables, so there may be residual confounding by severity of these comorbidities. We did not use the urine output criterion. We used only SCr and no other biomarkers for diagnosing and staging AKI. We could not differentiate between true AoCKD and progression of primary renal disease (no biomarkers, few renal biopsies). Follow up was limited to the length of admission to reduce potential bias associated with differential losses to follow up between groups.highlighted.

5. Conclusions

To our knowledge, this is the first study that compares the in-hospital outcomes of patients with previous normal and impaired renal function through KDIGO-2012 stages and criteria. The results showed that AKI KDIGO-2012 classification predicted in-hospital mortality in both P-AKI and AoCKD patients, but we found a differential effect of AKI KDIGO-2012 criteria on outcomes among AoCKD patients compared to P-AKI subjects. Several authors have proposed that certain specific conditions, such as CKD or advanced age, should be taken into account while applying AKI classifications [35,48]. RIFLE, AKIN and/or KDIGO-2012 were designed for and tested in patients with previously normal renal function, but considering the different outcomes observed among P-AKI and AoCKD subjects within the same AKI stage and criterion maybe one size does not fit all AKI patients. We consider that AoCKD may constitute a separate clinical syndrome, and due to the increasing prevalence of CKD, the development of adequate staging criteria for AoCKD could help prompt the diagnosis and administration of appropriate therapy.

Author Contributions: Conceptualization and methodology, I.A.-O., J.B.-B., A.M.-H. and A.C.-R.; formal analysis, I.A.-O. and A.C.-R.; investigation, I.A.-O., data curation, I.A.-O. and A.C.-R.; writing—original draft preparation, I.A.-O. and A.C.-R.; writing—review and editing, I.A.-O., J.B.-M. and A.C.-R.; supervision, J.B.-M., J.B.-B. and A.M.-H.

Acknowledgments: To J. Martín-Gago, staff and residents of the nephrology department of our hospital.

References

1. Sawhney, S.; Fraser, S.D. Epidemiology of AKI: Utilizing Large Databases to Determine the Burden of AKI. *Adv. Chronic. Kidney Dis.* **2017**, *24*, 194–204. [CrossRef] [PubMed]
2. Kidney Disease: Improving Global Outcomes (KDIGO); Acute Kidney Injury Work Group. KDIGO clinical practice guidelines for acute kidney injury. *Kidney Int. Suppl.* **2012**, *2*, 1–138.
3. Susantitaphong, P.; Cruz, D.N.; Cerda, J.; Abulfaraj, M.; Alqahtani, F.; Koulouridis, I.; Jaber, B.L.; Acute Kidney Injury Advisory Group of the American Society of Nephrology. World incidence of AKI: A meta-analysis. *Clin. J. Am. Soc. Nephrol.* **2013**, *8*, 1482–1493. [CrossRef] [PubMed]
4. Lameire, N.H.; Bagga, A.; Cruz, D.; de Maeseneer, J.; Endre, Z.; Kellum, J.A.; Liu, K.D.; Mehta, R.L.; Pannu, N.; van Biesen, W.; et al. Acute kidney injury: An increasing global concern. *Lancet* **2013**, *382*, 170–179. [CrossRef]
5. Collister, D.; Pannu, N.; Ye, F.; James, M.; Hemmelgarn, B.; Chui, B.; Manns, B.; Klarenbach, S. Alberta Kidney Disease Network. Health Care Costs Associated with AKI. *Clin. J. Am. Soc. Nephrol.* **2017**, *12*, 1733–1743. [CrossRef] [PubMed]
6. Murugan, R.; Kellum, J.A. Acute kidney injury: What's the prognosis? *Nat. Rev. Nephrol.* **2011**, *7*, 209–217. [CrossRef]
7. Chawla, L.S.; Amdur, R.L.; Shaw, A.D.; Faselis, C.; Palant, C.E.; Kimmel, P.L. Association between AKI and long-term renal and cardiovascular outcomes in United States veterans. *Clin. J. Am. Soc. Nephrol.* **2014**, *9*, 448–456. [CrossRef]
8. Omotoso, B.A.; Abdel-Rahman, E.M.; Xin, W.; Ma, J.Z.; Scully, K.W.; Arogundade, F.A.; Balogun, R.A. Acute kidney injury (AKI) outcome, a predictor of long-term major adverse cardiovascular events (MACE). *Clin. Nephrol.* **2016**, *85*, 1–11. [CrossRef]
9. Odutayo, A.; Wong, C.X.; Farkouh, M.; Altman, D.G.; Hopewell, S.; Emdin, C.A.; Hunn, B.H. AKI and Long-Term Risk for Cardiovascular Events and Mortality. *J. Am. Soc. Nephrol.* **2017**, *28*, 377–387. [CrossRef]
10. Chawla, L.S. Disentanglement of the acute kidney injury syndrome. *Curr. Opin. Crit. Care.* **2012**, *18*, 579–584. [CrossRef]
11. Palevsky, P.M. Renal replacement therapy in acute kidney injury. *Adv. Chronic. Kidney Dis.* **2013**, *20*, 76–84. [CrossRef] [PubMed]
12. Brienza, N.; Giglio, M.T.; Dalfino, L. Protocoled resuscitation and the prevention of acute kidney injury. *Curr. Opin. Crit. Care.* **2012**, *18*, 613–622. [CrossRef] [PubMed]

13. Alsabbagh, M.M.; Asmar, A.; Ejaz, N.I.; Aiyer, R.K.; Kambhampati, G.; Ejaz, A.A. Update on clinical trials for the prevention of acute kidney injury in patients undergoing cardiac surgery. *Am. J. Surg.* **2013**, *206*, 86–95. [CrossRef] [PubMed]

14. Chopra, T.A.; Brooks, C.H.; Okusa, M.D. Acute Kidney Injury Prevention. *Contrib. Nephrol.* **2016**, *187*, 9–23. [CrossRef] [PubMed]

15. Hayes, W. Stop adding insult to injury-identifying and managing risk factors for the progression of acute kidney injury in children. *Pediatr. Nephrol.* **2017**, *32*, 2235–2243. [CrossRef] [PubMed]

16. Kidney Disease: Improving Global Outcomes (KDIGO) CKD Work Group. KDIGO 2012 Clinical Practice Guideline for the Evaluation and Management of Chronic Kidney Disease. *Kidney Int. Suppl.* **2013**, *3*, 1–150.

17. Jha, V.; Garcia-Garcia, G.; Iseki, K.; Li, Z.; Naicker, S.; Plattner, B.; Saran, R.; Wang, A.Y.; Yang, C.W. Chronic kidney disease: Global dimension and perspectives. *Lancet* **2013**, *382*, 260–272. [CrossRef]

18. Quaggin, S.E. Kindling the Kidney. *N. Engl. J. Med.* **2016**, *374*, 281–283. [CrossRef]

19. Hsu, C.Y.; Ordonez, J.D.; Chertow, G.M.; Fan, D.; McCulloch, C.E.; Go, A.S. The risk of acute renal failure in patients with chronic kidney disease. *Kidney Int.* **2008**, *74*, 101–107. [CrossRef]

20. Bedford, M.; Farmer, C.; Levin, A.; Ali, T.; Stevens, P. Acute Kidney Injury and CKD: Chicken or Egg? *Am. J. Kidney Dis.* **2012**, *59*, 485–491. [CrossRef]

21. Palevsky, P.M. Chronic-on-acute kidney injury. *Kidney Int.* **2012**, *81*, 430–431. [CrossRef] [PubMed]

22. Heung, M.; Steffick, D.E.; Zivin, K.; Gillespie, B.W.; Banerjee, T.; Hsu, C.Y.; Powe, N.R.; Pavkov, M.E.; Williams, D.E.; Saran, R.; et al. Centers for Disease Control and Prevention CKD Surveillance Team. Acute Kidney Injury Recovery Pattern and Subsequent Risk of CKD: An Analysis of Veterans Health Administration Data. *Am. J. Kidney Dis.* **2016**, *67*, 742–752. [CrossRef] [PubMed]

23. Chawla, L.S.; Eggers, P.W.; Star, R.A.; Kimmel, P.L. Acute kidney injury and chronic kidney disease as interconnected syndromes. *N. Engl. J. Med.* **2014**, *371*, 58–66. [CrossRef] [PubMed]

24. Lim, P.; Khoo, O.T. Hypermagnesaemia in Presence of Magnesium Depletion in Acute-on-chronic Renal Failure. *Br. Med. J.* **1969**, *1*, 414–416. [CrossRef] [PubMed]

25. He, L.; Wei, Q.; Liu, J.; Yi, M.; Liu, Y.; Liu, H.; Sun, L.; Peng, Y.; Liu, F.; Venkatachalam, M.A.; et al. AKI on CKD: Heightened injury, suppressed repair, and the underling mechanisms. *Kidney Int.* **2017**, *92*, 1071–1083. [CrossRef] [PubMed]

26. Zager, R.A. Progression of Acute Kidney Injury to Chronic Kidney Disease: Clinical and Experimental Insights and Queries. *Nephron. Clin. Pract.* **2014**, *127*, 46–50. [CrossRef] [PubMed]

27. Zager, R.A. 'Biologic memory' in response to acute kidney injury: Cytoresistance, toll-like receptor hyper-responsiveness and the onset of progressive renal disease. *Nephrol. Dial. Transplant.* **2013**, *28*, 1985–1993. [CrossRef] [PubMed]

28. Goldfarb, M.; Rosenberger, C.; Abassi, Z.; Shina, A.; Zilbersat, F.; Eckardt, K.U.; Rosen, S.; Heyman, S.N.; Source, AJ. Acute-on-chronic renal failure in the rat: Functional compensation and hypoxia tolerance. *Am. J. Nephrol.* **2006**, *26*, 22–33. [CrossRef] [PubMed]

29. Singh, P.; Rifkin, D.E.; Blantz, R.C. Chronic kidney disease: An inherent risk factor for acute kidney injury? *Clin. J. Am. Soc. Nephrol.* **2010**, *5*, 1690–1695. [CrossRef]

30. Grams, M.E.; Sang, Y.; Ballew, S.H.; Gansevoort, R.T.; Kimm, H.; Kovesdy, C.P.; Naimark, D.; Oien, C.; Smith, D.H.; Coresh, J.; et al. A Meta-analysis of the Association of Estimated GFR, Albuminuria, Age, Race, and Sex with Acute Kidney Injury. *Am. J. Kidney Dis.* **2015**, *66*, 591–601. [CrossRef]

31. Zhou, Q.; Zhao, C.; Xie, D.; Xu, D.; Bin, J.; Chen, P.; Liang, M.; Zhang, X.; Hou, F. Acute and acute-on-chronic kidney injury of patients with decompensated heart failure: Impact on outcomes. *BMC Nephrol.* **2012**. [CrossRef] [PubMed]

32. Hsu, C.Y.; Chertow, G.M.; McCulloch, C.E.; Fan, D.; Ordoñez, J.D.; Go, A.S. Nonrecovery of Kidney Function and Death after Acute on Chronic Renal Failure. *Clin. J. Am. Soc. Nephrol.* **2009**, *4*, 891–898. [CrossRef] [PubMed]

33. Pannu, N.; James, M.; Hemmelgarn, B.R.; Dong, J.; Tonelli, M.; Klarenbach, S. Modification of outcomes after acute kidney injury by the presence of CKD. *Am. J. Kid. Dis.* **2011**, *58*, 206–213. [CrossRef] [PubMed]

34. Neyra, J.A.; Mescia, F.; Li, X.; Adams-Huet, B.; Yessayan, L.; Yee, J.; Toto, R.D.; Moe, O.W. Impact of acute kidney injury and CKD on adverse outcomes in critically ill septic patients. *Kidney Int. Rep.* **2018**, *3*, 1344–1353. [CrossRef] [PubMed]

35. Pan, H.C.; Wu, P.C.; Wu, V.C.; Yang, Y.F.; Huang, T.M.; Shiao, C.C.; Chen, T.C.; Tarng, D.C.; Lin, J.H.; Yang, W.S.; et al. A nationwide survey of clinical characteristics, management, and outcomes of acute kidney injury (AKI)-patients with and without preexisting chronic kidney disease have different prognoses. *Medicine (Baltimore)* **2016**, *95*, e4987. [CrossRef] [PubMed]

36. Khosla, N.; Soroko, S.B.; Chertow, G.M.; Himmelfarb, J.; Ikizler, T.A.; Paganini, E.; Mehta, R.L.; Program to Improve Care in Acute Renal Disease (PICARD). Preexisting chronic kidney disease: A potential for improved outcomes from acute kidney injury. *Clin. J. Am. Soc. Nephrol.* **2009**, *4*, 1914–1919. [CrossRef] [PubMed]

37. Prakash, J.; Rathore, S.S.; Arora, P.; Ghosh, B.; Singh, T.B.; Gupta, T.; Mishra, R.N. Comparison of clinical characteristics of acute kidney injury versus acute-on-chronic renal failure: Our experience in a developing country. *Hong Kong J. Nephrol.* **2015**, *17*, 14e20. [CrossRef]

38. Ali, T.; Khan, I.; Simpson, W.; Prescott, G.; Townend, J.; Smith, W.; Macleod, A. Incidence and outcomes in acute kidney injury: A comprehensive population-based study. *J. Am. Soc. Nephrol.* **2007**, *18*, 1292–1298. [CrossRef] [PubMed]

39. Bellomo, R.; Ronco, C.; Kellum, J.A.; Mehta, R.L.; Palevsky, P.; ADQI Workgroup. Acute renal failure—definition, outcome measures, animal models, fluid therapy and information technology needs: The Second International Consensus Conference of the Acute Dialysis Quality Initiative (ADQI) Group. *Crit. Care* **2004**, *8*, R204–R212. [CrossRef]

40. Ronco, C.; Levin, A.; Warnock, D.G.; Mehta, R.; Kellum, J.A.; Shah, S.; Molitoris, B.A.; AKIN Working Group. Improving outcomes from acute kidney injury (AKI): Report on an initiative. *Int. J. Artif. Organs.* **2007**, *30*, 373–376. [CrossRef]

41. Levey, A.S.; Bosch, J.P.; Lewis, J.B.; Greene, T.; Rogers, N.; Roth, D. A more accurate method to estimate glomerular filtration rate from serum creatinine: A new prediction equation. Modification of Diet in Renal Disease Study Group. *Ann. Intern. Med.* **1999**, *130*, 461–470. [CrossRef] [PubMed]

42. Siew, E.D.; Ikizler, T.A.; Matheny, M.E.; Shi, Y.; Schildcrout, J.S.; Danciu, I.; Dwyer, J.P.; Srichai, M.; Hung, A.M.; Smith, J.P.; et al. Estimating Baseline Kidney Function in Hospitalized Patients with Impaired Kidney Function. *Clin. J. Am. Soc. Nephrol.* **2012**, *7*, 712–719. [CrossRef] [PubMed]

43. Der Mesropian, P.J.; Kalamaras, J.S.; Eisele, G.; Phelps, K.R.; Asif, A.; Mathew, R.O. Long-term outcomes of community-acquired versus hospital-acquired acute kidney injury: A retrospective analysis. *Clin. Nephrol.* **2014**, *81*, 81–174. [CrossRef] [PubMed]

44. Charlson, M.E.; Pompei, P.; Ales, K.L.; MacKenzie, C.R. A new method of classifying prognostic comorbidity in longitudinal studies: Development and validation. *J. Chronic. Dis.* **1987**, *40*, 373–383. [CrossRef]

45. Hatakeyama, Y.; Horino, T.; Nagata, K.; Matsumoto, T.; Terada, Y.; Okuhara, Y. Transition from acute kidney injury to chronic kidney disease: A single centre cohort study. *Clin. Exp. Nephrol.* **2018**, *22*, 1281–1293. [CrossRef] [PubMed]

46. Machado, M.N.; Nakazone, M.A.; Maia, L.N. Acute kidney injury based on KDIGO (Kidney Disease Improving Global Outcomes) criteria in patients with elevated baseline serum creatinine undergoing cardiac surgery. *Rev. Bras. Cir. Cardiovasc.* **2014**, *29*, 299–307. [CrossRef]

47. Sawhney, S.; Marks, A.; Fluck, N.; Levin, A.; Prescott, G.; Black, C. Intermediate and long-term outcomes of survivors of acute kidney injury episodes: A large population-based cohort study. *Am. J. Kid. Dis.* **2017**, *69*, 18–28. [CrossRef] [PubMed]

48. Chao, C.T.; Wu, VC.; Lai, C.F.; Shiao, C.C.; Huang, T.M.; Wu, P.C.; Tsai, I.J.; Hou, C.C.; Wang, W.J.; Tsai, H.B.; et al. Advanced age affects the outcome-predictive power of RIFLE classification in geriatric patients with acute kidney injury. *Kidney Int.* **2012**, *82*, 920–927. [CrossRef]

17

Outcome Prediction of Acute Kidney Injury Biomarkers at Initiation of Dialysis in Critical Units

Vin-Cent Wu [1], **Chih-Chung Shiao** [2,3], **Nai-Hsin Chi** [4], **Chih-Hsien Wang** [4],
Shih-Chieh Jeff Chueh [5], **Hung-Hsiang Liou** [6], **Herbert D. Spapen** [7,*], **Patrick M. Honore** [8,*]
and Tzong-Shinn Chu [1,9,*]

[1]   Division of Nephrology, National Taiwan University Hospital, No. 7 Chung-Shan South Road,
       Zhong-Zheng District, Taipei 100, Taiwan; q91421028@ntu.edu.tw
[2]   Division of Nephrology, Department of Internal Medicine, Saint Mary's Hospital Luodong,
       No. 160 Chong-Cheng South Road, Loudong, Yilan 265, Taiwan; chungyy2001@yahoo.com.tw
[3]   Saint Mary's Junior College of Medicine, Nursing and Management College, No. 100, Ln. 265, Sec. 2,
       Sanxing Rd., Sanxing Township, Yilan 266, Taiwan
[4]   Surgery Department, National Taiwan University Hospital, No. 7 Chung-Shan South Road,
       Zhong-Zheng District, Taipei 100, Taiwan; chinaihsin@ntuh.gov.tw (N.-H.C.); wchemail@gmail.com (C.-H.W.)
[5]   Glickman Urological and Kidney Institute, Cleveland Clinic Lerner College of Medicine, Cleveland Clinic,
       Cleveland, 9500 Euclid Ave., Cleveland, OH 44195, USA; jeffchueh@gmail.com
[6]   Division of Nephrology, Department of Internal Medicine, Hsin-Jen Hospital, Dialysis Center,
       Hsin-Ren Clinics, No. 395, Chung-Shan Road, New Taipei City 231, Taiwan; hh258527@ms23.hinet.net
[7]   ICU Department, Universitair Ziekenhuis Brussel, Vrije Universiteit Brussel, 101, Laarbeeklaan,
       1090 Jette, Belgium
[8]   ICU Department, CHU Brugmann University Hospital, 4 Place Arthur Van Gehucthen, 1020 Brussels, Belgium
[9]   NSARF Group (National Taiwan University Hospital Study Group of ARF), Taipei 100, Taiwan
[*]   Correspondence: herbert.spapen@uzbrussel.be (H.D.S.); Patrick.Honore@CHU-Brugmann.be (P.M.H.);
       tschu@ntu.edu.tw (T.-S.C.)

Abstract: The ideal circumstances for whether and when to start RRT remain unclear. The outcome predictive ability of acute kidney injury (AKI) biomarkers measuring at dialysis initializing need more validation. This prospective, multi-center observational cohort study enrolled 257 patients with AKI undergoing renal replacement therapy (RRT) shortly after admission. At the start of RRT, blood and urine samples were collected for relevant biomarker measurement. RRT dependence and all-cause mortality were recorded up to 90 days after discharge. Areas under the receiver operator characteristic (AUROC) curves and a multivariate generalized additive model were applied to predict outcomes. One hundred and thirty-five (52.5%) patients died within 90 days of hospital discharge. Plasma c-terminal FGF-23 (cFGF-23) had the best discriminative ability (AUROC, 0.687) as compared with intact FGF-23 (iFGF-23) (AUROC, 0.504), creatinine-adjusted urine neutrophil gelatinase-associated lipocalin (AUROC, 0.599), and adjusted urine cFGF-23 (AUROC, 0.653) regardless whether patients were alive or not on day 90. Plasma cFGF-23 levels above 2050 RU/mL were independently associated with higher 90-day mortality (HR 1.76, $p = 0.020$). Higher cFGF-23 levels predicted less weaning from dialysis in survivors (HR, 0.62, $p = 0.032$), taking mortality as a competing risk. Adding cFGF-23 measurement to the AKI risk predicting score significantly improved risk stratification and 90-day mortality prediction (total net reclassification improvement = 0.148; $p = 0.002$). In patients with AKI who required RRT, increased plasma cFGF-23 levels correlated with higher 90-day overall mortality after discharge and predicted worse kidney recovery in survivors. When coupled to the AKI risk predicting score, cFGF-23 significantly improved mortality risk prediction. This observation adds evidence that cFGF-23 could be used as an optimal timing biomarker to initiate RRT.

Keywords: acute kidney injury; biomarker; fibroblast growth factor-23; kidney injury molecule-1; mortality; neutrophil gelatinase-associated lipocalin; renal replacement therapy

1. Background

Renal replacement therapy (RRT) is life-saving in patients with acute kidney injury (AKI) but is not devoid of serious complications and severe adverse events [1]. Patients who, even temporarily, require RRT also may develop more frequently long-term or end-stage renal disease (ESRD) and have a higher mortality risk [2]. The need for and the optimal timing to initiate RRT are crucial yet unresolved issues [1,3].

Nephrologists continuously look out for kidney specific biomarkers that assist in fine-tuning of diagnosis, treatment, and prognosis of AKI [4]. Few biomarkers were validated as outcome-specific biomarkers in critically ill patients at initiation of RRT. Urine neutrophil gelatinase-associated lipocalin (NGAL) was one of the first biomarkers to be validated for predicting short-term mortality in patients with advanced AKI [5] and recently became part of the indicators to decide early start of dialysis [6]. Interleukin-18 (IL-18) at the commencement of dialysis could also predict hospital mortality in critically ill patients [7]. Adding plasma interleukin-8 to a parsimonious clinical model (i.e., age, mean arterial pressure, mechanical ventilation, and bilirubin) augmented prediction of renal recovery and AKI mortality compared with using only the clinical variables [8].

Fibroblast growth factor 23 (FGF-23), a peptide initially recognized for its phosphaturic role in rare genetic or acquired hypophosphatemia disorders [9], is one of the most recently proposed kidney biomarkers. FGF-23 acts as a hormone that significantly influences phosphate, vitamin D, and bone mineral homeostasis [10]. Several research groups have proposed cFGF-23 as a biomarker for predicting early occurrence of AKI, evaluating prognosis of chronic kidney disease (CKD), and estimating cardiovascular morbidity and mortality [11–15].

An important area of AKI research particularly focuses on reinforcing current dialysis requiring AKI by adding measurement of (a) sensitive biomarker (s) to assess the impact of RRT on relevant patient outcome variables. Within this perspective, we designed a study to evaluate the predictive capacity of various structural and functional kidney biomarkers (including the novel markers cFGF-23 and iFGF-23) and disease severity scores, measured at initiation of RRT, on survival and renal function recovery in a cohort of AKI patients.

2. Methods

2.1. Registration of Clinical Trials

This study was approved by the University's Institutional Review Board (201409024RINB in National Taiwan University Hospital, 01-X16-059 in Buddhist Tzu Chi General Hospital, and TYGH104007 in Taoyuan General Hospital) and written informed consent was obtained from all subjects participating in the trial. The trial was registered prior to patient enrollment at clinicaltrials.gov (NCT01503710, Principal investigator: V.-C.W, Date of registration: 28 February 2012).

2.2. Study Population

The study was conducted by the National Taiwan University Study Group on Acute Renal Failure (NSARF) and based on a prospectively created AKI database [16–20]. From August 2011 until January 2015, 257 AKI patients who required RRT after intensive care unit (ICU) admission were prospectively enrolled. Exclusion criteria included: age <18 years, previous nephrectomy, renal transplantation or RRT treatment, ICU or hospital length of stay of respectively <2 days and >180 days during the index hospitalization, and AKI caused by urologic surgery induced injury, vasculitis, obstruction, glomerulonephritis, interstitial nephritis, hemolytic uremic syndrome, or thrombotic thrombocytopenic purpura.

2.3. Data Collection

Baseline characteristics, including demographic data, co-morbidities, the cause of AKI. For the risk prediction before initializing dialysis, the individual AKI risk predicting score was calculated [21]. The worst physiological values and biochemical data on the index day were recorded.

Baseline serum creatinine (sCr) was the nadir value obtained after the previous admission in those who had more than one admission within 1 year before the index admission, or estimated with the Modification of Diet in Renal Disease equation (assuming an average eGFR of 75 mL/min/1.73 m^2) [22]. Peak sCr was defined as the highest sCr before RRT initiation in the ICU. Indication for dialysis and organ failure were defined as previously reported [16,23,24] (Supplemental Data file).

RRT modalities in each patient were initially chosen by the attending physician and adapted according to hemodynamic evaluation and evolution by the critical care nephrologist (Supplemental Data file).

2.4. Measurements of Kidney Biomarkers

The urine samples, collected in separate polypropylene tubes containing sodium azide at dialysis initiation, were stored at -80 °C until required. Each specimen was centrifuged (800× g at 4 °C for 5 min) and the supernatant was collected for ELISA analysis.

Kidney biomarker levels were assessed with a human FGF-23 C-terminal/intact-terminal ELISA kit (Immutopics; San Clemente, CA, USA), a human KIM-1, and a lipocalin-2/NGAL ELISA kit (R&D Systems, Inc., Minneapolis, MN, USA).

The cFGF-23 and iFGF-23 values were expressed in relative units (RU)/mL and pg/mL, respectively. The coefficient of variation was 4.4% for iFGF-23 and 4.0% for cFGF-23. The lower limits for detection of cFGF-23, iFGF-23, KIM-1 and NGAL were 0.156 RU/mL, 0.2 pg/mL, 0.046 ng/mL, and 0.04 ng/mL, respectively were completed as described by the manufacturer's protocol and performed in duplicate. 1,25 di hydroxyvitamin D was measured using DiaSorin radioimmunoassay assays kit (Stillwater, MN, USA) and total 25-hydroxyvitamin D was measured using an electro-chemiluminescence (Elecsys® Vitamin D total, Cobas, Roche©). Urine creatinine levels were measured with the Jaffe assay, with standardization of the isotope dilution mass spectrometry traceable reference.

2.5. Outcome Definitions

Primary clinical endpoints were 90-day mortality after hospital discharge and dialysis dependency at 90 days in survivors. Secondary end-points included a 90-day composite outcome (ongoing dialysis or 90-day mortality after discharge), in-hospital mortality, and a composite outcome at discharge (ongoing dialysis or mortality at discharge). All patients were followed until death or for a time span exceeding 90 days after discharge, whichever occurred first. Successful withdrawal from dialysis was defined as surviving without dialysis at the end of study.

2.6. Statistical Analysis

All the univariate significant and non-significant relevant covariates, including age, sex, baseline comorbidities, indication for dialysis, etiology of AKI, kidney function profile (e.g., baseline eGFR and candidate biomarkers, candidate biomarkers and SOFA score at dialysis initiation, dialysis modality, and some of their interactions were put on the variable lists to be selected (Table 1). Two-sample student's t-test was used to analyze continuous data and χ^2 test or Fisher's exact test was used to analyze categorical data. The accumulated hazard ratio was modeled by Cox regression models and adjusted for the covariates for the outcomes of interest (Supplemental Data file). The significance levels for entry (SLE) and for stay (SLS) were set to 0.15 for being conservative. Then, with the aid of substantive knowledge, the best candidate final logistic regression model was identified manually by dropping the covariates with $p > 0.05$ one at a time until all regression coefficients were significantly different from 0.

Table 1. Clinical characteristics of patient grouped by 90 days outcome.

	All	90-Day Survival	90-Day Mortality	p	90-Day Composite Outcome (−)	90-Day Composite Outcome (+)	p
	(n = 257)	(n = 122)	(n = 135)		(n = 76)	(n = 181)	
Patient characteristics							
Age	65.7 ± 16.6	63.4 ± 16.0	67.8 ± 16.9	0.035	61.3 ± 17.5	67.6 ± 15.9	0.005
Gender (male (%))	167 (65.0%)	82 (67.2%)	85 (63.0%)	0.514	54 (71.1%)	113 (62.4%)	0.200
Baseline creatinine (mg/dL)	2.0 ± 1.6	2.5 ± 1.9	1.5 ± 1.1	<0.001	1.8 ± 1.3	2.1 ± 1.7	0.220
eGFR (MDRD) (mL/min/1.73 m²)	55.6 ± 41.0	48.3 ± 44.2	62.2 ± 36.9	0.006	63.3 ± 47.6	52.3 ± 37.6	0.428
Co-morbidities							
Diabetes mellitus	115 (44.7%)	61 (50.0%)	54 (40.0%)	0.132	33 (43.4%)	82 (45.3%)	0.891
Cirrhosis	9 (3.5%)	3 (2.5%)	6 (4.4%)	0.505	2 (2.6%)	7 (3.9%)	0.999
COPD	15 (5.8%)	5 (4.1%)	10 (7.4%)	0.297	5 (6.6%)	10 (5.5%)	0.777
CAD	54 (21.0%)	24 (19.7%)	30 (22.2%)	0.648	18 (23.7%)	36 (19.9%)	0.505
CVA	24 (9.3%)	9 (7.4%)	15 (11.1%)	0.392	4 (5.3%)	20 (11.0%)	0.166
Congestive heart failure				0.683			0.780
0	67 (26.1%)	33 (27.0%)	34 (25.2%)		19 (25.0%)	48 (26.5%)	
I	100 (38.9%)	43 (35.2%)	57 (42.2%)		28 (36.8%)	72 (39.8%)	
II	51 (19.8%)	24 (19.7%)	27 (20.0%)		14 (18.4%)	37 (20.4%)	
III	31 (12.1%)	17 (13.9%)	14 (10.4%)		12 (15.8%)	19 (10.5%)	
Laboratory data at ICU admission							
BUN (mg/dL)	48.0 ± 33.5	58.1 ± 34.5	38.9 ± 29.9	<0.001	48.9 ± 36.6	47.7 ± 32.2	0.783
pH	7.4 ± 0.1	7.4 ± 0.8	7.4 ± 0.1	0.659	7.4 ± 0.1	7.4 ± 0.1	0.612
FiO₂	0.5 ± 0.2	0.5 ± 0.2	0.5 ± 0.2	0.916	5 ± 0.2	0.5 ± 0.2	0.218
SBP (mmHg)	121.0 ± 28.4	129.8 ± 28.8	113.0 ± 25.6	<0.001	126.0 ± 25.6	118.8 ± 29.3	0.063
GCS	11.9 ± 4.2	12.3 ± 4.0	11.6 ± 4.4	0.164	11.9 ± 4.1	11.9 ± 4.3	0.948
SOFA	8.9 ± 3.5	8.3 ± 3.1	9.5 ± 3.7	0.008	8.7 ± 3.4	9.1 ± 3.6	0.410
APACHE II	16.3 ± 6.2	15.6 ± 6.0	9.5 ± 3.8	0.094	15.0 ± 6.4	16.9 ± 6.0	0.025
MODS	5.9 ± 3.7	5.5 ± 3.4	6.4 ± 3.8	0.040	5.7 ± 3.3	6.0 ± 3.8	0.507

Table 1. *Cont.*

	All	90-Day Survival	90-Day Mortality	p	90-Day Composite Outcome (−)	90-Day Composite Outcome (+)	p
	(n = 257)	(n = 122)	(n = 135)		(n = 76)	(n = 181)	
Etiology of AKI							
Shock	150 (58.4%)	56 (5.9%)	94 (69.6)	<0.001	40 (52.6%)	110 (60.8%)	0.268
Sepsis	98 (38.1%)	26 (23.8%)	69 (51.1%)	<0.001	22 (28.9%)	76 (42.0%)	0.067
Drug-induced	3 (1.2%)	0 (0%)	3 (2.2%)	0.249	0 (0%)	3 (1.7%)	0.557
Rhabdomyolysis	9 (3.5%)	5 (4.1%)	4 (3.0%)	0.740	4 (5.3%)	5 (2.8%)	0.457
Pigmentation	6 (2.3%)	4 (3.3%)	2 (1.5%)	0.427	4 (5.3%)	2 (1.1%)	0.065
Contrast	37 (14.4%)	22 (18.0%)	15 (11.1%)	0.154	13 (17.1%)	24 (13.3%)	0.440
Other	26 (10.1%)	16 (13.1%)	10 (7.4%)	0.150	7 (9.2%)	19 (10.5%)	0.825
At initiating dialysis							
Admission to dialysis (days)	40.3 ± 27.1	42.0 ± 31.8	37.1 ± 47.5	0.335	45.8 ± 33.9	36.8 ± 43.1	0.106
Mechanical Ventilation	185 (72.0%)	74 (60.7%)	111 (82.2%)	<0.001	49 (64.5%)	136 (75.1%)	0.095
Emergency Surgery	100 (38.9%)	49 (40.2%)	51 (37.8%)	0.703	33 (43.4%)	67 (37.0%)	0.400
IABP	27 (10.5%)	10 (8.2%)	17 (12.6%)	0.310	7 (9.2%)	20 (11.0%)	0.824
Urine output (mL/24 h)	591.7 ± 790.3	750.3 ± 1013.0	448.3 ± 472.1	0.002	869.7 ± 1188.7	474.9 ± 503.1	<0.001
AKI risk prediction score	22.6 ± 6.9	20.2 ± 6.5	24.9 ± 6.5	<0.001	20.8 ± 6.4	23.4 ± 7.0	0.004
Body weight (kg)	66.8 ± 14.3	68.6 ± 15.9	67.8 ± 16.9	0.055	70.0 ± 15.9	65.5 ± 13.4	0.021
IE	8.2 ± 15.0	4.7 ± 8.3	11.3 ± 18.7	<0.001	5.24 ± 9.32	9.43 ± 16.75	0.041
SOFA	10.9 ± 3.9	9.1 ± 3.2	12.6 ± 3.8	<0.001	9.4 ± 3.3	11.6 ± 4.0	<0.001
APACHE II	17.8 ± 6.4	15.6 ± 5.4	19.8 ± 6.7	<0.001	15.5 ± 5.7	18.7 ± 6.5	<0.001
MODS	8.1 ± 4.1	6.5 ± 3.7	9.5 ± 3.9	<0.001	7.0 ± 3.6	8.6 ± 4.2	0.005
Phosphate (mg/dL)	4.5 ± 1.7	4.8 ± 1.6	4.3 ± 1.8	0.085	4.8 ± 1.5	4.4 ± 1.8	0.333
25 OH Vit D, ng/mL	11.7 ± 5.6	10.8 ± 5.5	12.9 ± 5.9	0.471	11.2 ± 7.1	12.0 ± 5.2	0.812
1,25 diOH Vit D, pg/mL	27.3 ± 6.5	25.5 ± 6.4	29.7 ± 6.4	0.545	28.9 ± 6.8	26.6 ± 6.6	0.545

Table 1. *Cont.*

	All	90-Day Survival	90-Day Mortality	p	90-Day Composite Outcome (−)	90-Day Composite Outcome (+)	p
	(n = 257)	(n = 122)	(n = 135)		(n = 76)	(n = 181)	
Kidney function marker							
BUN (mg/dL)	82.4 ± 47.2	82.7 ± 51.5	82.5 ± 45.4	0.922	82.3 ± 51.5	82.5 ± 45.4	0.978
Creatinine (mg/dL)	2.0 ± 1.6	4.1 ± 2.2	4.2 ± 2.4	0.745	4.1 ± 2.2	4.2 ± 2.4	0.745
Urine NGAL (ng/mL)	197.5 ± 85.3	191.0 ± 93.3	203.5 ± 77.1	0.254	189.2 ± 97.6	201.0 ± 79.7	0.330
Urine NGAL/Cre	6.9 ± 11.1	6.8 ± 12.5	6.9 ± 9.7	0.912	5.0 ± 6.9	7.7 ± 12.4	0.085
Urine KIM1 (ng/mL)	6.0 ± 5.8	5.8 ± 5.8	6.2 ± 5.8	0.529	5.9 ± 6.5	5.7 ± 5.4	0.139
Urine KIM1/Cre	0.1 ± 0.2	0.1 ± 0.2	0.1 ± 0.1	0.993	0.1 ± 0.1	0.1 ± 0.2	0.699
Urine cFGF-23/Cre	877.4 ± 994.3	671.4 ± 924.9	1063.5 ± 1021.2	<0.001	699.1 ± 1015.0	952.2 ± 978.6	0.062
Plasma iFGF-23 (pg/mL)	304.2 ± 468.0	395.1 ± 635.6	269.0 ± 385.2	0.265	320.4 ± 551.8	300.2 ± 449.5	0.875
Plasma cFGF-23 (RU/mL)	2630.1 ± 2259.5	1926.7 ± 1745.4	3265.9 ± 2479.0	<0.001	1925.3 ± 1917.3	2926.1 ± 2330.0	0.001
Indication for dialysis							
Azotemia	123 (47.9%)	58 (47.5%)	65 (48.1%)	0.999	32 (42.1%)	91 (50.3%)	0.274
Fluid overload	111 (43.2%)	51 (41.8%)	60 (44.4%)	0.706	30 (39.5%)	81 (44.8%)	0.491
Electrolyte disorders	18 (7.0%)	10 (8.2%)	8 (5.9%)	0.626	7 (9.2%)	11 (6.1%)	0.423
Metabolic acidosis	46 (17.9%)	17 (13.9%)	29 (21.5%)	0.143	11 (14.5%)	35 (19.3%)	0.380
Oliguria	166 (64.6%)	69 (56.6%)	97 (71.9%)	0.013	43 (56.6%)	123 (68.0%)	0.088
Uremic encephalopathy	12 (4.7%)	9 (7.4%)	3 (2.2%)	0.074	6 (7.9%)	6 (3.3%)	0.191
Dialysis modality							
CVVH	62 (21.1%)	16 (13.1)	46 (34.1)	<0.001	15 (19.7%)	47 (26.0%)	0.296
IHD	62 (29.2%)	47 (38.5%)	28 (20.7%)		27 (35.5%)	48 (26.5%)	
SLED	120 (46.7%)	59 (48.5%)	61 (45.2%)		34 (44.7%)	86 (47.5%)	
Relevant outcome parameters							
Hospital length of stay (days)	54.7 ± 50.4	52.3 ± 41.1	56.9 ± 57.6	0.459	59.0 ± 46.3	52.9 ± 52.0	0.383
Duration of hospital dialysis (days)	82.4 ± 60.7	42.0 ± 31.8	37.1 ± 47.5	0.335	45.8 ± 33.9	36.8 ± 43.1	0.745

Abbreviations: AKI, acute kidney injury; APACHE:, Acute Physiology and Chronic Health Evaluation, BMI, body mass index; CABG, coronary artery bypass graft; BUN, blood urea nitrogen; COPD, chronic obstructive pulmonary disease; CPB, cardiopulmonary bypass; Cre, creatinine; CVA, cerebrovascular accident; CVVH, continuous venovenous hemofiltration; eGFR, estimated glomerular filtration rate; FGF-23, Fibroblast growth factor-23; GCS, Glasgow Coma Scale; IABP: intra-aortic balloon pump; IE, inotropic equivalent; ICU, intensive care unit; IHD, intermittent hemodialysis; KIM-1, Kidney Injury Molecule-1; LVEF, Left ventricular ejection fraction; MDRD, Modification of Diet in Renal Disease; MODS, Multiple Organ Dysfunction Syndrome; NGAL, neutrophil gelatinase-associated lipocalin; SLED, sustained low efficiency dialysis; SOFA, Sequential Organ Failure Assessment; Vit D, vitamin D.

Area under the receiver operating characteristic (AUROC) curves were generated to evaluate biomarker performance. We use the methods of Hanley & McNeil (PMID, 6878708) for the calculation of the Standard Error of the Area Under the Curve (AUC) and of the difference between two AUCs. A generalized additive model (GAM) (with spline), incorporating the subject-specific (longitudinal) random effects, was plotted with adjustment for other clinical parameters to assess outcome-predictive effects of candidate biomarkers in individual patients [25,26].

Nonlinear effects of continuous covariates were explored with simple and multiple GAMs, which determine appropriate cut-off point(s) for discriminating candidate biomarkers, if necessary, during the stepwise variable selection procedure. The optimal cut-off value was defined as the log odd equaling zero [27].

Because of the high mortality rate among dialysis patients, competing-risk regression using the Fine and Gray model by considering the subdistribution hazard was also performed [28].

Net re-classification improvement (NRI) and integrated discrimination improvement (IDI) were used to evaluate the ability of candidate biomarkers for more accurate stratification of individuals into higher or lower risk categories (re-classification). Regarding 90-day mortality, an increase in NRI was calculated in a model containing both the AKI risk predicting score [21] and the cFGF-23 measurements, and the result was compared with the AKI risk predicting score alone. We defined 0–20%, 20–80%, and >80% as risk categories and re-classified patients with mortality by decision curve analysis and scatter plot (Supplemental Data file). A $p < 0.05$ was considered significant.

3. Results

3.1. Clinical Characteristics

Two hundred and fifty-seven patients (mean age 65.7 years; 167 (65%) male) with AKI who required RRT were studied. Average SOFA, APACHE II, and MODS scores were respectively 8.9, 16.3, and 5.9.

The main causes of AKI were shock (58.4%), sepsis (38.1%) and contrast nephrotoxicity (14.4%). Nine patients (3.5%) had stage 1 AKI, 58 (22.6%) patients had stage 2 AKI, and 190 (73.9%) patients had stage 3 AKI at RRT initiation. The most frequent indication for RRT was oliguria (64.6%), followed by azotemia (47.9%) and fluid overload (43.2%) (Table 1).

3.2. Hospital and 90-Day Outcomes

The in-hospital mortality rate, composite outcome at discharge, 90-day mortality rate and 90-day composite outcome rate were respectively 48.2%, 67.3%, 52.5%, and 70.4%. Table 1 shows baseline characteristics, pre-RRT and outcome parameters of patients categorized by 90-day mortality and 90-day composite outcome, respectively. Patients who did not survive at 90 days or with a 90–day composite outcome were older, had lower urine output, higher disease severity, risk predicting scores and received higher doses of inotropic equivalents than survivals (Table 1).

Importantly, only higher plasma cFGF-23 levels enabled to differentiate patients with both 90-day mortality/composite outcomes from those without events ($p = 0.001$).

3.3. Discriminative Power of Biomarkers for 90-Day Relevant Outcomes

Levels of SOFA (AUROC, 0.706), AKI risk predicting score (0.677), sCr (0.619), cFGF-23 (0.687), plasma iFGF-23 (0.504), creatinine-adjusted urine NGAL (0.599), adjusted urine cFGF-23 (0.653) and adjusted urine KIM-1 (0.547) at initiation of dialysis could predict 90-day mortality. Plasma cFGF-23 demonstrated better discriminative ability than NGAL for mortality at 90 days ($p = 0.001$ by AUROC comparison) (Figure 1, p at Table S1).

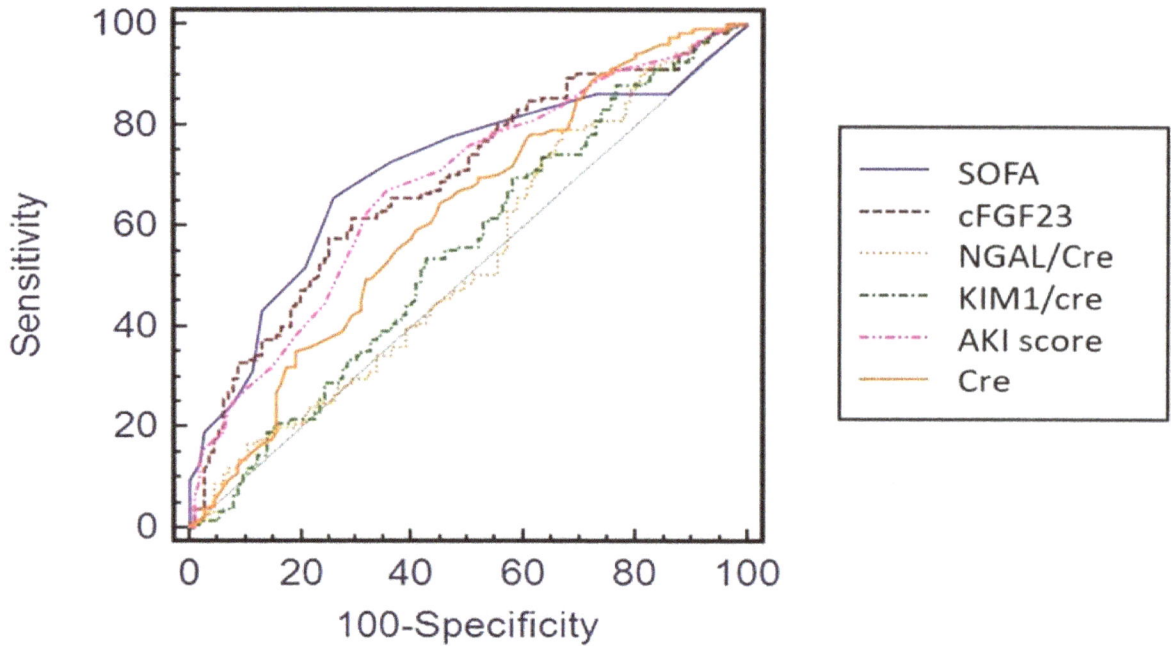

Figure 1. Comparisons of predictive powers for 90-day mortality among different variables. Note: the comparison was performed using the area under the receiver operator characteristic curves (AUROCs). Abbreviations: Cre, creatinine; cFGF-23, c-terminal fibroblast growth factor-23; KIM-1, Kidney Injury Molecule-1; NGAL, neutrophil gelatinase-associated lipocalin; SOFA, Sequential Organ Failure Assessment; KDIGO, Kidney Disease Improving Global Outcomes; AKI, acute kidney injury.

The GAM plot showed a positive correlation between increased plasma cFGF-23 levels at start of dialysis and the log of the odds of 90-day mortality and composite outcome. After adjusting all variables listed in Table 1 for nonlinear effects, plasma cFGF-23, at a cut-off value of 2050 RU/mL by the GAM model, demonstrated independently good prediction of both 90-day mortality (Figure 2A) and 90-day composite outcome (Figure 2B).

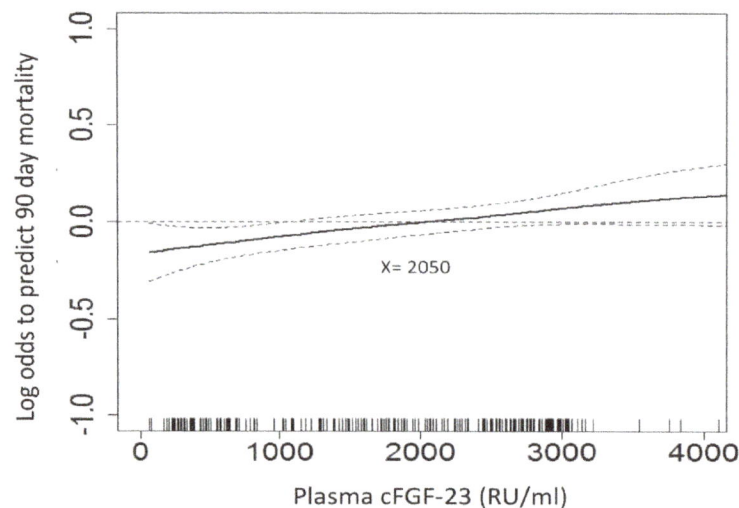

(A)

Figure 2. *Cont.*

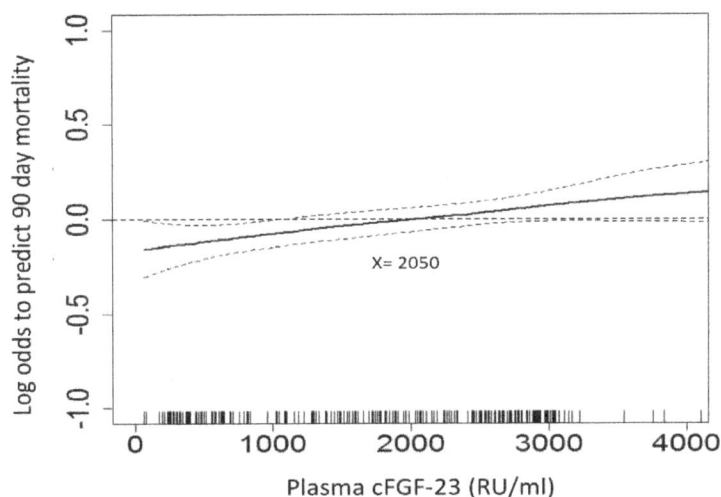

(B)

Figure 2. Generalized additive model (GAM) plot for the probability of (**A**) 90-day mortality, and (**B**) 90-day composite outcome against serum cFGF-23 levels at initiation of dialysis. Note: The GAM plot was incorporated with the subject-specific (longitudinal) random effects expressed as the logarithm of the odds (logit). The probability of outcome events was constructed with cFGF-23 levels averaging zero over the range of the data, i.e., cFGF-23 = 2050 ng/mL. All the relevant covariates, including characteristics, comorbidities, laboratory data, at intensive care unit (ICU) admission, etiology of acute kidney injury (AKI), indication for dialysis, dialysis modality, SOFA score, and plasma cFGF-23 at dialysis, and some of their interactions, such as interventions listed in Table 1, were put on a selected variable list to predict the outcome of interest.

3.4. Plasma cFGF-23 and Outcome

Using a cut-off value of 2050 RU/mL, patients were divided in a "high" and a "low" cFGF-23 group. Subjects with high cFGF-23 had lower baseline sCr, but higher phosphate concentrations at dialysis initiation, higher in-hospital and 90-day mortality, lower dialysis weaning rate and higher composite outcome results (Table 2).

Table 2. Clinical characteristics of patients with high versus low plasma cFGF-23 levels.

Serum cFGF23 Categories	Low cFGF-23	High cFGF-23	p
	(n = 116)	(n = 141)	
Patient characteristics			
Age (years)	65.8 ± 16.0	65.7 ± 17.2	0.973
Gender (male)	77 (66.4%)	90 (63.8%)	0.695
Baseline creatinine (mg/dL)	2.2 ± 1.9	1.8 ± 1.3	0.039
eGFR (MDRD) (mL/min/1.73 m^2)	54.4 ± 42.5	56.5 ± 39.8	0.690
Comorbidities			
Diabetes mellitus	33 (43.4%)	82 (45.3%)	0.891
Cirrhosis	1 (0.9%)	8 (5.7%)	0.044
COPD	7 (6.0%)	8 (5.7%)	0.999
CAD	27 (23.3%)	27 (19.1%)	0.445
CVA	12 (10.3%)	12 (8.5%)	0.670

Table 2. *Cont.*

Serum cFGF23 Categories	Low cFGF-23 (n = 116)	High cFGF-23 (n = 141)	p
Congestive heart failure			0.265
0	32 (27.6%)	35 (24.8%)	
I	37 (31.9%)	63 (44.7%)	
II	27 (23.3%)	24 (17.0%)	
III	15 (12.9%)	16 (11.3%)	
IV	0 (0%)	8 (5.5%)	
Laboratory data at ICU admission			
BUN (mg/dL)	48.3 ± 36.1	47.8 ± 31.4	0.897
pH	7.4 ± 0.1	7.4 ± 0.1	0.354
FiO2	0.5 ± 0.2	0.5 ± 0.2	0.609
SBP	126.1 ± 29.2	116.7 ± 27.0	0.008
GCS	11.9 ± 4.3	11.9 ± 4.2	0.984
SOFA	8.2 ± 3.6	9.6 ± 3.3	0.001
APACHE II	15.9 ± 6.0	16.6 ± 6.4	0.405
MODS	5.7 ± 3.5	6.1 ± 3.8	0.328
Etiology of AKI			
Shock	66 (56.9%)	84 (59.6%)	0.704
Sepsis	40 (34.5%)	58 (41.1%)	0.303
Rhabdomyolysis	7 (6.0%)	2 (1.4%)	0.083
Drug-induced	2 (1.7%)	1 (0.7%)	0.591
Pigmentation	5 (4.3%)	1 (0.7%)	0.094
Contrast	17 (14.7%)	20 (14.2%)	0.999
Others	12 (10.3%)	14 (9.9%)	0.999
At initiating dialysis			
Admission to dialysis (days)	35.5 ± 34.1	42.6 ± 45.4	0.163
Mechanical ventilation	78 (67.2%)	107 (75.9%)	0.128
Emergency Surgery	45 (38.8%)	55 (39.0%)	0.999
IABP	13 (11.2%)	14 (9.9%)	0.839
Urine output (mL/24 h)	650.9 ± 642.9	542.9 ± 892.8	0.277
AKI risk prediction score	21.5 ± 6.7	23.5 ± 6.9	0.021
Body weight (kg)	67.2 ± 15.4	66.5 ± 13.3	0.728
IE	7.14 ± 11.5	9.1 ± 17.4	0.310
SOFA	10.6 ± 4.3	11.2 ± 3.6	0.218
APACHE II	17.8 ± 6.7	11.8 ± 6.2	0.980
MODS	7.8 ± 4.4	8.4 ± 3.8	0.222
Phosphate, mg/dL	4.1 ± 1.7	4.9 ± 1.7	0.021
25 OH Vit D, ng/mL	11.0 ± 5.8	12.5 ± 5.6	0.617
1,25 diOH Vit D, pg/mL	29.7 ± 6.9	25.0 ± 5.5	0.149
Kidney function marker			
BUN (mg/dL)	81.2 ± 45.8	83.4 ± 48.4	0.714
Creatinine (mg/dL)	4.2 ± 2.4	4.1 ± 2.3	0.677
Urine KIM1 (ng/mL)	5.9 ± 5.9	6.1 ± 5.7	0.800
Urine KIM1/Cre	0.13 ± 0.18	0.14 ± 0.14	0.715
Urine NGAL (ng/mL)	196.5 ± 86.1	198.2 ± 85.0	0.916
Urine NGAL/Cre	7.0 12.9	6.8 ± 9.4	0.877
Urine cFGF-23/Cre	523.4 ± 747.2	1173.3 ± 1077.6	<0.001
Plasma iFGF-23 (pg/mL)	257.6 ± 243.0	325.50 ± 542.3	0.536

Table 2. *Cont.*

Serum cFGF23 Categories	Low cFGF-23 (*n* = 116)	High cFGF-23 (*n* = 141)	*p*
Indication for dialysis			
Azotemia	56 (48.3%)	67 (47.5%)	0.999
Fluid overload	48 (41.4%)	63 (44.7%)	0.615
Electrolyte disorders	7 (60%)	11 (7.8%)	0.631
Metabolic acidosis	22 (19.0%)	24 (17.0%)	0.745
Oliguria	73 (62.9%)	93 (66.0%)	0.694
Uremic complication	7 (6.0%)	5 (3.5%)	0.386
Dialysis modality			0.011
CVVH	44 (37.9%)	31 (22.0%)	
IHD	21 (18.1%)	41 (29.1%)	
SLED	51 (44.0%)	69 (48.9%)	
Outcomes of interest			
Hospital length of stay (days)	49.0 ± 43.0	59.4 ± 55.5	0.101
Duration of hospital dialysis (days)	39.9 ± 34.4	39.0 ± 45.5	0.862
Hospital mortality	42 (36.2%)	82 (58.2%)	<0.001
Composite outcome at discharge	69 (59.5%)	104 (73.8%)	<0.001
90-day mortality	45 (38.8%)	90 (63.8%)	<0.001
90-day weaning from dialysis	47 (40.5%)	29 (20.6%)	<0.001
90-day composite outcome	69 (59.5%)	112 (79.4%)	<0.001

Abbreviations: AKI, acute kidney injury; APACHE; Acute Physiology and Chronic Health Evaluation, BMI, body mass index; CABG, coronary artery bypass graft; Cre, creatinine; BUN, blood urea nitrogen; COPD, chronic obstructive pulmonary disease; CPB, cardiopulmonary bypass; Cre, creatinine; CVA, cerebrovascular accident; CVVH, continuous venovenous hemofiltration; eGFR, estimated glomerular filtration rate; FGF-23, Fibroblast growth factor-23; GCS, Glasgow Coma Scale; IABP: intra-aortic balloon pump; IE, inotropic equivalent; ICU, intensive care unit; IHD, intermittent hemodialysis; KIM-1, Kidney Injury Molecule-1; LVEF, Left ventricular ejection fraction; MDRD, Modification of Diet in Renal Disease; MODS, Multiple Organ Dysfunction Syndrome; NGAL, neutrophil gelatinase-associated lipocalin; SLED, sustained low efficiency dialysis; SOFA, Sequential Organ Failure Assessment; Vit D, vitamin D.

A high cFGF-23 level represented an independent risk factor for in-hospital mortality (OR, 1.80, $p = 0.049$), composite outcome at discharge (OR, 1.80, 95% CI = 1.01–3.24; $p = 0.043$), 90–day mortality (OR, 2.19, 95% CI = 1.20–4.00; $p = 0.011$), and 90-day composite outcome (OR, 2.39, 95% CI = 1.31–4.35; $p = 0.005$) after adjusting for age, gender, baseline eGFR, and factor interaction with cFGF-23 and SOFA score. Importantly, no interaction was observed between the cFGF-23 level and underlying diabetes mellitus, baseline eGFR, age, and AKI risk predicting score at dialysis initiation (all $p > 0.05$) (Table 3).

Table 3. Logistic regression model for mortality and composite outcomes at hospital discharge and 90 days after discharge. Significant risks were shown.

Independent Variables	Hospital Mortality			Composite Outcome at Discharge		
	OR	95% CI	*p*	OR	95% CI	*p*
Age (per year)	1.03	1.01–1.04	0.007	1.03	1.01–1.04	0.004
SOFA (per score)	1.26	1.15–1.39	<0.001	1.12	1.03–1.22	0.011
High cFGF-23	1.80	1.01–3.24	0.043	1.80	1.01–3.19	0.045
	90-Day Mortality			**90-Day Composite Outcome**		
Age (per year)	1.03	1.01–1.05	0.001	1.03	1.01–1.05	0.001
SOFA (per score)	1.30	1.17–1.44	0.037	1.17	1.07–1.27	<0.001
High cFGF-23	2.19	1.20–4.00	0.011	2.39	1.31–4.35	0.005

Abbreviations: cFGF-23, c-terminal fibroblast growth factor-23; CI, confidence interval; HR, hazard ratio; SOFA, Sequential Organ Failure Assessment. All the univariate significant and non-significant relevant covariates, including age, sex, baseline comorbidities, indication for dialysis, etiology of AKI, kidney function profile (e.g., baseline eGFR and candidate biomarkers), cFGF-23 and SOFA score at dialysis initiation, dialysis modality, and some of their interactions were put on the variable lists to be selected (Table 1).

Cox proportional hazard regression analysis revealed that patients undergoing RRT who displayed high cFGF-23 levels had a higher 90-day mortality during the follow-up period with an adjusted HR of 1.76 (95% CI, 1.22–2.53; p = 0.020) as compared with patients with lower cFGF-23 values (Figure 3A). There was no interaction of the baseline comorbidities with high cFGF-23 to predict 90-day composite outcome. (Table S2) Taking mortality as a competing risk factor for dialysis, high cFGF-23 levels also predicted less weaning from dialysis in surviving patients (HR, 0.62, p = 0.032) (Figure 3B).

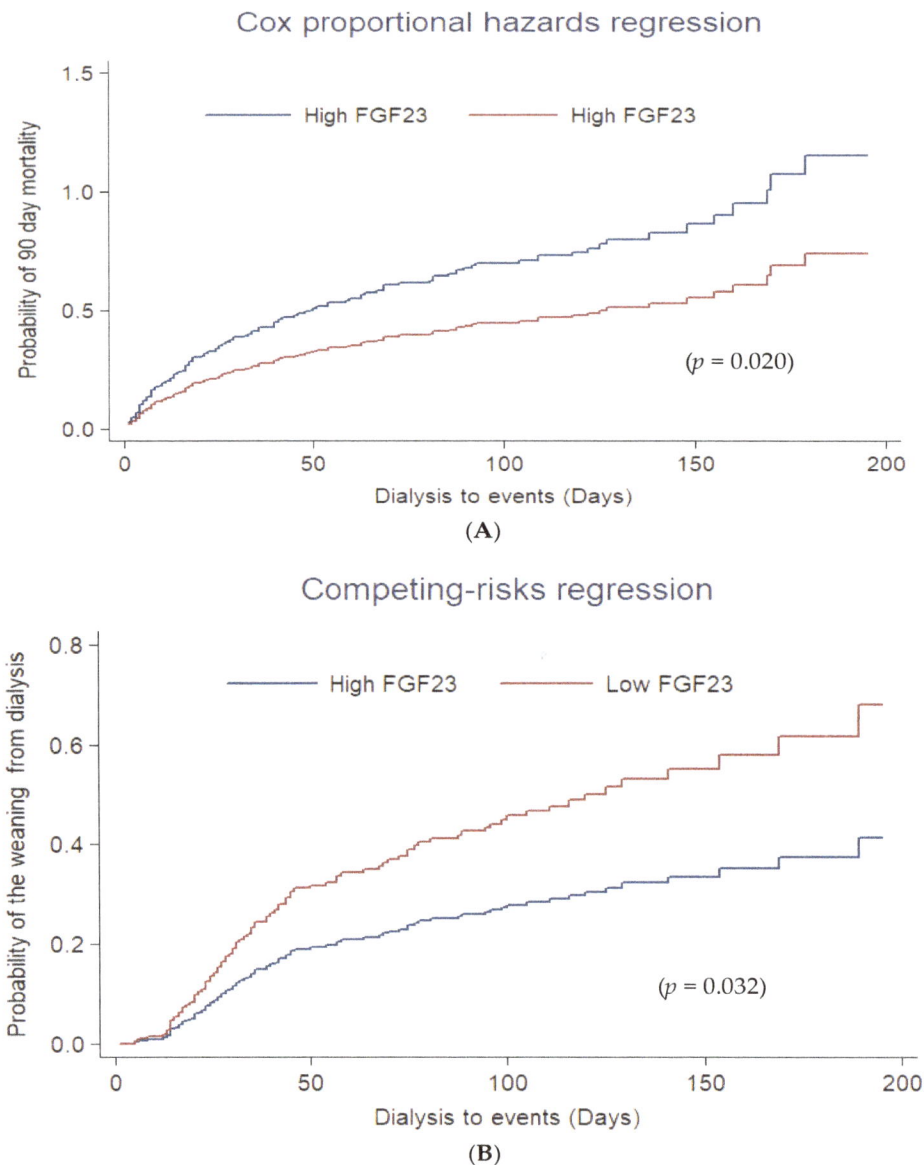

Figure 3. Cox proportional hazard plots stratified by serum cFGF-23 level for assessing probability of 90-day mortality (**A**) and the weaning from dialysis (**B**) by competing analysis and with mortality as a risk factor. Abbreviations: cFGF-23, c-terminal fibroblast growth factor-23; Using a cut-off value of 2050 RU/mL of cFGF-23 at initializing dialysis, patients were divided in a "high" and a "low" cFGF-23 group; all the relevant covariates, including characteristics, comorbidities, laboratory data, at ICU admission, etiology of AKI, indication for dialysis, dialysis modality, SOFA score, and plasma cFGF-23 at dialysis, and some of their interactions, such as interventions listed in Table 1, were put on a selected variable list to predict the outcome of interest.

The relationship of cFGF-23 with these variables was also underscored by a GAM analysis adjusted for SOFA score, gender, and age, which showed that cFGF-23 levels correlated with iFGF-23 ($p = 0.013$) and SOFA score ($p < 0.001$), but not with sCr ($p = 0.116$), phosphate ($p = 0.591$), 25-hydroxy Vit D ($p = 0.485$) and 1, 25 dihydroxy vit D ($p = 0.638$) concentrations at initiating RRT (Figure S1).

3.5. Addition of cFGF-23 to AKI Risk Predicting Score at Start of Dialysis

Adding cFGF-23 to the AKI risk predicting score at dialysis initiation significantly increased risk stratification (total NRI = 0.148; 95% CI = 0.057–0.239; $p = 0.002$) for detection of 90-day mortality. This effect was primarily determined by death (NRI event = 0.068, 95% CI = 0.043–0.087; $p = 0.025$) and survival (NRI event = 0.069; 95% CI = 0.039–0.097; $p = 0.029$). Similarly, the total IDI was significant. (0.051, 95% CI = 0.024–0.079; $p < 0.001$) (Figures S2 and S3).

4. Discussion

At initializing dialysis, the discriminative power of AKI biomarkers for 90-day mortality is fair. At dialysis initiation, the discrimination of cFGF-23 is better than NGAL, KIM-1, iFGF-23 and creatinine predicting patients' outcome. With mortality as competing risk, higher cFGF-23 levels also predicted lesser kidney recovery in survivors. More importantly, cFGF-23 had better predictive power than creatinine-adjusted urine NGAL and its integration into the AKI risk predicting score significantly enhanced the accuracy of risk stratification. At a cut-off level above 2050 RU/mL, cFGF-23 could predict of AKI mortality after adjusting for different clinical and disease severity parameters. Thus, cFGF-23 could be used as an early determinant of prognosis in ICU patients subjected at initializing RRT and also as an early determinant of the timing of dialysis initiation.

An increasing body of evidence has shown that cFGF-23 levels are increased in patients with AKI [11,14,29–32]. No significant interaction was observed between cFGF-23 and baseline CKD, sepsis grading in predicting mortality. The SOFA score was independently associated with increased cFGF-23 levels, which underpins the potential use of cFGF-23 in a critical care setting. We dare suggest that a higher plasma cFGF-23 not only corresponds with more severe AKI, but also reflects a higher degree of systemic inflammation.

Several mechanisms may explain increased FGF-23 levels in AKI: (1) increased production by osteocytes and possibly osteoblasts, that escapes regulation by parathyroid hormone, vitamin D signaling, and dietary phosphate restriction [33,34]; (2) increased ectopic production of FGF-23 by damaged renal tubules [33,35]; (3) tubular dysfunction resulting in FGF-23 resistance [36]; (4) and decreased clearance of circulating FGF-23 [14]. Whilst circulating FGF-23 levels rise rapidly during AKI [14] and a causal role for FGF-23 in the pathogenesis of left ventricular hypertrophy has previously been unveiled, suggesting that chronically elevated FGF-23 levels contribute directly to cardiac mortality in patients with CKD [37].

The ideal circumstances for whether and when to start RRT remain unclear [4]. We found significantly elevated cFGF-23 levels at the start of dialysis in non-survivors, whilst other structural and functional renal biomarkers failed to discriminate. Elevated plasma cFGF-23 was related to the degree of organ failure at initializing RRT [33]. In fact, high cFGF-23 concentrations predicted worse outcome equally well as the SOFA score in critically ill patients with advanced AKI [38]. Moreover, in patients without AKI, plasma cFGF-23 levels were significantly higher in the more severely ill patients [14]. This underscores that high cFGF-23 levels are correlated with increased systemic inflammation and/or stress secondary to illness or major surgery [33]. Although both serum and urine cFGF-23 could predict AKI mortality after ICU admission [12], many patients were oliguric at initializing dialysis, that will highlight the role of serum cFGF-23. In surviving patients, high cFGF-23 levels also predicted a lesser possibility for RRT withdrawal. Early prediction of renal recovery is likely to be helpful with regard to post-discharge care after critical illness and subsequent progression to CKD and ESRD.

Taken together, the ability of cFGF-23 to predict adverse outcomes might be related more to the systemic inflammatory status than to tubular damage. Based on our findings, a prognostic model can be constructed that allows to predict individual mortality risk as well as potential kidney recovery in surviving patients before starting RRT. The addition of cFGF-23 to a clinical AKI risk predicting score resulted in greater discrimination, and enhanced the ability to anticipate a higher number of subsequent deaths. Given the lack of appropriate or reliable biomarkers in patients receiving RRT, plasma cFGF-23 tentatively may serve as a novel outcome-specific marker in critical care nephrology. In patients with augmented plasma cFGF-23 concentration to arrive 2050 RU/mL, the clinician should evaluate the traditional AKI risk score or parameters to decide commencing dialysis.

Whether the cFGF-23 assay provides comparable sensitivity to that for iFGF-23 in patients with different stages of AKI or illness severity is still debated [13]. Although measurements obtained with iFGF-23 and cFGF-23 assays reflect the same circulating moiety, it has been suggested that the levels of iFGF23 also increased in patients who developed severe AKI, but the magnitude was lower than cFGF23 [13]. This is also supported by the present study showing that a plasma cFGF-23 concentration exceeding 2050 RU/mL at initializing RRT was significantly associated with worse patient outcome at a higher discriminative power than iFGF-23. The levels of adjusted urine cFGF23 also increased in patients who did not survive, but the magnitude was lower than serum cFGF23.

Several limitations of our study must be highlighted. Our cFGF-23 cutoff value was somewhat higher than that in other AKI studies [11–15], probably because most patients already had advanced AKI when admitted to the ICU. Furthermore, the predicting power of cFGF-23 in patients without AKI but with high inflammation status needs further validation. Finally, the exact mechanism underlying increased cFGF-23 concentrations in AKI patients as well as possible other intrinsic biological effects of cFGF-23 in this particular population remain to be explored. As previously studies few biomarkers were ever validated and they could only modestly predictive of renal recovery [8]; we do acknowledge also that the AUCs of cFGF-23 were relatively modest in AKI-D patients with critical status, however adding cFGF-23 to a parsimonious model augmented prediction of mortality and kidney recovery.

5. Conclusions

At initializing dialysis, the discriminative power of AKI biomarkers for 90-day mortality is fair. Our study showed that cFGF-23, measured at initiation of RRT in critical patients with AKI, may be a novel and distinct marker for predicting 90-day mortality after discharge and less weaning from RRT in survivors. Its predictive discrimination was superior to other established biomarkers of kidney injury, in particular creatinine, NGAL and Kim-1. Adding cFGF-23 to the traditional AKI risk predicting score may allow better risk stratification and enhance prognostic power. cFGF-23 could further be used as a surrogate marker to decide the best timing to initiate RRT.

Supplementary Materials:
Figure S1: Scatter plots with an adjusted spline of cFGF23 with (A) iFGF23 ($p = 0.013$), (B) phosphate ($p = 0.591$) (C) creatinine ($p = 0.116$) (D) 25 OH Vitamin D ($p = 0.485$) and (E) 1,25 OH, Vitamin D ($p = 0.638$) (F) KDIGO-AKI score ($p = 0.820$) (G) SOFA ($p < 0.001$) at initiation of dialysis, Figure S2: Decision curve analysis (DCA) plot to assess 90 day mortality using cFGF-23 in addition to AKI risk prediction score, Figure S3: The correlation of AKI risk predicting score and AKI risk predicting score with cFGF-23 predicting 90 day mortality, Table S1: p value comparison of the receiver operating characteristic (ROC) curve for discriminative ability, Table S2: Interaction of baseline co-morbidity with high cFGF-23 to predict 90-day composite outcome.

Author Contributions: V.-C.W., C.-C.S., S.-C.J.C., H.-H.L. and T.-S.C. conceived the review topic, analysis and interpretation and wrote the manuscript. H.D.S., N.-H.C., C.-H.W. and P.M.H. revised and approved the final version of the manuscript.

Acknowledgments: We also express our sincere gratitude to all staff of the Taiwan Clinical Trial Consortium, TCTC, and extracorporeal membrane oxygenation team in NTUH. All authors read and approved the final version of the manuscript.

Abbreviations

AKI	acute kidney injury
APACHE II	Acute Physiology and Chronic Health Evaluation II
AUROC	area under the receiver operator characteristic curve
CKD	chronic kidney disease
ESRD	end-stage renal disease
ICU	intensive care unit
KIM-1	Kidney Injury Molecule-1
MODS	Multiple Organ Dysfunction Score
NGAL	neutrophil gelatinase-associated lipocalin
RRT	renal replacement therapy
RU	relative units
sCr	serum creatinine
SOFA	Sequential Organ Failure Assessment

References

1. Shiao, C.C.; Wu, P.C.; Huang, T.M.; Lai, T.S.; Yang, W.S.; Wu, C.H.; Lai, C.F.; Wu, V.C.; Chu, T.S.; Wu, K.D.; et al. Long-term remote organ consequences following acute kidney injury. *Crit. Care* **2015**, *19*, 438. [CrossRef] [PubMed]

2. Wu, V.C.; Shiao, C.C.; Chang, C.H.; Huang, T.M.; Lai, C.F.; Lin, M.C.; Chiang, W.C.; Chu, T.S.; Wu, K.D.; Ko, W.J.; et al. Long-term outcomes after dialysis-requiring acute kidney injury. *Biomed. Res. Int.* **2014**, *2014*, 365186. [CrossRef] [PubMed]

3. Wald, R.; Bagshaw, S.M. The timing of renal replacement therapy initiation in acute kidney injury: Is earlier truly better? *Crit. Care Med.* **2014**, *42*, 1933–1934. [CrossRef] [PubMed]

4. Klein, S.J.; Brandtner, A.K.; Lehner, G.F.; Ulmer, H.; Bagshaw, S.M.; Wiedermann, C.J.; Joannidis, M. Biomarkers for prediction of renal replacement therapy in acute kidney injury: A systematic review and meta-analysis. *Intensive Care Med.* **2018**, *44*, 323–336. [CrossRef] [PubMed]

5. Kumpers, P.; Hafer, C.; Lukasz, A.; Lichtinghagen, R.; Brand, K.; Fliser, D.; Faulhaber-Walter, R.; Kielstein, J.T. Serum neutrophil gelatinase-associated lipocalin at inception of renal replacement therapy predicts survival in critically ill patients with acute kidney injury. *Crit. Care* **2010**, *14*, R9. [CrossRef] [PubMed]

6. Zarbock, A.; Kellum, J.A.; Schmidt, C.; Van Aken, H.; Wempe, C.; Pavenstadt, H.; Boanta, A.; Gerss, J.; Meersch, M. Effect of Early vs Delayed Initiation of Renal Replacement Therapy on Mortality in Critically Ill Patients With Acute Kidney Injury: The Elain Randomized Clinical Trial. *JAMA* **2016**, *315*, 2190–2199. [CrossRef] [PubMed]

7. Lin, C.Y.; Chang, C.H.; Fan, P.C.; Tian, Y.C.; Chang, M.Y.; Jenq, C.C.; Hung, C.C.; Fang, J.T.; Yang, C.W.; Chen, Y.C. Serum interleukin-18 at commencement of renal replacement therapy predicts short-term prognosis in critically ill patients with acute kidney injury. *PLoS ONE* **2013**, *8*, e66028. [CrossRef] [PubMed]

8. Pike, F.; Murugan, R.; Keener, C.; Palevsky, P.M.; Vijayan, A.; Unruh, M.; Finkel, K.; Wen, X.; Kellum, J.A. Biomarker Enhanced Risk Prediction for Adverse Outcomes in Critically Ill Patients Receiving RRT. *Clin. J. Am. Soc. Nephrol.* **2015**, *10*, 1332–1339. [CrossRef] [PubMed]

9. Consortium, A. Autosomal dominant hypophosphataemic rickets is associated with mutations in FGF23. *Nat. Genet.* **2000**, *26*, 345–348.

10. Berndt, T.; Kumar, R. Phosphatonins and the regulation of phosphate homeostasis. *Annu. Rev. Physiol.* **2007**, *69*, 341–359. [CrossRef] [PubMed]

11. Ali, F.N.; Hassinger, A.; Price, H.; Langman, C.B. Preoperative plasma FGF23 levels predict acute kidney injury in children: Results of a pilot study. *Pediatr. Nephrol.* **2013**, *28*, 959–962. [CrossRef] [PubMed]

12. Leaf, D.E.; Jacob, K.A.; Srivastava, A.; Chen, M.E.; Christov, M.; Juppner, H.; Sabbisetti, V.S.; Martin, A.; Wolf, M.; Waikar, S.S. Fibroblast Growth Factor 23 Levels Associate with AKI and Death in Critical Illness. *J. Am. Soc. Nephrol.* **2017**, *28*, 1877–1885. [CrossRef] [PubMed]

13. Leaf, D.E.; Christov, M.; Juppner, H.; Siew, E.; Ikizler, T.A.; Bian, A.; Chen, G.; Sabbisetti, V.S.; Bonventre, J.V.; Cai, X.; et al. Fibroblast growth factor 23 levels are elevated and associated with severe acute kidney injury and death following cardiac surgery. *Kidney Int.* **2016**, *89*, 939–948. [CrossRef] [PubMed]

14. Christov, M.; Waikar, S.S.; Pereira, R.C.; Havasi, A.; Leaf, D.E.; Goltzman, D.; Pajevic, P.D.; Wolf, M.; Juppner, H. Plasma FGF23 levels increase rapidly after acute kidney injury. *Kidney Int.* **2013**, *84*, 776–785. [CrossRef] [PubMed]

15. Donate-Correa, J.; de Fuentes, M.M.; Mora-Fernandez, C.; Navarro-Gonzalez, J.F. Pathophysiological implications of fibroblast growth factor-23 and Klotho and their potential role as clinical biomarkers. *Clin. Chem.* **2014**, *60*, 933–940. [CrossRef] [PubMed]

16. Wu, V.C.; Ko, W.J.; Chang, H.W.; Chen, Y.S.; Chen, Y.W.; Chen, Y.M.; Hu, F.C.; Lin, Y.H.; Tsai, P.R.; Wu, K.D. Early renal replacement therapy in patients with postoperative acute liver failure associated with acute renal failure: Effect on postoperative outcomes. *J. Am. Coll. Surg.* **2007**, *205*, 266–276. [CrossRef] [PubMed]

17. Wu, V.C.; Ko, W.J.; Chang, H.W.; Chen, Y.W.; Lin, Y.F.; Shiao, C.C.; Chen, Y.M.; Chen, Y.S.; Tsai, P.R.; Hu, F.C.; et al. Risk factors of early redialysis after weaning from postoperative acute renal replacement therapy. *Intensive Care Med.* **2008**, *34*, 101–108. [CrossRef] [PubMed]

18. Shiao, C.C.; Wu, V.C.; Li, W.Y.; Lin, Y.F.; Hu, F.C.; Young, G.H.; Kuo, C.C.; Kao, T.W.; Huang, D.M.; Chen, Y.M.; et al. Late initiation of renal replacement therapy is associated with worse outcomes in acute kidney injury after major abdominal surgery. *Crit. Care* **2009**, *13*, R171. [CrossRef] [PubMed]

19. Wu, V.C.; Wang, C.H.; Wang, W.J.; Lin, Y.F.; Hu, F.C.; Chen, Y.W.; Chen, Y.S.; Wu, M.S.; Lin, Y.H.; Kuo, C.C.; et al. Sustained low-efficiency dialysis versus continuous veno-venous hemofiltration for postsurgical acute renal failure. *Am. J. Surg.* **2010**, *199*, 466–476. [CrossRef] [PubMed]

20. Huang, T.M.; Wu, V.C.; Young, G.H.; Lin, Y.F.; Shiao, C.C.; Wu, P.C.; Li, W.Y.; Yu, H.Y.; Hu, F.C.; Lin, J.W.; et al. Preoperative proteinuria predicts adverse renal outcomes after coronary artery bypass grafting. *J. Am. Soc. Nephrol.* **2011**, *22*, 156–163. [CrossRef] [PubMed]

21. Demirjian, S.; Chertow, G.M.; Zhang, J.H.; O'Connor, T.Z.; Vitale, J.; Paganini, E.P.; Palevsky, P.M. Network VNARFT. Model to predict mortality in critically ill adults with acute kidney injury. *Clin. J. Am. Soc. Nephrol.* **2011**, *6*, 2114–2120. [CrossRef] [PubMed]

22. Wu, V.C.; Huang, T.M.; Lai, C.F.; Shiao, C.C.; Lin, Y.F.; Chu, T.S.; Wu, P.C.; Chao, C.T.; Wang, J.Y.; Kao, T.W.; et al. Acute-on-chronic kidney injury at hospital discharge is associated with long-term dialysis and mortality. *Kidney Int.* **2011**, *80*, 1222–1230. [CrossRef] [PubMed]

23. Lin, Y.F.; Ko, W.J.; Wu, V.C.; Chen, Y.S.; Chen, Y.M.; Hu, F.C.; Shiao, C.C.; Wu, M.S.; Chen, Y.W.; Li, W.Y.; et al. A modified sequential organ failure assessment score to predict hospital mortality of postoperative acute renal failure patients requiring renal replacement therapy. *Blood Purif.* **2008**, *26*, 547–554. [CrossRef] [PubMed]

24. Shiao, C.C.; Ko, W.J.; Wu, V.C.; Huang, T.M.; Lai, C.F.; Lin, Y.F.; Chao, C.T.; Chu, T.S.; Tsai, H.B.; Wu, P.C.; et al. U-curve association between timing of renal replacement therapy initiation and in-hospital mortality in postoperative acute kidney injury. *PLoS ONE* **2012**, *7*, e42952. [CrossRef] [PubMed]

25. Wu, V.C.; Lo, S.C.; Chen, Y.L.; Huang, P.H.; Tsai, C.T.; Liang, C.J.; Kuo, C.C.; Kuo, Y.S.; Lee, B.C.; Wu, E.L.; et al. Endothelial progenitor cells in primary aldosteronism: A biomarker of severity for aldosterone vasculopathy and prognosis. *J. Clin. Endocrinol. Metab.* **2011**, *96*, 3175–3183. [CrossRef] [PubMed]

26. Wu, V.C.; Lai, C.F.; Shiao, C.C.; Lin, Y.F.; Wu, P.C.; Chao, C.T.; Hu, F.C.; Huang, T.M.; Yeh, Y.C.; Tsai, I.J.; et al. Effect of diuretic use on 30-day postdialysis mortality in critically ill patients receiving acute dialysis. *PLoS ONE* **2012**, *7*, e30836. [CrossRef] [PubMed]

27. Hin, L.Y.; Lau, T.K.; Rogers, M.S.; Chang, A.M. Dichotomization of continuous measurements using generalized additive modelling—Application in predicting intrapartum caesarean delivery. *Stat. Med.* **1999**, *18*, 1101–1110. [CrossRef]

28. Wu, V.C.; Chang, C.H.; Wang, C.Y.; Lin, Y.H.; Kao, T.W.; Lin, P.C.; Chu, T.S.; Chang, Y.S.; Chen, L.; Wu, K.D.; et al. Risk of Fracture in Primary Aldosteronism: A Population-Based Cohort Study. *J. Bone Miner. Res.* **2017**, *32*, 743–752. [CrossRef] [PubMed]

29. Zhang, M.; Hsu, R.; Hsu, C.Y.; Kordesch, K.; Nicasio, E.; Cortez, A.; McAlpine, I.; Brady, S.; Zhuo, H.; Kangelaris, K.N.; et al. FGF-23 and PTH levels in patients with acute kidney injury: A cross-sectional case series study. *Ann. Intensive Care.* **2011**, *1*, 21. [CrossRef] [PubMed]

30. Leaf, D.E.; Wolf, M.; Waikar, S.S.; Chase, H.; Christov, M.; Cremers, S.; Stern, L. FGF-23 levels in patients with AKI and risk of adverse outcomes. *Clin. J. Am. Soc. Nephrol.* **2012**, *7*, 1217–1223. [CrossRef] [PubMed]

31. Leaf, D.E.; Waikar, S.S.; Wolf, M.; Cremers, S.; Bhan, I.; Stern, L. Dysregulated mineral metabolism in patients with acute kidney injury and risk of adverse outcomes. *Clin. Endocrinol.* **2013**, *79*, 491–498. [CrossRef] [PubMed]

32. Brown, J.R.; Katz, R.; Ix, J.H.; de Boer, I.H.; Siscovick, D.S.; Grams, M.E.; Shlipak, M.; Sarnak, M.J. Fibroblast growth factor-23 and the long-term risk of hospital-associated AKI among community-dwelling older individuals. *Clin. J. Am. Soc. Nephrol.* **2014**, *9*, 239–246. [CrossRef] [PubMed]

33. Neyra, J.A.; Moe, O.W.; Hu, M.C. Fibroblast growth factor 23 and acute kidney injury. *Pediatr. Nephrol.* **2015**, *30*, 1909–1918. [CrossRef] [PubMed]

34. Shimada, T.; Muto, T.; Urakawa, I.; Yoneya, T.; Yamazaki, Y.; Okawa, K.; Takeuchi, Y.; Fujita, T.; Fukumoto, S.; Yamashita, T. Mutant FGF-23 responsible for autosomal dominant hypophosphatemic rickets is resistant to proteolytic cleavage and causes hypophosphatemia in vivo. *Endocrinology* **2002**, *143*, 3179–3182. [CrossRef] [PubMed]

35. Spichtig, D.; Zhang, H.; Mohebbi, N.; Pavik, I.; Petzold, K.; Stange, G.; Saleh, L.; Edenhofer, I.; Segerer, S.; Biber, J.; et al. Renal expression of FGF23 and peripheral resistance to elevated FGF23 in rodent models of polycystic kidney disease. *Kidney Int.* **2014**, *85*, 1340–1350. [CrossRef] [PubMed]

36. Hassan, A.; Durlacher, K.; Silver, J.; Naveh-Many, T.; Levi, R. The fibroblast growth factor receptor mediates the increased FGF23 expression in acute and chronic uremia. *Am. J. Physiol. Renal Physiol.* **2016**, *310*, F217–F221. [CrossRef] [PubMed]

37. Faul, C.; Amaral, A.P.; Oskouei, B.; Hu, M.C.; Sloan, A.; Isakova, T.; Gutierrez, O.M.; Aguillon-Prada, R.; Lincoln, J.; Hare, J.M.; et al. FGF23 induces left ventricular hypertrophy. *J. Clin. Investig.* **2011**, *121*, 4393–4408. [CrossRef] [PubMed]

38. Chang, C.H.; Fan, P.C.; Chang, M.Y.; Tian, Y.C.; Hung, C.C.; Fang, J.T.; Yang, C.W.; Chen, Y.C. Acute kidney injury enhances outcome prediction ability of sequential organ failure assessment score in critically ill patients. *PLoS ONE* **2014**, *9*, e109649. [CrossRef] [PubMed]

Permissions

The contributors of this book come from diverse backgrounds, making this book a truly international effort. This book will bring forth new frontiers with its revolutionizing research information and detailed analysis of the nascent developments around the world.

We would like to thank all the contributing authors for lending their expertise to make the book truly unique. They have played a crucial role in the development of this book. Without their invaluable contributions this book wouldn't have been possible. They have made vital efforts to compile up to date information on the varied aspects of this subject to make this book a valuable addition to the collection of many professionals and students.

This book was conceptualized with the vision of imparting up-to-date information and advanced data in this field. To ensure the same, a matchless editorial board was set up. Every individual on the board went through rigorous rounds of assessment to prove their worth. After which they invested a large part of their time researching and compiling the most relevant data for our readers.

The editorial board has been involved in producing this book since its inception. They have spent rigorous hours researching and exploring the diverse topics which have resulted in the successful publishing of this book. They have passed on their knowledge of decades through this book. To expedite this challenging task, the publisher supported the team at every step. A small team of assistant editors was also appointed to further simplify the editing procedure and attain best results for the readers.

Apart from the editorial board, the designing team has also invested a significant amount of their time in understanding the subject and creating the most relevant covers. They scrutinized every image to scout for the most suitable representation of the subject and create an appropriate cover for the book.

The publishing team has been an ardent support to the editorial, designing and production team. Their endless efforts to recruit the best for this project, has resulted in the accomplishment of this book. They are a veteran in the field of academics and their pool of knowledge is as vast as their experience in printing. Their expertise and guidance has proved useful at every step. Their uncompromising quality standards have made this book an exceptional effort. Their encouragement from time to time has been an inspiration for everyone.

The publisher and the editorial board hope that this book will prove to be a valuable piece of knowledge for researchers, students, practitioners and scholars across the globe.

List of Contributors

Chung-Kuan Wu
Institute of Clinical Medicine, National Yang-Ming University, Taipei 11221, Taiwan
Division of Nephrology, Department of Internal Medicine, Shin-Kong Wu Ho-Su Memorial Hospital, Taipei 11101, Taiwan
School of Medicine, Fu-Jen Catholic University, New Taipei 24205, Taiwan

Chia-Lin Wu
Institute of Clinical Medicine, National Yang-Ming University, Taipei 11221, Taiwan
Division of Nephrology, Department of Internal Medicine, Changhua Christian Hospital, Changhua 50006, Taiwan
School of Medicine, Chung-Shan Medical University, Taichung 40201, Taiwan

Tzu-Cheng Su
Department of Pathology, Changhua Christian Hospital, Changhua 50006, Taiwan

Yu Ru Kou
Department of Physiology, School of Medicine, National Yang-Ming University, Taipei 11221, Taiwan

Chew-Teng Kor
Internal Medicine Research Center, Changhua Christian Hospital, Changhua 50006, Taiwan

Tzong-Shyuan Lee
Department of Physiology, College of Medicine, National Taiwan University, Taipei 10617, Taiwan

Der-Cherng Tarng
Institute of Clinical Medicine, National Yang-Ming University, Taipei 11221, Taiwan
Department of Physiology, School of Medicine, National Yang-Ming University, Taipei 11221, Taiwan
Division of Nephrology, Department of Medicine, Taipei Veterans General Hospital, Taipei 11217, Taiwan

Ana Isabel Connor
Division of Clinical Pharmacy, UCSD Skaggs School of Pharmacy and Pharmaceutical Sciences, San Diego, CA 92093, USA

Linda Awdishu
Division of Clinical Pharmacy, UCSD Skaggs School of Pharmacy and Pharmaceutical Sciences, San Diego, CA 92093, USA
Department of Medicine, Division of Nephrology, UCSD School of Medicine, San Diego, CA 92093, USA

Etienne Macedo and Ravindra L. Mehta
Department of Medicine, Division of Nephrology, UCSD School of Medicine, San Diego, CA 92093, USA

Josée Bouchard
Department of Medicine, University of Montreal, Montreal, QC H3T 1J4, Canada

Glenn M. Chertow
Department of Medicine, Division of Nephrology, Stanford University School of Medicine, Palo Alto, CA 94034, USA

Lisa Gianesello, Monica Ceol, Liliana Terrin, Giovanna Priante and Dorella Del Prete
Laboratory of Histomorphology and Molecular Biology of the Kidney, Clinical Nephrology, Department of Medicine — DIMED, University of Padua, 35128 Padua, Italy

Loris Bertoldi and Giorgio Valle
CRIBI Biotechnology Centre, University of Padua, 35131 Padua, Italy

Franca Anglani
Laboratory of Histomorphology and Molecular Biology of the Kidney, Clinical Nephrology, Department of Medicine — DIMED, University of Padua, 35128 Padua, Italy
CRIBI Biotechnology Centre, University of Padua, 35131 Padua, Italy

Luisa Murer
Pediatric Nephrology, Dialysis and Transplant Unit, Department of Women's and Children's Health, Padua University Hospital, 35128 Padua, Italy

Licia Peruzzi
Pediatric Nephrology Unit, Regina Margherita Children's Hospital, 10126 CDSS Turin, Italy

Mario Giordano
Pediatric Nephrology Unit, University Hospital, 70126 Bari, Italy

Fabio Paglialonga
Pediatric Nephrology, Dialysis and Transplant Unit, Fondazione IRCCS, Ca' Granda Ospedale Maggiore Policlinico, 20122 Milan, Italy

Vincenzo Cantaluppi and Claudio Musetti
Nephrology and Kidney Transplantation Unit, Department of Translational Medicine, University of Piemonte Orientale (UPO), 28100 Novara, Italy

Adrianna Douvris, Khalid Zeid, Rima Abou Arkoub and Gurpreet Malhi
Department of Medicine, University of Ottawa, Ottawa, ON K1H 7W9, Canada

Swapnil Hiremath, Pierre Antoine Brown, Manish M. Sood and Edward G. Clark
Division of Nephrology, Department of Medicine and Kidney Research Centre, Ottawa Hospital Research Institute, University of Ottawa, Ottawa, ON K1H 7W9, Canada

Joana Gameiro, Jose Agapito Fonseca, Sofia Jorge and Jose Antonio Lopes
Division of Nephrology and Renal Transplantation, Department of Medicine Centro Hospitalar Lisboa Norte, EPE, Av. Prof. Egas Moniz, 1649-035 Lisboa, Portugal

Jae Won Shin, Mi Rireu Park and Jae Hyun Lee
Department of Pediatrics, Yonsei University College of Medicine, Yonsei-ro 50, Seodaemun-gu, Seoul 03722, Korea

Keum Hwa Lee and Jae Il Shin
Department of Pediatrics, Yonsei University College of Medicine, Yonsei-ro 50, Seodaemun-gu, Seoul 03722, Korea
Division of Pediatric Nephrology, Severance Children's Hospital, Seoul 03722, Korea
Institute of Kidney Disease Research, Yonsei University College of Medicine, Seoul 03722, Korea

In Suk Sol
Department of Pediatrics, Severance Hospital, Yonsei University College of Medicine, Seoul 03722, Korea
Department of Pediatrics, Hallym University Chuncheon Sacred Heart Hospital, Sakju-ro 77, Gangwon-do, Chuncheon 24253, Korea

Jung Tak Park
Institute of Kidney Disease Research, Yonsei University College of Medicine, Seoul 03722, Korea
Department of Internal Medicine, Yonsei University College of Medicine, Seoul 03722, Korea

Ji Hong Kim
Department of Pediatrics, Yonsei University College of Medicine, Yonsei-ro 50, Seodaemun-gu, Seoul 03722, Korea
Department of Pediatrics, Gangnam Severance Hospital, Yonsei University College of Medicine, Eonjuro 211, Gangnam-gu, Seoul 06273, Korea

Kyung Won Kim
Department of Pediatrics, Severance Hospital, Yonsei University College of Medicine, Seoul 03722, Korea

Yoon Hee Kim
Department of Pediatrics, Severance Hospital, Yonsei University College of Medicine, Seoul 03722, Korea
Department of Pediatrics, Gangnam Severance Hospital, Yonsei University College of Medicine, Eonjuro 211, Gangnam-gu, Seoul 06273, Korea

Laura M. Vilander, Suvi T. Vaara and Ville Pettilä
Division of Intensive Care Medicine, Department of Anesthesiology, Intensive Care and Pain Medicine, University of Helsinki and Helsinki University Hospital, 00014 Helsinki, Finland

Mari A. Kaunisto
Institute for Molecular Medicine Finland (FIMM), HiLIFE, University of Helsinki, 000014 Helsinki, Finland

Ya-Lien Cheng, George Kuo and Ya-Chung Tian
Kidney Research Center, Department of Nephrology, Chang Gung Memorial Hospital, College of Medicine, Chang Gung University, Taoyuan 333, Taiwan

Cheng-Chia Lee, Chih-Hsiang Chang and Yi-Jung Li
Kidney Research Center, Department of Nephrology, Chang Gung Memorial Hospital, College of Medicine, Chang Gung University, Taoyuan 333, Taiwan
Graduate Institute of Clinical Medical Sciences, College of Medicine, Chang Gung University, Taoyuan 333, Taiwan

Shao-Wei Chen
Graduate Institute of Clinical Medical Sciences, College of Medicine, Chang Gung University, Taoyuan 333, Taiwan
Department of Cardiothoracic and Vascular Surgery, Chang Gung Memorial Hospital, Linkou branch, College of Medicine, Chang Gung University, Taoyuan 333, Taiwan

Yi-Ting Chen
Department of Biomedical Sciences, College of Medicine, Chang Gung University, Taoyuan 333, Taiwan

Ronak Jagdeep Shah
Division of Nephrology and Hypertension, Mayo Clinic, Rochester, MN 55905, USA

Lisa E. Vaughan and Felicity T. Enders
Division of Biomedical Statistics and Informatics, Mayo Clinic, Rochester, MN 55905, USA

Dawn S. Milliner
Division of Nephrology and Hypertension, Mayo Clinic, Rochester, MN 55905, USA
Division of Pediatric Nephrology, Mayo Clinic, Rochester, MN 55905, USA

John C. Lieske
Division of Nephrology and Hypertension, Mayo Clinic, Rochester, MN 55905, USA
Division of Laboratory Medicine and Pathology, Mayo Clinic, Rochester, MN 55905, USA

June-sung Kim, Youn-Jung Kim, Seung Mok Ryoo, Chang Hwan Sohn, Dong Woo Seo, Shin Ahn, Kyoung Soo Lim and Won Young Kim
Department of Emergency Medicine, Asan Medical Center, University of Ulsan College of Medicine, Seoul 05505, Korea

Hyung-Chul Lee, Hyun-Kyu Yoon, Karam Nam, Youn Joung Cho, Tae Kyong Kim, Won Ho Kim and Jae-Hyon Bahk
Department of Anesthesiology and Pain Medicine, Seoul National University Hospital, Seoul National University College of Medicine, Seoul 03080, Korea

Tak Kyu Oh, In-Ae Song and Young-Tae Jeon
Department of Anesthesiology and Pain Medicine, Seoul National University Bundang Hospital, Gumi-ro 173 Beon-gil, Bundang-gu, Seongnam 13620, Korea

Young-Jae Cho
Division of Pulmonary and Critical Care Medicine, Department of Internal Medicine, Seoul National University Bundang Hospital, Gumi-ro 173 Beon-gil, Bundang-gu, Seongnam 13620, Korea

Cheong Lim
Department of Thoracic and Cardiovascular Surgery, Seoul National University Bundang Hospital, Gumi-ro 173 Beon-gil, Bundang-gu, Seongnam 13620, Korea

Hee-Joon Bae
Department of Neurology, Stroke Center, Seoul National University Bundang Hospital, Gumi-ro 173 Beon-gil, Bundang-gu, Seongnam 13620, Korea

You Hwan Jo
Department of Emergency Medicine, Seoul National University Bundang Hospital, Gumi-ro 173 Beon-gil, Bundang-gu, Seongnam 13620, Korea

Fay J. Dickson
Hull University Teaching Hospitals, Anlaby Road, Hull HU3 2JZ, UK

John A. Sayer
Translational and Clinical Research Institute, Faculty of Medical Sciences, Newcastle University, Central Parkway, Newcastle upon Tyne NE1 3BZ, UK
The Newcastle upon Tyne NHS Hospitals Foundation Trust, Newcastle upon Tyne NE7 7DN, UK
NIHR Newcastle Biomedical Research Centre, Newcastle upon Tyne NE4 5PL, UK

Sébastien Rubin, Arthur Orieux, Claire Rigothier and Christian Combe
Service de Néphrologie, Transplantation, Dialyse, Aphérèses, Hôpital Pellegrin, Centre Hospitalier Universitaire de Bordeaux, 33076 Bordeaux CEDEX, France

Benjamin Clouzeau, Didier Gruson and Alexandre Boyer
Service de Médecine Intensive Réanimation, Hôpital Pellegrin, Centre Hospitalier Universitaire de Bordeaux, 33076 Bordeaux Cedex, France

Charat Thongprayoon
Division of Nephrology and Hypertension, Mayo Clinic, Rochester, MN 55905, USA

Wisit Cheungpasitporn
Division of Nephrology, Department of Medicine, University of Mississippi Medical Center, Jackson, MS 39216, USA

Ploypin Lertjitbanjong and Kanramon Watthanasuntorn
Department of Internal Medicine, Bassett Medical Center, Cooperstown, NY 13326, USA

Narothama Reddy Aeddula
Division of Nephrology, Department of Medicine, Deaconess Health System, Evansville, IN 47747, USA

Tarun Bathini
Department of Internal Medicine, University of Arizona, Tucson, AZ 85721, USA

Narat Srivali
Division of Pulmonary and Critical Care Medicine, St. Agnes Hospital, Baltimore, MD 21229, USA

Michael A. Mao
Division of Nephrology and Hypertension, Mayo Clinic, Jacksonville, FL 32224, USA

Kianoush Kashani
Division of Nephrology and Hypertension, Mayo Clinic, Rochester, MN 55905, USA
Division of Pulmonary and Critical Care Medicine, Department of Medicine, Mayo Clinic, Rochester, MN 55905, USA

Isabel Acosta-Ochoa, Alicia Mendiluce-Herrero and Armando Coca-Rojo
Department of Nephrology, Hospital Clinico Universitario, 47003 Valladolid, Spain

Juan Bustamante-Munguira
Department of Cardiac Surgery, Hospital Clinico Universitario, 47003 Valladolid, Spain

Jesús Bustamante-Bustamante
Department of Medicine, Dermatology and Toxicology, School of Medicine, University of Valladolid, 47005 Valladolid, Spain

Vin-Cent Wu
Division of Nephrology, National Taiwan University Hospital, No. 7 Chung-Shan South Road, Zhong-Zheng District, Taipei 100, Taiwan

Chih-Chung Shiao
Division of Nephrology, Department of Internal Medicine, Saint Mary's Hospital Luodong, No. 160 Chong-Cheng South Road, Loudong, Yilan 265, Taiwan Saint Mary's Junior College of Medicine, Nursing and Management College, No. 100, Ln. 265, Sec. 2, Sanxing Rd., Sanxing Township, Yilan 266, Taiwan

Nai-Hsin Chi and Chih-Hsien Wang
Surgery Department, National Taiwan University Hospital, No. 7 Chung-Shan South Road, Zhong-Zheng District, Taipei 100, Taiwan

Shih-Chieh Jeff Chueh
Glickman Urological and Kidney Institute, Cleveland Clinic Lerner College of Medicine, Cleveland Clinic, Cleveland, 9500 Euclid Ave., Cleveland, OH 44195, USA

Hung-Hsiang Liou
Division of Nephrology, Department of Internal Medicine, Hsin-Jen Hospital, Dialysis Center, Hsin-Ren Clinics, No. 395, Chung-Shan Road, New Taipei City 231, Taiwan

Herbert D. Spapen
ICU Department, Universitair Ziekenhuis Brussel, Vrije Universiteit Brussel, 101, Laarbeeklaan, 1090 Jette, Belgium

Patrick M. Honore
ICU Department, CHU Brugmann University Hospital, 4 Place Arthur Van Gehucthen, 1020 Brussels, Belgium

Tzong-Shinn Chu
Division of Nephrology, National Taiwan University Hospital, No. 7 Chung-Shan South Road, Zhong-Zheng District, Taipei 100, Taiwan NSARF Group (National Taiwan University Hospital Study Group of ARF), Taipei 100, Taiwan

Index